"In his always engaging and vivid style of prose, Simon Chapman provides a comprehensive exploration of the critical, yet often unsexy topic of quitting smoking. He brings his vast and varied academic expertise and real-world experiences, accumulated over his illustrious career, to this nuanced examination of how the greatest numbers of people truly quit smoking. This has clear implications for how to most rapidly and effectively bring an end to the massive, yet wholly preventable, tobacco-caused death and disease that the human race continues to endure."
-- *Joanna Cohen, Bloomberg Professor of Disease Prevention, Johns Hopkins University Bloomberg School of Public Health*

"This is a splendid read for anyone interested in what really works to reduce smoking, and what helps to keep Big Tobacco in business. In Simon Chapman's typically trenchant style, it tells you everything you want to know (and some people won't want to know) about the myths and realities of smoking cessation and other aspects of tobacco policy. All this alongside lessons learned from a lifetime's work on tobacco. Top class – don't miss it."
-- *Mike Daube AO, Emeritus Professor in Public Health, Curtin University*

"Simon Chapman's latest book offers academic and non-academic readers a deep, provocative, historical, current and evidence-based perspective on elements influencing both smoking and the policies which drive it down. This stunning book should promote understanding of the complex relationships between tobacco and pharmaceutical companies, public health practitioners and public policy makers, and smokers who want and must decide how to quit."
-- *Esteve Fernández, Professor of Public Health, University of Barcelona, and Director of the WHO Collaborating Centre for Tobacco Control, Catalan Institute of Oncology*

"While the broad evidence that people change from problem drug or alcohol use mostly on their own is still met with scepticism, everybody knows ex-smokers from daily life experience who quit

without professional help. Yet, the success stories of this majority of successful quitters and their lay strategies, which could motivate others and inspire population-level measures, are hardly part of the public discourse dominated by the disease concept. Simon Chapman addresses this blind spot and dissects convincingly the agenda of tobacco and treatment industries with their focus on discrediting self-change friendly policies regardless of empirical evidence. The book is an excellent manual to assist necessary changes of perspective and thinking out of the box. To be read before the patient information leaflet!"
-- *Dr Harald Klingemann, Senior Research Fellow, Bern University of Applied Sciences*

"'I'm here to help you.' Who could argue with that? But when people build a business model based on helping individuals, there is little incentive to get rid of the problem. Recent decades have seen the growth of a smoking cessation industry, dedicated to helping individuals quit. With the advent of e-cigarettes, this now includes tobacco producers themselves. Yet as Simon Chapman shows in his fascinating forensic analysis, a narrative has taken hold in tobacco control that is unsupported by evidence, and worse, is a distraction from tackling the real issue. This book will be essential reading, not just for the tobacco control community, but for anyone tackling trade in harmful commodities."
-- *Martin McKee CBE, Professor of European Public Health, London School of Hygiene and Tropical Medicine, Research Director European Observatory on Health Systems and Policies*

"The tobacco pandemic has resulted from a 'ludicrous exceptionalist' status for tobacco products that governments have wholly failed to address, while devoting endless resources to elaborate, well-intentioned efforts to convince, one by one, people who smoke that they must not try it alone and need 'help' to quit. Simon Chapman's witty and well-argued book suggests cessation programs have perhaps made it even more difficult to become tobacco-free, while distracting from the real issue of better implementing what works to achieve further population-level

reductions in tobacco use. There is something in this book for everyone who thinks critically about how to bring the tobacco pandemic to an end."
-- *Ruth Malone, Professor in Social Behavioral Sciences, University of California San Francisco. Editor Tobacco Control since 2009*

"Simon Chapman has had a distinguished career in public health science, where he has been a strong advocate for both upstream policy and personal agency in behavior change at the population level. This book documents his two-decade struggle against those who argue that quitting smoking is so difficult that the only way that many smokers can quit is by switching to another source of nicotine – a business-friendly approach to cessation services. He documents how these advocates have consistently ignored the two-thirds of quitters who continue to achieve nicotine abstinence on their own. This book is a must read for those interested in the politicization of science."
-- *John Pierce, Distinguished Professor Emeritus, University of California San Diego*

"Simon Chapman is a giant in tobacco control. Fiercely empirical, he shows that Big Pharma has brainwashed too many of us into thinking that drugs are the only way to get off nicotine. Chapman is indispensable reading for anyone wanting to help the billion-odd smokers end their addiction. A powerful and important book!"

— *Robert Proctor Professor of the History of Science at Stanford University. Author of Golden Holocaust: origins of the cigarette catastrophe and the case for abolition. Berkeley: University of California Press, 2011*

Quit Smoking Weapons of Mass Distraction

PUBLIC AND SOCIAL POLICY SERIES

Gaby Ramia, Series Editor

The Public and Social Policy series publishes books that pose challenging questions about policy from national, comparative and international perspectives. The series explores policy design, implementation and evaluation; the politics of policy making; and analyses of particular areas of public and social policy.

Australian social attitudes IV: the age of insecurity
Ed. Shaun Wilson and Markus Hadler

Buying and selling the poor: inside Australia's privatised welfare-to-work market
Siobhan O'Sullivan, Michael McGann and Mark Considine

Globalisation, the state and regional Australia
Amanda Walsh

Markets, rights and power in Australian social policy
Ed. Gabrielle Meagher and Susan Goodwin

One planet, one health
Ed. Merrilyn Walton

Risking together: how finance is dominating everyday life in Australia
Dick Bryan and Mike Rafferty

Wind turbine syndrome: a communicated disease
Simon Chapman and Fiona Crichton

Quit Smoking Weapons of Mass Distraction

Simon Chapman

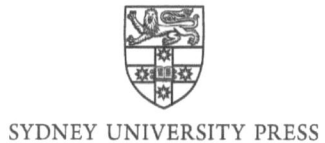

SYDNEY UNIVERSITY PRESS

First published by Sydney University Press
© Simon Chapman 2022
© Sydney University Press 2022

Reproduction and communication for other purposes
Except as permitted under the Act, no part of this edition may be reproduced, stored in a retrieval system, or communicated in any form or by any means without prior written permission. All requests for reproduction or communication should be made to Sydney University Press at the address below:

Sydney University Press
Fisher Library F03
University of Sydney NSW 2006
Australia
sup.info@sydney.edu.au
sydneyuniversitypress.com.au

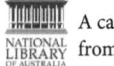 A catalogue record for this book is available from the National Library of Australia.

ISBN 9781743328538 paperback
ISBN 9781743328545 epub
ISBN 9781743328590 pdf

Cover design by Miguel Yamin.

We acknowledge the traditional owners of the lands on which Sydney University Press is located, the Gadigal people of the Eora Nation, and we pay our respects to the knowledge embedded forever within the Aboriginal Custodianship of Country.

Contents

Acknowledgements xi

Abbreviations xiii

Introduction xv

1 How do most people quit other addictions? 1
2 How we study quitting smoking: a critical look 12
3 Quitting unassisted: before and after "evidence-based" methods 56
4 The modest impact of most popular interventions 79
5 "Don't try to quit cold turkey" 107
6 Vaping to quit: the latest mass distraction 145
7 Insights from qualitative research with unassisted quitters 203
8 Strategies for reducing smoking across populations 229
9 Controlling tobacco supply and the endgame 265

References 298
Index 354

Acknowledgements

It is over 45 years since I first became engaged with questions about how best to reduce tobacco use across populations and the diseases that this causes. Across this time I have met, often worked with and become close friends with many of the best minds in international tobacco control. Seventeen years of that time were spent being deputy editor (1992–97) and then editor (1998–2008) of *Tobacco Control*, the world's first research journal entirely dedicated to reducing tobacco use and the diseases it causes. During those years, it was a rare day when I was not reading and editing one or more of the thousands of papers that were submitted to the journal, even on Christmas Day. There are very few long-term researchers active across the many disciplinary and sub-topic fields of tobacco control whose most important work I've not read.

Trying to list and thank everyone who has ever influenced my thinking about tobacco control is an almost boundless task. But the following people are those to whom across different times – including during the writing of this book – I owe a huge collective debt in many ways: Mary Assunta, Emily Banks, David Bareham, Lisa Bero, John Bevins, Stella Bialous, Ron Borland, Fiona Byrne, Cynthia Callard, Tom Carroll, Stacy Carter, Joanna Cohen, Greg Connolly, John Cornwall, Elif Dağlı, Mike Daube, the late Ron Davis, Tom Eissenberg, Sherry Emery, Michael Farrell, Cecilia Farren, Esteve Fernández, Becky Freeman, Coral Gartner, Anna Gilmore, Gary Giovino, Stan Glantz, the late Nigel Gray, Paul Grogan, Prakash Gupta, Wayne Hall, Abby Haynes, Marita Hefler, David Hill, Janet Hoek, Bobbie Jacobson, the late Konrad Jamrozik, Anne

Jones, Melissa Jones, Luk Joossens, Harald and Justyna Klingemann, Kylie Lindorff, Ruth Malone, Bernie McKay, Judith Mackay, Ross MacKenzie, Martin McKee, Wasim Maziak, Robert Moodie, Michael Moore, Matt Myers, Andrew Penman, Matthew Peters, Richard Peto, Chris Picton, John Pierce, Charlotta Pisinger, Angela Pratt, Robert Proctor, Nicola Roxon, Rob Sanson-Fisher, Michelle Scollo, Stan Shatenstein, David Simpson, Andrea Smith, Maurice Swanson, Prakit Vathesatogkit, Melanie Wakefield, Raoul Walsh, Ken Warner, Ann Westmore, Sarah White and Pin Pin Zheng.

Thanks also go to seven Australian and international colleagues for their critical reading of parts of or the entire manuscript, to my long-time editor at Sydney University Press, the wonderful Agata Mrva-Montoya and to Jo Lyons who edited the final text.

I also want to thank two people I will always regard as my career mentors: Henry Mayer (1919–91), professor of politics at the University of Sydney, and Steve Leeder, the head of department in the early stage of my academic career. Henry was a man with a true European renaissance intellect who called me out of the blue one day after reading an early paper I'd written. Over the next few years, we would lunch and talk and he would send me large envelopes each week stuffed with notes about what I needed to read across a sometimes bewildering range of often esoteric material. Steve gave me every encouragement and a very long leash from which to explore whatever I felt interesting and important. That was the best supervisory and mentoring gift I could have ever received.

But my greatest thanks must go to my parents and several teachers who, perhaps without knowing they were doing it, must have done everything right to foment in me a deep instinct for scepticism. For as long as I can remember, my immediate response to anything redolent with dogma or orthodoxy has been to quietly and then sometimes loudly interrogate it. In 2013 when I was given the Australian Skeptic of the Year award, I couldn't have been more pleased.

This is my tenth and probably last book. I've deeply enjoyed writing it and hope its readers will get the same satisfaction. As always, thanks to Trish and my amazing family for all the love we share, and especially to Ali for taking the public health advocacy baton at full speed.

30 March 2022

Abbreviations

ACS	American Cancer Society
AIHW	Australian Institute of Health and Welfare
BAT	British American Tobacco
BATA	British American Tobacco Australia
CI	confidence interval
CO	carbon monoxide
CSIRO	Commonwealth Scientific and Industrial Research Organisation
ECs	electronic cigarettes
EVALI	e-cigarette- or vaping product-use associated lung injury
HCP	healthcare provider
HSI	Heaviness of Smoking Index
HTP	heated tobacco products
ITT	illicit tobacco trade
JTI	Japan Tobacco International
NGP	next generation products
NIH	National Institutes of Health, USA
NHMRC	National Health and Medical Research Council (Australia)
NRT	nicotine replacement therapy
NVPs	nicotine vaping products
OR	odds ratio
OTC	over-the-counter
PBS	Pharmaceutical Benefits Scheme (Australia).

PHE	Public Health England
PMI	Philip Morris International
PNG	Papua New Guinea
QALY	Quality-Adjusted Life Years
RCT	randomised controlled trial
RR	risk ratio
SSMs	stop smoking medications
TGA	Therapeutic Goods Administration (Australia).
USFDA	United States Food and Drug Administration
WHO	World Health Organization
WHO FCTC	WHO Framework Convention on Tobacco Control

Dollar figures are in Australian dollars unless otherwise specified as US$ (A$1 = US$0.72)

Introduction

I can't recall smoking my first full cigarette. I was probably around 14 or 15, had long been intrigued about smoking and had taken occasional drags on friends' furtive offerings away from the sight of parents. I thought a lot about the cachet I would instantly be given once people knew I was a smoker. I knew it would add to the usual gormless adolescent preoccupations of being respected as cool and edgy by friends.

In my teenage years in the 1960s, cigarette advertising wallpapered every media outlet in Australia. My tastes in music and fashion were very different to the sons of central western district farmers at the boys school I attended in country New South Wales. It was a similar story with smoking. Those who smoked mostly bought popular brands like Rothmans, Craven A or Viscount. When it came time for me to buy my first cigarettes, I needed to ask for a brand and I thought carefully about the statement I hoped I might make to others by my choice. My first brand was Country Life, a minor brand that I vaguely recall thinking would somehow stand out more than the brands that others smoked.

I hid them in a cavity in our garage roof and quietly got the pack down when I was going to a party or meeting up with friends at the local swimming pool. The ability to produce a pack of cigarettes in the right circumstances was important; you needed to have cigarettes and other rich clandestine signifiers at hand when an impression needed to be made. I also carried condoms long before I ever had an opportunity to use them, and I had an older friend who was happy to go into pubs to buy me cans of beer when these purchases were also needed to impress others. The first

Country Life pack took me months to finish. I found actually smoking them rather than just showing them around pretty unpleasant.

At university I continued to smoke. I remember buying brands I calculated would add some intrigue. There was a specialist tobacconist in Sydney's Potts Point which stocked evocative brands I'd encountered in novels or seen in ponderous European art-house films: Senior Service, Camel, Gauloises, Gitanes, Sobranie Black Russian and Abdulla. I bought all of these at different times. I smoked every day and more than I did at school, but a pack would still usually last me all week.

My early personal interest in cigarettes as an identity-signalling prop later morphed into an academic interest when I'd finished with smoking. As an undergraduate, I'd read Erving Goffman's 1956 sociological classic *The presentation of self in everyday life* and thought about what his ideas meant for the appeal of smoking and cigarette brand choice. My 1984 PhD on the semiotics of tobacco advertising was co-supervised by Henry Mayer, then Professor of Government at the University of Sydney. Mayer is described in the *Australian Dictionary of Biography* as "the founding father of the study of mass communication in Australia" (Goot 2014). When we first met, he encouraged me to read French essayist Roland Barthes' *Mythologies* (London: Paladin, 1973) and to think about the application of anthropologist Claude Lévi-Strauss' work on totemism to the way that advertising communicated with consumers and provided almost totemic identification and loyalty to different brands. Judith Williamson's *Decoding advertisements* (London: Marion Boyars, 1978) and Varda Langholz Leymore's *Hidden myth: structure and symbolism in advertising* (London: Heinemann, 1975) were also very influential on my thinking.

My PhD thesis was titled *Cigarette advertising as myth: a re-evaluation of the relationship of advertising to smoking*. An edited version of it was later published as *Great expectorations: advertising and the tobacco industry* (London: Co-media, 1986). A central part of it looked at different Australian cigarette-brand advertising, and the ways in which the themes and propositions in branding offered promises that could alleviate a variety of problems (insecurity, isolation, ordinariness, wanting to stand out from or merge with a peer group, concerns about smoking and health, people thinking you were not very smart if you smoked, and so on). Advertising proposed to smokers that they were winners, not losers; leaders not followers; or followers not leaders for those who walked to the beat of that drum.

Quitting cigarettes

But for all their value in conspicuously badging my evolving identity to others in those early years, right from the beginning I never really enjoyed cigarettes. I knew and accepted what was said about smoking being bad for your health. But I also thought everything except the first puff tasted acrid and unpleasant. So when I started working for the NSW Health Commission when I was 24, I saw this as a great excuse to stop buying them. For a few years I'd still occasionally take a cigarette when one was offered but rarely finished it.

Unlike some ex-smokers, I don't remember the day when I stopped. I also don't recall going without smoking as being in any way difficult or unpleasant. There was no sudden stop. I just drifted out of it and didn't think of myself anymore as someone who smoked. I didn't miss smoking, and experienced nothing remotely like withdrawal when I tried to stop. In fact, I didn't have to *try* to stop, I just decided I would. Despite smoking for about 10 years at least weekly and often daily from the age of 16, it was likely that I was not addicted to nicotine, and like the seldom-mentioned experience of many ex-smokers, I had experienced little if any difficulty or stress in quitting. This book will discuss how widespread my way of stopping has always been in a surprisingly large proportion of former smokers, while the smoking-cessation industry relentlessly frames quitting as being hugely protracted and difficult.

Toward the end of the 1970s, I became immersed in tobacco control through my work and especially through efforts with colleagues to politicise government inaction on tobacco industry advertising and promotion (Chapman 1980). While I was mainly engaged in advocacy to end tobacco advertising, population-wide smoking cessation – how to maximise the number of smokers throughout the population who quit – was also something with which I became very interested.

In those days – as now to a lesser extent – talk in my work environment about quitting smoking was preoccupied with interventions directed at individuals, either alone or in small groups. The Seventh-day Adventist Church had long run its 5-Day Plan (since 1959). Efforts were made to get smokers to go along to meetings across five days with the target of quitting on the fifth day. There were folksy tips about drinking lots of water between meals, distracting yourself by eating carrot sticks and avoiding situations where one usually smoked, as well as opaque references to a higher power. Predictably, the non-smoking, non-drinking, non-gambling and vegetarian church also counselled smokers to not drink alcohol when trying to quit. But nothing in this advice was supported by anything that today would pass as credible, robust evidence about efficacy or effectiveness in smoking cessation.

When we in the Health Commission enquired with the Adventists about how frequently their courses were run and how many people might be able to attend, the information we received was very vague. It seemed that what was on offer was quite a lot less than any vision of a proliferation of courses being run each week across Sydney's vast suburbs, let alone beyond into country areas. No numbers were forthcoming on whether attendance at the few courses on offer could be counted on two hands or was something far more substantial, with packed halls and long waiting lists. Beyond claims about percentages of smokers who had quit smoking on the last night of their courses, I never saw anything remotely approaching any formal evaluation of what they were doing in Australia, although several papers had been published in the USA showing lasting success in quitting in a small minority of attendees, for example (Thompson and Wilson 1966).

With such reticence about the reach of what they were doing, it seemed obvious that there was likely almost zero match between the vast number of smokers across Sydney who wanted to stop smoking and the ability of the local 5-Day Plan organisers to accommodate even a miniscule fraction of these numbers. This was a fundamental early insight that quickly took root in my instinctive assessment of claims being made and informed the way I came to think of organised efforts and products designed to help smokers quit.

Introduction

Early Australian efforts at promoting quitting

From the early years of the 20th century, there has been a long history in Australia, as elsewhere, of urgings and later advice to smokers to quit. In the early decades, this was mostly delivered by Christian temperance movement groups, with core messages that smoking defiled the temple of the body and displeased God. There was early emphasis on preventing youth (especially boys) from smoking, with parliamentary acts preventing sales to youth passed in NSW (1903), South Australia (1904), Queensland (1905), Victoria (1906) and Western Australia (1917). The boy scout movement promoted founder Robert Baden-Powell's view that smoking stunted the body and befuddled the brain (Walker 1984, Tyrrell 1999). Powell wrote

> When a lad smokes before he is fully grown up it is almost sure to make his heart feeble, and the heart is the most important organ in a lad's body (Roher 2007).

In the 1950s, considerable news coverage was given to early epidemiology examining the association between smoking and lung cancer, starting with two seminal case-control studies from England (Doll and Hill 1950) and the USA (Wynder and Graham 1950). The US-based *Reader's Digest*, which enjoyed wide subscriber-based circulation in Australia, covered these studies (Parssinen 2017). Australia's peak health advisory group, the National Health and Medical Research Council (NHMRC), first raised smoking with the Minister of Health in 1957, recommending, "States should commence publicity campaigns (i) to warn non-smokers against acquiring the habit of smoking (ii) to induce habitual smokers to cease smoking or to reduce consumption" (NHMRC 1957).

The NHMRC's recommendation had profoundly little impact on government policy. Sixteen years later in 1973, and seven years after the USA became the first nation to do so, Australia legislated our first timid cigarette-pack warning – "Warning: Smoking is a health hazard" in a tiny font at the base of packs in a colour that was easily lost against the pack colours (Chapman and Carter 2003). Nearly one in three 10–12-year-old Sydney schoolchildren thought "hazard" meant "habit", a confusion that undoubtedly would have delighted tobacco industry lobbyists at the time in their negotiations with government over the preferred wording (Long 1975).

Governments had published sporadic anti-smoking posters and pamphlets in the 1960s. In the early 1970s, the Anti-Cancer Council of Victoria (now Cancer Council Victoria), led by tobacco control pioneer Nigel Gray (1928–2014), produced and broadcast a number of satirical anti-smoking television advertisements that were run only a few times because of budgetary constraints, but attracted widespread public attention because of efforts by advertising authorities to ban them (Cancer Council Victoria 2020). The consumer magazine *Choice*, which commenced publication in April 1960, gave early priority to warning about the health effects of smoking. Its May 1961 issue included analysis of the effect of cigarette filters in removing "solids" from smoke that was inhaled through the filter (*Choice* magazine 1961). The filters performed woefully, as shown in a simple YouTube demonstration (TLB Productions 2007) of the residual black particulate matter ('tar') deposited on tissue paper when exhaled after being just held in the mouth and after being drawn deep into the lungs.

There was also considerable news media attention given to the harm caused by smoking, as well as to the dissembling activities of a small number of local (Chapman 2003a) and visiting doctors (Chapman 2003b) who assisted the tobacco industry in its global "smoker reassurance" efforts (Francey and Chapman 2000). Tobacco retail trade magazines from the 1950s described strategies used by tobacconists to assuage nervous smokers' concerns about health problems (Tofler and Chapman 2003). They frequently proposed that diseases such as lung cancer were caused by industrial and motor vehicle pollution, not smoking.

I have large folders of photocopied Australian newspaper clippings dating from the 1950s about smoking and health. As an expert witness in litigation, I was provided these by law firms acting for plaintiffs dying from mesothelioma, a cancer of mesothelial tissue, associated especially with exposure to asbestos, who were suing asbestos companies for negligence (Heenan 2006). Many of these plaintiffs were also smokers and the asbestos companies were seeking to argue a defence of contributory negligence in asbestos-exposed plaintiffs who "chose" to

Introduction

smoke, despite the widespread negative publicity. With smoking in men being very widespread in the 1950s and '60s, this was the situation of many of the mesothelioma victims. While this news coverage was dominated by items covering health risks of smoking, there were also many which focused on the "controversy" about whether smoking was in fact risky. There has been a good deal of publicity seen by millions of Australians about the risks of smoking in the 70 years since 1950. Much of this influenced a lot of people to quit smoking. In those early days there was no regular surveying of how many smokers quit which commenced in Australia in the 1970s, so there is no fine-grained data to assist in analyses of how effective news publicity alone was in driving down smoking.

Australia's first mass-reach quit-smoking campaign

From 1981 to February 1983, I was head of the New South Wales Health Commission's Anti-Smoking Project Group, with a roving brief to find innovative ways of promoting quitting. The portentous-sounding "group" I headed never consisted of anyone but me and a part-time librarian Edith Falk, whose job it was to build up and disseminate a collection of reports and scientific papers about smoking and how to quit. During this time, the NSW Labor health minister Laurie Brereton, had been persuaded about the importance of running large scale, mass-reach anti-smoking campaigns by an early pioneer, health administrator Bernie McKay, who led Australia's first significantly budgeted quit-smoking campaign on the North Coast of NSW (Egger, Fitzgerald et al. 1983). The success of this campaign saw it rolled out statewide after McKay was promoted to secretary of the NSW Department of Health in 1982 and lost no time in elevating the North Coast approach to statewide reach.

In 1982, a set of TV, radio and print advertisements were produced by Sydney advertising creative director John Bevins, who had worked on the North Coast campaign and earlier on the pioneering advertisements commissioned by the Anti-Cancer Council of Victoria. An evaluation team was also assembled, led by John Pierce at the University of Sydney. For the first time, Sydney residents regularly saw prime-time, highly professional quit-smoking advertising (Pierce, Dwyer et al. 1986) in what was called the *Quit. For Life* campaign. A collection of most of these advertisements can be seen on YouTube (Chapman 2020b).

We must provide help!

I was part of the team that implemented the campaign in 1983–84. While it was being planned, voices up and down the bureaucratic tree began insisting that it would be simply unacceptable to raise concerns about smoking in TV advertising and encouraging quitting across the community, without providing "help" to these smokers to do so. This was the first time I'd encountered the idea that if you were wanting to quit, you would benefit from being professionally assisted while you attempted to stop. There was furious agreement with this idea from many of those who had been brought in to advise and work on the campaign.

In fact, it went further than this. Never far from the surface of conversations about quitting was the idea that the best way to quit was to immerse yourself in some new form of innovative talk therapy or procedure – often to have something *done to you* – that would supposedly greatly increase your chances of quitting for good. We were seeing an early manifestation of clinical psychologists broadening their canvas from the individual in front of them to problems that affected vast numbers of the population.

Plans got underway to open a dedicated quit-smoking centre during the *Quit. For Life* media campaign, providing various forms of assistance to those wanting help. The idea was that the centre's staff would offer a smorgasbord of quit assistance from which smokers could choose. Renee Bittoun, who ran a quit-smoking service at Sydney's St Vincent's Hospital and had tried to help media mogul Kerry Packer quit smoking after he'd been admitted to hospital in October 1990 after a heart attack, headed the centre. A psychologist from the University of New South Wales, Chris Clarke, who was interested in a new aversive experimental strategy called "rapid smoking" (Danaher 1977) was also in attendance. With the rapid smoking approach, participants smoked several cigarettes in quick succession to try to maximise unpleasant reactions and taste. This procedure was designed to condition smokers to experience unpleasant, aversive associations with smoking when

Introduction

they lit up. Pioneering Russian physiologist Ivan Pavlov's work on classical conditioning had paved the way for this type of "great idea".

A publication from the time describing the centre lists six treatment options: hypnosis-assisted therapy; "non-cult" meditation; relaxation; rapid smoking; 14-day withdrawal; and self-control ("this consisted of attention centring on non-cult meditation combined with an abbreviated deep muscle relaxation procedure. It was explained that learning how to combat smoking-related thoughts and images, and physical tensions would provide the self-control necessary to not smoke") (Bittoun and Clarke 1985).

This was at a time well before any considerations of robust evidence were in the forefront of government and professional recommendations about how to quit. I recall being in a meeting called to discuss who might be suitable to provide "non-cult" hypnotherapy to those who chose it from the clinic's menu. The yellow pages business phone directory located several of these and some were contacted. Some turned out to be little more than theatrical stage hypnotherapists. There were no clinical accreditation procedures for hypnotherapy in those days, let alone for "non-cult meditation" or "relaxation".

"Relaxation" sessions had enjoyed a period of being fashionable in health promotion professional circles in the 1970s in Australia. I can recall attending staff development courses on a miscellany of issues which often featured periods where softly spoken psychologists would ask everyone to lie on the floor with their shoes off, in the loose clothing we had been requested to wear for the day. Over about 20 minutes, the supine participants would be invited to concentrate on thoughts about progressively relaxing different parts of our bodies, often to the gentle sounds of a tape playing whisper-soft bird, water or rustling tree sounds. I don't remember dangling crystals or mists of heated essential oils, but you get the picture.

At the end of each session, which sometimes saw participants fall asleep and start to snore, people would sit up and beatifically assure the relaxation session leader that they had been transformed from being stressed and tight to being blissfully relaxed and centred and ready for the stressful challenges of the day.

Somewhere among all this, someone must have thought they had a ripe audience in naïve health promotion leaders from the period for the idea that these rituals could somehow help many thousands of people stop smoking. Yes, it was that amateur – all in the self-evident, unquestioning line of duty to the rapidly emerging dogma that smokers serious about quitting should always be helped. Almost anything was worth trying, it seemed.

The quit-smoking centre was at Sydney Hospital, on the edge of the central business district. It operated for three months, during which time "over 3,500" smokers attended at least one session of the various interventions being offered. Two months after attendance, they were mailed a questionnaire and 2,491 (said to represent 69% of those who attended) were returned. Of these, 738 claimed to have stopped smoking (30% of those returning questionnaires, and 21% of those who ever attended) (Bittoun and Clarke 1985).

In 1983, around 67% of Sydney's then 3.355 million population was aged 20 years and over and smoking prevalence was 35%. This meant there were some 786,000 over-20-year-old smokers in Sydney. The 738 smokers who said they had quit after attending the centre thus represented one in 1,065 or 0.09% of Sydney's smokers. And that's before we consider questions of the reliability of self-reported quit data provided to those conducting the interventions, the absence of any biochemical validation of whether they had truly stopped smoking, and of considerable relapse rates that would have still occurred after two months (JR Hughes, Keely et al. 2004) – see Chapter 2. And it was also before anyone asked the obvious question: how many of the people who attended the clinics would have quit anyway, sooner or later, had they never attended the clinic.

Nascent scepticism starts to foment

Because I had begun working in tobacco control, had quit myself and knew plenty of others who also had stopped smoking, I sometimes asked people how they had gone about stopping. My daily, increasing gut instinct in those very early years of my career in tobacco control was that the growing number of people I knew who used to smoke but no longer did had nearly all stopped smoking without any formal or professional help. This was borne out in a 1975 paper by Nigel Gray and

Introduction

David Hill who reported that by the age of 45, half of those who had ever smoked in Australia had quit (Gray and Hill 1975). The corollary of that instinct was that the galloping momentum among many of my work colleagues to steer people into "professionally" mediated cessation was a castle being enthusiastically built on very wet and avoidable sand.

In the late 1970s, I was very influenced by the writings of Ivan Illich. His *Medical nemesis: the expropriation of health* (London: Marion Boyars, 1976) explored the issue of iatrogenic medicine – the ways in which the practice of medicine can harm health. He identified three forms of iatrogenesis: (1) clinical, or the direct harm done by various medical treatments; (2) social, or the medicalisation of ordinary life; and (3) cultural, or the loss of traditional ways of preventing and dealing with health problems. I began to wonder if the professionalisation of smoking cessation was an example of this medicalisation, and whether it was undermining "agency" in many smokers to feel confident that they could quit on their own. US critic Stanton Peele's 1989 book *Diseasing of America: how we allowed recovery zealots and the treatment industry to convince us we are out of control* (Peele 1989) further consolidated my thinking in the 1990s. I discuss this in Chapter 5.

A 1977 collection of essays by Illich and others called *Disabling professions* (London: Marion Boyars, 1977) included a piece by American medical sociologist Irving Zola, who wrote about the growing medicalisation of society and the ways in which this often disempowered people to do things they had long done without help. These works were early articulations of a theme that today attracts enormous attention in public health, clinical and health services scholarship: the idea that *far less* medical and professional intervention can often result in *better* outcomes for a wide range of health problems.

I began thinking a lot about the application of these perspectives to tobacco control. At the core of what both interested and disturbed me was those back-of-an-envelope calculations I'd done for the Sydney quit-smoking centre which showed the utterly hopeless mismatch between one-on-one or small group approaches to quitting and the vast numbers of smokers who had an interest in quitting. If we were going to make serious inroads into reducing smoking, the approaches to doing this would need to be able to reach correspondingly huge numbers of people, before questions of the effectiveness of those policies and programs were even considered.

Individuals or populations?

When I began running this perspective past colleagues, I found a polarised reaction. There were many who immediately got it. These were people who instinctively understood that with a problem as widespread as smoking, the very first criterion in evaluating the sense in running potential strategies was whether a policy or program could even *reach* millions of smokers, before questions of how effective these might be were evaluated. If it was obvious that a particular program could never attract the attention of – let alone involve – even tiny fractions of smokers, such programs could never hope to make a small impression in reducing smoking across a population.

Those who thought quit clinics were serious ways of helping lots of people quit smoking were almost invariably clinicians or those employed in the helping professions. Their training and experience involved trying to assist individuals or sometimes small groups of individuals to change. An eye-moistening parable I often used in teaching public health is useful here in distinguishing individual from population-wide perspectives.

A parent and child are walking on a beach and see thousands of fish being washed up on the shoreline by a strong tide. Many of the fish are dead and the rest flap helplessly on the sand. The parent begins to throw surviving fish back into the water, liberating them from their fate one at a time. The child questions the parent, asking what the point is of saving a few fish when inevitably, for each one saved, hundreds or thousands more will immediately take their place, being washed ashore with each wave. The parent replies that while the child's observation is true, each fish that is saved by their actions will be in no doubt that being helped to live was a good thing.

I told this parable to emphasise that personal acts of generosity, helpfulness, care and attention can make important differences to others. Very relevant here is the concept of the "rule of rescue" (McKie and Richardson 2003), which sees political and resource allocation priority always given to efforts to save identifiable, named individuals, rather than unnamed "statistical" individuals whose lives might be saved or their quality of life enhanced in years to come by policy decisions taken today. Civilised societies always value individuals and so dropping everything and sparing no expense to cure or save them is always valued.

Rescuing individuals – or for our purposes here, assisting people to stop smoking – is nearly always virtuous. People running small interventions in the community such as quit clinics undeniably help some of those who attend their clinics to stop. But a population perspective focuses on the comparative utility of individuals saving fish one at a time, versus efforts to mitigate the factors that are causing so many fish to be washed ashore in the first place, and adopting policies that might trigger large numbers of smokers to quit without enormous investments in labour or drugs.

Many tobacco control policies reach *every* smoker (for example, widespread smoking restrictions in indoor settings, advertising bans, graphic pack health warnings, taxation increases, plain packaging). Mass-reach interventions like major, well-funded public awareness campaigns are likewise seen by most smokers and might collectively inspire large numbers to try to quit. In Chapter 8, I'll look at what areas of tobacco control are worth serious government investment and action if a population focus is the canvas.

Over the 47 years of my career, I often saw well-meaning but hopelessly inconsequential small-scale quit-assistance efforts bobbing up in many nations. Between 1982 and 2014, I worked as a consultant or advisor on tobacco control to the World Health Organization, the Union for International Cancer Control (formerly International Union Against Cancer), and Consumers International on 25 occasions in 17 nations. On every one of these occasions, the numbers of those attending the meetings or training workshops I was organising or helping with were dominated by people with clinical orientations.

When we did our introductions on the first mornings and people were asked to say what they did in tobacco control, by far the most common response was that those attending ran smoking cessation clinics in hospitals or community settings, often only occasionally as an add-on to their primary clinical roles. Many kept no records of smoker throughput (how many attended their clinics) or even short-term quit outcomes, let alone well-down-the-track impacts. Yet in many of these nations, there was only the most rudimentary level of tobacco control law, regulation or policy in place. Tobacco control in these nations was often the sum total of the effort of these few individuals trying to coax small numbers of smokers into quitting.

Frankly, the aggregated contributions of these few individually focused people in reducing smoking across whole populations was nothing but spitting into the wind of huge forces which were recruiting people into smoking, keeping them there with industry chemists optimising nicotine addiction (Henningfield, Pankow et al. 2004) and wrecking policies that might seriously slow all this down. Every day, untold thousands of people took their first puff of a cigarette, driven by the marketing efforts of the tobacco industry and by governments which failed to control these promotions.

Early provocations

I began writing about this total futility in 1985, when I was awarded an Australian NHMRC travelling fellowship to London to study the natural history of smoking cessation. Seeing burgeoning examples of quit-smoking clinics in England, I published a deliberately provocative paper in *The Lancet* called "Stop-smoking clinics: a case for their abandonment" (Chapman 1985). I walked readers through the arithmetical mismatch between the reach and impact of these clinics and any population-wide ambition to reduce smoking throughout England. The paper upset several early leaders in English tobacco control and while I was not run out of the country, I experienced my first taste of the renowned English cold shoulder.

In later years, seeing a major consolidation of resources devoted to assisted smoking cessation (particularly in England – see Chapter 4), I returned several times to this issue, publishing next a short piece in *The Lancet* titled, "The inverse impact law of smoking cessation in 2009" (Chapman 2009). In this I wrote:

Introduction

Acknowledging Julian Tudor Hart (Hart 1971), I propose the inverse impact law of smoking cessation. This law states that the volume of research and effort devoted to professionally and pharmacologically mediated cessation is in inverse proportion to that examining how ex-smokers actually quit. Research on cessation is dominated by ever-finely tuned accounts of how smokers can be encouraged to do anything but go it alone when trying to quit – exactly opposite of how a very large majority of ex-smokers succeeded. The virtual silence about this undeniably positive news reflects the dominance of those whose careers depend on continuing to offer and evaluate labour-intensive regimens and the influence of the drug industry which has a vested interest in prolonging cessation and in repeat attempts after relapse.

I followed this in 2010 with a longer piece with Ross MacKenzie in *PLOS Medicine*, looking at the huge research neglect of unassisted cessation, and summarising the factors that together seemed responsible for this neglect (Chapman and MacKenzie 2010). By March 2022, the paper had been accessed over 58,000 times and cited 300 times. I summarise that paper in Chapter 3.

These papers saw me get a lot of invitations to speak at meetings about my argument. As had occurred 25 years earlier when I published my original *Lancet* piece, key figures in British tobacco control seemed intensely irritated by what I was arguing. I give some examples of this in Chapter 5 where I examine the almost cult-like dogma that so many in tobacco control, particularly in Britain, embrace and defend.

Outline of this book

For as long as people have smoked tobacco, there have also been many who decided to stop doing it. No one has ever attempted to estimate the total, aggregated number of people across the centuries who once smoked and then no longer did. For almost all of that time, quitting was something that was never studied or counted. I've never seen an estimate of total quitting numbers for even the 60-year post-1960 period when quitting accelerated. But as I will consider in Chapter 3, such a figure in global aggregate would number in the hundreds of millions.

Considered against this historical backdrop, "modern" professionalised, pharmaceutical and, most recently, vaping approaches to quitting are all very recent phenomena that have occurred within the five minutes before midnight on a 24-hour clock of the full history of smoking cessation. If we were able to estimate the total number of people who have ever smoked and the total number who later stopped smoking completely, the proportion who were assisted in quitting by the actions of any kind of therapist or interventionist, or by consuming a potion, a pill or nicotine replacement (pharmaceutical, or most recently, from e-cigarettes) would be a small minority.

I have often asked my public health classes, groups of friends around a dinner table and many individuals if they ever smoked but have now quit. I then ask them *how* they quit. Overwhelmingly, most ex-smokers say they quit without taking any drug, wearing a nicotine patch, seeing a therapist or attending a special clinic. Try that exercise yourself a few times and you will almost certainly have the same experience.

Unassisted quitting is not a phenomenon that is unique to smoking. It is also very common among other dependencies, and this is important to understand. So in Chapter 1, we'll step away from smoking and briefly consider how people with other addictions and compulsive behaviours end their dependencies. I'll summarise the evidence about unassisted cessation of problematic alcohol, opiate and cannabis use and problem gambling.

Before turning the focus onto how most people stop smoking, in Chapter 2 I'll next review the strengths and weaknesses of different types of evidence that are often used to make claims about success rates in quitting smoking. We'll also look carefully at the great variability in what is meant by smoking cessation – stopping, quitting or remission from smoking, and the core issue of relapse in that understanding. This chapter will lay the bedrock for the subsequent chapters where we will look at the track record of various assisted routes to quitting, and especially the contribution of these to population-wide quitting. I will move from considering the weakest form of evidence – testimonials and anecdotes from those who swear by a particular way of quitting – to looking at stronger forms: randomised controlled trials, cross-sectional

Introduction

"snapshot" and time-series surveys, and cohort studies of large groups of randomly selected smokers who are followed across time to see how many keep smoking, quit and relapse back to smoking.

There are several important biases in studies of smoking cessation: self-selection bias, competing-interest bias, recall bias, positive outcome bias and indication bias. I'll summarise what we need to know about each of these in interpreting claims for smoking cessation.

I'll also look at the problem of determining both the whys and hows of successful quitting, including complex questions of attribution: of how clear we can be about what motivated people to quit and what should be best considered the "how" of ex-smokers' success in completely stopping smoking.

Chapter 3 will examine what we know about how many millions of smokers quit in the eras both before and after the availability of nicotine replacement therapy (NRT), prescribed drugs like bupropion (Zyban™) and varenicline (Champix™), and most recently e-cigarettes. The introduction of these drugs in the modern era of smoking cessation dates from the 1980s when public discussions of quitting began becoming increasingly "medicalised" as a problem best needing treatment. I'll summarise some of the most important studies looking at the questions of whether the availability of these aids changed both quit attempts and quit successes in real-world settings.

Chapter 4 will look at the track record of various approaches to promoting smoking cessation that have been promoted as having potentially mass-reach impact. These include establishing and promoting networks of specialised quit clinics (particularly in England), efforts to increase doctors' rates of actively assisting their smoking patients to quit, telephone quitlines, apps and online quit programs, "contingency payments" (paying smokers to quit), and quit and win lotteries.

This chapter will conclude with a look at the evidence about the extent to which interventions that are frequently described and evaluated in research journals and presented at research conferences are ever "upscaled" to become serious ways capable of assisting significant numbers of smokers to quit. When we read a report that shows a particular intervention has been a success, it is perhaps natural to assume that it will soon happen that governments, non-government public health organisations or the private sector will pounce on this good news and start offering the intervention to large numbers of smokers who are clamouring to participate.

As we will see, this is far from the case. In brief, very few behavioural interventions of the type we trip over daily in the pages of research journals ever go on to become routinely adopted into policies and practices which actually reach and affect mass numbers of people who might benefit from that exposure. Most intervention research papers delivered at health conferences and published in journals describe interventions that only those who were exposed in the research project ever experience. They rarely become a routine part of day-to-day communicative, workplace, educational or clinical environments, which was the whole idea in trialling these interventions in the first place. For this reason, much published intervention research is very inconsequential and a distraction from the year-on, year-out ways that see most smokers actually go about and succeed in quitting.

Chapter 5 will look at the way those promoting assisted quitting have attempted to sell and defend their message to smokers and the news media. Here, we'll take a critical look at the core subtexts of the ways in which advocates for assisted smoking cessation, the pharmaceutical industry and vaping advocates have sought to frame the benefits of assisted cessation. First, I'll forensically examine the arguments on which the entire pitch for smokers *needing* assistance rests. The first of these is the "hardening hypothesis", which posits that today's smokers are dominated by hardcore, intractable smokers who are deeply addicted to nicotine, have repeatedly failed to quit and are highly unlikely to do so without a leg-up from pharmacological assistance and/or professional support.

Another aspect of often unchallenged folk and professional wisdom is the widely held belief that quitting is often extremely difficult, as attested by the many failed attempts or relapses back to smoking that often characterise smokers' efforts to quit. As we'll see, one of the best kept secrets about quitting is that a very sizable proportion of those who quit find it unexpectedly easy to stop. I'll look at why this is such a closely held secret for many working in tobacco control.

Another dominant narrative is that to quit, a smoker needs to transit through several "stages of change" before they have any real chance of quitting successfully. A first stage has been called the "precontemplation" stage. This is where smokers aren't considering quitting at all. Many smokers progress to a next stage where they "contemplate" quitting, but don't take any serious steps to do so. Next comes the preparation, action to quit and maintenance of quitting stages. And then, for many, the relapse stage followed by recycling at a later time through it all again.

The trouble with all this is there is widespread evidence that many people leapfrog several of these stages and suddenly quit, often permanently, without following the neat model pathway laid out in what has been called the transtheoretical theory of behaviour change (Prochaska and Velicer 1997).

Those promoting assisted quitting have frequently denigrated cold turkey as the very worst way of trying to quit by using a number of interrelated strategies. These include the bizarre exclusion and cursory dismissal of unassisted quitting from reviews of "evidence-based cessation", implying that there is no "evidence" to support unaided quitting as the method that yields (by far) the most long-term successful quitting numbers in whole populations. Clinical guidelines on how clinicians can best promote quitting among their patients routinely give no mention of unassisted quitting.

This chapter will also discuss factors and actors that have and continue to drive the commodified "specialisation" of smoking cessation. It will explore how the medicalisation of quitting over the past 40 years has been an entirely predictable development against the background of the burgeoning commodified medicalisation of common, ordinary human problems which have previously not been medically labelled as pathologies and supervised by clinicians. The dominance of the interventionist paradigm in mainstream tobacco-control thinking dovetails strongly with this medicalisation. The chapter will look at the promotion of, not just cessation medication, but maintenance (long-term or lifetime) medication, multiple medication and even pre-quit medication.

The two principal actors driving the narrative of "don't try to quit unaided" are first corporations benefitting from as many quit attempts as possible, ringing their cash registers every time a medication is used or an e-cigarette powered on; and second, professional and commercial interventionists wedded to the "take something or do something" school of behaviour change who often find natural alliance with the industries which make such products.

In Chapter 6, I'll look critically at the latest kids on the block in commodified smoking cessation: electronic cigarettes and other novel nicotine products. The hype about these products is that they are massively disrupting the entire approach to tobacco control because of the twin claims that they are all but completely benign and unparalleled in being useful for quitting smoking. The use of these products has grown rapidly in many nations since around 2010. I'll look closely at the claims that are made for them about smoking cessation by their advocates and the rather different reality of what we know about how successful they have been. The evidence to date on claims that they are spectacularly effective in helping people quit is sadly the latest outing of an old quit proselytising emperor, this time in new, still threadbare but very flavoursome clothes. My view is that the rise of vaping is just the latest chapter in the history of smoking cessation's mass distractions. As the saying goes, "Same, same but different."

Chapter 7 reproduces two edited open-access papers from a wider body of work arising from a three-year Australian NHMRC grant I led and worked on with five others, titled *The natural history of unassisted smoking cessation in Australia*. This grant produced seven research papers which formed the basis of the PhD thesis I co-supervised of Andrea Smith, awarded in 2018. The first paper is a systematic review of what the qualitative research literature available on unassisted quitting prior to September 2013 reported about the main themes elicited from successful quitters on why they "went it alone" when quitting. The second paper reports original work we conducted with successful ex-smokers in Sydney, and in particular about why these people had chosen not to quit using medications or professional help. This qualitative analysis of the accounts of unassisted quitting remains one of the most detailed examinations of how and why those who take this route out of smoking decide to do it.

Chapter 8 urges that we look at the big picture instead of being preoccupied with the impact of single interventions and policies. We should instead reflect on the huge rhino in the room of smoking cessation: that there have long been more ex-smokers than smokers, that most of them have quit unassisted and that they all were motivated to stop smoking by a complex synergy of factors that played out over years, not just in the final days or weeks before they ended their smoking.

This chapter will briefly summarise the available evidence on policies and mass-reach interventions that have driven smoking prevalence down in many nations which have taken tobacco control seriously. Often these policies have been implemented at glacial pace and interventions given only token funding, greatly reducing their reach. Part of the reason for this is that policies, interventions and assumptions of mass distraction have diverted funding attention and workforce focus away from research, policies and interventions that together promote the idea that smokers have agency or self-efficacy to try to succeed in quitting. We know that these policies collectively can drive smoking down across whole populations but are being sidelined by those in tobacco control who still can't or won't see the wood for the trees.

The final chapter in the book looks at policies to control and regulate the supply of tobacco. I compare how tobacco products are sold from literally any retail outlet that chooses to do so, while other products and services have long been subject to strictly enforced regulations around selling and access. The access to scheduled pharmaceutical products is the obvious comparison.

I end the book by looking at so-called endgame arguments for phasing out the sale of combustible tobacco and regulating nicotine vaping products in the ways that other addictive drugs have been regulated for decades.

1
How do most people quit other addictions?

> It does appear that the generally accepted professional and public impression that nicotine addiction, heroin addiction, and obesity are almost hopelessly difficult conditions to correct is flatly wrong. People can and do cure themselves of smoking, obesity and heroin addiction. They do so in large numbers and for long periods of time, in many cases apparently permanently (Schachter 1982).

Before turning to the focus of this book – how most ex-smokers stop smoking unassisted and the censorious reception that profane, heretical broadcasting of this too loudly can attract – I want to provide a brief overview of parallels with other dependencies or addictions. So, in this chapter, I will summarise the evidence about how the many people who once had other problem dependencies but no longer do, moved away from the fabled clutches of these without treatment or any formal support.

Within the addictions research field there has been a small group of pioneers of this research who have studied the natural histories of various substance and behavioural dependencies. They have shone light on what the research literature says about this phenomenon which is variously referred to as spontaneous remission, natural recovery, maturing out and unassisted change or cessation. These pioneers include Patrick Biernacki (Biernacki 1986), George Vaillant (Vaillant 1995), Jim Orford (Orford 1985), Harald Klingemann, Linda and Mark Sobell (Klingemann, Sobell et al. 2010) and Stanton Peele (Peele 1989). As we will see, there are some similarities here with what happens with the major phenomenon of unassisted recovery from smoking.

There have been several reviews of the early literature on unassisted remission from problematic substance use. Rossana Mariezcurrena published a narrative, descriptive review of the available literature in 1994, with sections on alcohol, drugs, tobacco and obesity (Mariezcurrena 1994). Walters' 2000 review of the quantitative literature on unassisted remission across several fields of substance dependence reported on just 11 papers, some of which covered more than one dependency (Walters 2000). He summarised a table in his paper on the prevalence of spontaneous remission in these dependencies as being "4.3% to 56.4% ... attributed to differences in the length of follow-up (range 1 to 27 years) and the time frame used to determine spontaneous remission (range 6 months to 3 years). The mean general prevalence of spontaneous remission for studies utilising a broad definition of remission was 26.2% in follow-ups averaging 5.3 years, with a mean rate of 31.4% for alcohol ($n = 8$ studies), 37.9% for illicit drugs ($n = 2$), and 13.4% for tobacco ($n = 5$)."

A 2010 systematic review of studies published between 1990 and 2009 on unassisted remission from amphetamines, cocaine, cannabis and opioids found just 10 studies of opioid and three for cannabis dependence. Definitions of remission varied and most did not clearly assess remission from dependence. Using conservative criteria for remission, rates varied between cannabis dependence (17.3%), amphetamines (16.4%), opioid (9.2%) and cocaine dependence (5.3%) (Calabria, Degenhardt et al. 2010).

Alcohol

In Australia in 2019, 6.7% of the adult population reported drinking more than 11 standard drinks on the one occasion, with 30% in the 18–24 year age group having done this (and 14.6% having done this at least monthly) (Australian Institute of Health and Welfare 2020f).

1 How do most people quit other addictions?

That this measure of harmful drinking declines dramatically with age, suggests that a very large number of people who regularly drank heavily early in their drinking histories mature out of it. Here's a selection of research support for that proposition.

In 1989, Statistics Canada conducted a random-digit-dialling telephone survey of 11,634 people living in 10 Canadian provinces, called the National Alcohol and Drugs Survey. A 78.7% participation rate was obtained. In 1993, the Institute of Social Research at Toronto's York University conducted a similar survey. Both surveys assured respondents of anonymity and reported data on the proportion of drinkers aged 20 and over who declared that they had experienced problem drinking but had recovered for more than a year. Linda Sobell and colleagues summarised the findings of the two surveys in a 1996 paper (Sobell, Cunningham et al. 1996).

The two surveys found that 75.5% (in the national survey) and 77.7% (in the Ontario survey) of those who had experienced but resolved problem drinking for more than a year had done so without any formal help or treatment. The definition of help here included attendance at Alcoholics Anonymous or any other support group; seeing a psychologist, psychiatrist or social worker; attending a psychiatric hospital; receiving help via a minister, priest or rabbi; receiving help from a doctor or nurse; attendance at a hospital or emergency department, alcohol/drug-addiction agency, a detoxification centre or halfway house; or attending a drink-driving referral program.

These were the first times that large-scale population data on this plainly widespread phenomenon – three in four recovered problem drinkers – had been gathered and reported. But as we will see below, unassisted recovery had been described by clinicians and those following the life courses of alcoholics since at least 1953 (Lemere 1953). Below are summaries of the key findings of a selection of these.

Roizen et al (1978) reviewed the literature available at that time on problem drinkers who had declined or been refused treatment, concluding, "In spite of the climate of opinion in which spontaneous improvements are often regarded as rare ... remission in the sense of six months of abstinence can be expected in 15 percent of cases" (Roizen, Cahalan et al. 1978, 201).

A small 1979 Scottish study of 19 "definite alcoholics" and 41 "problem drinkers", all without current drinking problems, found none reported receiving treatment of any sort, but attributed their change to life events like marriage, job change or illness, or to family or doctor advice or improvement of financial problems (Saunders and Kershaw 1979).

Similar factors were reported in a Texas study by Tuchfeld of those who'd given up drinking without any formal treatment (Tuchfeld 1981). Tuchfeld was careful to conclude that describing cessation of alcohol as "spontaneous" risked missing the importance of "internal psychological commitment" to stopping drinking being "usually activated by social phenomena ... by significant alterations in social and leisure activities". Indeed, much of the research literature emphasises the same key factors in those who successfully end their dependencies without professional help.

George Vaillant's pioneering 1983 book *The natural history of alcoholism* and its 1995 update *The natural history of alcoholism revisited* (Vaillant 1995) contain a great deal of information on the life-course of alcoholism and problem drinking. His 1995 revised book reviews all known longitudinal studies at the time of treated and untreated alcoholics and explores in great depth difficulties of studying those with this problem.

Loss to follow-up is a major problem in researching people with serious alcohol problems. In cohorts followed for many years, the often chaotic lives of alcoholics caused by frequent intoxication, job losses, incarceration, hospitalisation, homelessness, poverty and early death all greatly confound any strong conclusions being drawn about the proportions of alcoholics who ever recover, about what factors predict continuing alcoholism and what predicts those who become abstinent or asymptomatic drinkers after earlier alcoholism.

This may suggest that investigation of unassisted recovery with alcoholics may be biased by over-representation of those in follow-up research whose lives may have been somewhat less chaotic and disrupted than those who failed to recover.

Relapse is also a major problem in investigating abstinence after alcoholism, with long-term follow-up of abstinent former alcoholics being very uncommon. Vaillant reports a study with a mean eight-year follow-up which found that 45% of alcoholics relapsed after two years of abstinence, but only 9% after six years (Vaillant 1995, 235).

His review of 10 long-term follow-up studies concluded that "the best outcomes were from [three] untreated community samples … the worst outcomes, if one includes deaths, were received by alcoholics who received inpatient treatment" while noting that the latter "represented a more severely ill population with poorer prognosis". They were also older, and therefore more likely to die.

In summary, Vaillant's review identifies so many fundamental caveats about differentiating the progression of treated and untreated alcoholics that nowhere in his 446-page book does he ever come close to making any definitive statements that might resolve the question.

A 2019 systematic review of international research on untreated remission of alcohol problems found 124 estimates from 27 different studies, with the authors finding large variations across these studies in the ways in which both "treatment" and alcohol problems were defined, making it problematic to come up with any "across all studies" figure for untreated remission (Mellor, Lancaster et al. 2019). The same authors later conducted an online survey on a Facebook-recruited convenience sample of 719 people who had resolved an alcohol problem in Australia. Almost half (49.8%) of all people who resolved their alcohol problem did so without any access to alcohol treatment (specialist alcohol treatment, mutual-aid services or digital support services). However, this estimate dropped to 12.8% when accessing mental health treatment was included in the definition of "treatment" (Mellor, Lancaster et al. 2019).

Opiates

Perhaps more than any other category of drug, opiate narcotics have a popular reputation as being perishingly difficult to stop using once a person develops a lasting narcotics addiction. But as we shall see, there are a huge number of former narcotic-dependent people who have permanently stopped using these drugs, often after prolonged periods of addiction.

Patrick Biernacki's 1986 book *Pathways from heroin addiction: recovery without treatment* (Biernacki 1986) was an early myth-busting review of the hitherto largely unexplored phenomenon of people moving away from heroin use without any professional assistance. He commenced his book by asking a similar question to the one I began exploring for tobacco around the same time (Chapman 1985, Chapman 1986):

> Since opiates were introduced into the United States more than two centuries ago, millions of people have used them, and more than tens of thousands have become addicted to them (Brecher 1972). Are we to conclude that, without therapeutic intervention, all these people were destined to remain addicted for their entire lives? Or is it possible that many of them ... came to a point where they voluntarily stopped using and recovered on their own – what I term "natural" recovery? (Biernacki 1986, 6).

Biernacki noted the very similar way that heroin dependency was viewed to alcoholism at the time (and still is very much today) by addiction theorists and therapeutic practitioners:

> These theories are absolute (and pessimistic) in the belief that without major social reform or dramatic therapeutic intervention, drug addiction is an unalterable affliction ... From their perspective, alcoholism, like opiate addiction, is thought to be an unalterable condition if allowed to take its "natural" course. Recovery is attained only as a result of some form of treatment ... These highly deterministic perspectives are tenaciously maintained by their subscribers (Biernacki 1986, 18).

Biernacki's book explores information provided to his research team by 101 former opiate-dependent people who had been addicted for at least a year, and who were located and interviewed across two years from August 1978. Duration of their narcotics use ranged from one to two years, and up to 15 or more, with the number of years since last use also covering those time periods. Because of the stigmatised, illegal and subterranean nature of narcotic use in the USA at that time, his subjects were located by snowball sampling where those interviewed recommend others to be approached to take part (Biernacki and Waldorf 1981), often via contactable former narcotics users who were or had used treatment facilities. The challenges of obtaining the subjects for interview are fully described in an extensive appendix to the book.

He explores his informants' resolution to stop using narcotics, their steps to break away, why they chose not to avail themselves of any treatment or support program (all 101 had never used such services), moving away from the world of narcotics using friends and acquaintances, and establishing new relationships, interests and identities, and becoming "ordinary".

As with Vaillant's book on recovery from alcoholism, because of the inherent difficulties in locating former narcotics users and obtaining their consent to be involved in research, Biernacki's study does not allow any conclusions to be drawn about how common "natural" unassisted recovery is with narcotics. But it most certainly shows that natural recovery from narcotics is a real phenomenon, understudied as much then as it continues to be today.

American armed forces heroin users after the Vietnam War

One of the most famous of all studies in the natural recovery field is that by Robins, Davis and Nurco of American armed forces personnel who served in Vietnam and used narcotics (mainly heroin and opium) (Robins, Davis et al. 1974). The study involved interviewing and urine testing for narcotics on a sample of 470 enlisted personnel drawn from 13,760 who had returned from Vietnam in September 1971. Nineteen percent of these men were still enlisted when being interviewed, with the remainder being at the time civilians for an average of seven months.

Forty-three percent of those interviewed had used narcotics in Vietnam, with 46% of these saying that they had been addicted. But only 7% said they were still addicted since their return to the USA, with only 1% having positive urines. Of those who were "narcotic virgins" on arrival in Vietnam, more than two-thirds stopped all narcotics use when they left Vietnam.

Unfortunately, the paper says nothing about *how* these narcotics users stopped using, but there is also no mention of any treatment facilities provided either in Vietnam or by the armed services for those who returned to the US who may have had addiction problems. This absence may suggest that those who did stop using narcotics on their return from Vietnam mostly recovered without assistance.

Cannabis

I went through my 20s in the 1970s. There was a lot of cannabis being smoked in that decade. I smoked it socially about once every couple of weeks for perhaps five or six years and associated with few people of my age who didn't. When I started taking my career seriously, as had happened with my cigarette smoking I decided I didn't want to continue using dope and have not touched it in decades. Smoking dope wasted a lot of productive time which I increasingly valued. I also began to see many stoners as being very limited in their conversation and didn't want to feel that I might seem like that to others as well. Researchers on this well-recognised phenomenon have long referred to it as "maturing out" (Winick 1962).

As with smoking cigarettes, I subsequently found across the next decades that my story of smoking dope and then stopping uneventfully was very common and unremarkable. For many, smoking dope was something you did when you were young but then you "grew out of it" as you took on more responsibilities in study, work and your family life. But, as with smoking, I was never a heavy user.

So much for an anecdote, but what does the research literature have to say about the natural history of cannabis use?

The Australian Institute of Health and Welfare's (AIHW) 2019 National Drug Strategy Household Survey found 32% of adults reported ever having used cannabis, but that only 11.6% reported using it in the past 12 months (Australian Institute of Health and Welfare 2020b). Cannabis use decreased from a peak in the 30–39 year age group (47.2% any lifetime use; 13.7% use in the last 12 months; 7% use in the last month; 4.7% use in the last week) to (respectively) 8.9%, 2.9%, 1.6% and 1.3% in the 60+ age group, the youngest of whom would have been born in 1959. While there are certainly birth cohort differences in cannabis use in these two age groups, the reductions are also compatible with the maturing-out hypothesis. In over 40 years working in Australian public health, I have never heard of anything but small, fringe "treatment" services for quitting cannabis use. The overwhelming majority of former users almost certainly stopped getting stoned without help.

Beyond observations like those above about many Australian cannabis users maturing out of use as they aged, the research on questions about both why and how cannabis users stop is disappointingly sparse and thin, beyond work that notes correlates of different patterns of or changes in use, such as changing neighbourhood and friendship networks (Pollard, Tucker et al. 2014), transition to adulthood (Schulenberg, Merline et al. 2005, Kelly and Vuolo 2018), getting married (Leonard and Homish 2005), onset of pregnancy (Chen and Kandel 1998) or having a psychosis-like experience (Sami, Notley et al. 2019). A 2019 German retrospective cohort study of 6,467 current or former cannabis users aged 15 to 46 years (mean age 22.5) who had used the drug for at least three years found 16.3% had not used it in the previous year. No information on why they stopped or how they went about it was reported, and the young age of most of those in the study means we know nothing about transitions past an age when cannabis use is still at its peak (Seidel, Pedersen et al. 2019).

Missing from the literature is any substantial examination of motivations to stop using cannabis or of how users went about stopping. Indeed, intense searching of research publication databases failed to find a single paper or even a section within a paper examining or even speculating about how millions of people who once used cannabis but no longer do so transitioned to non-use. Perhaps the answer lies in something unstated but almost taken for granted: that for many, regular cannabis use in teenage and early adult life is something that people grow out of with few difficulties or much effort, and that most users do not have a dependency problem.

Problem gambling

"Gambling disorder" has been classified by the American Psychiatric Association as a behavioural disorder since 2014. Nine criteria are set out, and for diagnosis to be met at least four of these must apply. The disorder can be episodic or persistent. When diagnosis has been made and a person does not meet any of the criteria for 12 months or more, sustained remission is said to apply (American Psychiatric Association 2018).

The prevalence of pathological problem gambling in the Australian population was estimated in 2010 by the government's Productivity Commission at 0.7% of adults (then 115,000) with a further 1.7% (280,000) experiencing moderate-risk problem gambling (Australian Productivity Commission 2010). However, a 1996 review of global studies on the prevalence of pathological gambling argued that most published estimates greatly over-estimated the prevalence because of failure to distinguish between people ever having experienced problem gambling and those currently experiencing it (Walker and Dickerson 1996).

Rates of recovery, treatment seeking and natural recovery from pathological gambling were estimated from two United States national surveys: the National Epidemiologic Survey on Alcohol and Related Conditions, and the Gambling Impact and Behavior Study (Slutske 2006). Both surveys found that the rates of recovery and treatment seeking were about 40% and 10% respectively, and that most who at any time in their life had experienced pathological gambling and recovered did so without any formal treatment.

An Australian paper drawing on the Australian Twin Register database found that 104 out of 4,764 people had ever experienced problem gambling, and that 82% of these had moved out of their gambling problems without any treatment (92% of men and 57% of women) (Slutske, Blaszczynski et al. 2009). Notwithstanding this, a 2012 review in *Australian Family Physician* made no mention of natural recovery, recommending that doctors refer patients to community support groups (Rodda, Lubman et al. 2012).

Many who have had personal histories of alcoholism, narcotics dependency and problem gambling have experienced many years of traumatic impact on their lives. They may have experienced devastating financial losses, family and friendship breakdown, job loss, imprisonment and significant health problems. Their problems have often deeply alienated them from family and friends, and they experience social stigma.

Over the last 50 or so years, tobacco smoking has become deeply denormalised (Chapman and Freeman 2008) in many nations as smoking prevalence plummets, and places and occasions where smoking is not permitted become ubiquitous. While smoking might be said to have become increasingly stigmatised, particularly when smokers impose their smoking on others (Colgrove, Bayer et al. 2011), the level of stigmatisation of smoking is incomparably less than the stigma that applies to problem drinking, narcotic dependence and serious problem gambling. So while we have seen that there are commonalities between how most people uncouple from these dependencies and the way that most smokers quit, there are also important differences.

Chief among these is that ex-smokers are typically anything but ashamed of their achievement in quitting. Many are very forthcoming about it and happy to describe their experience. Those who have recovered from serious and chronic drinking problems are often similarly proud of their achievements, but probably many more are reticent about it because of the more enduring and powerful stigma involved, and anxieties that telling people about significant past phases of life where one was a problem drinker might trigger circumspection in others.

As we will see in Chapter 7, smokers who have quit unassisted have many deep insights into why and how they went about it and what they see as key factors explaining their success. Their insights are rarely embraced by those trying to promote quit attempts. This is largely because those with fundamental vested interests in commodifying and professionally mediating smoking cessation are naturally drawn to study smokers who use their products and services, and to both de-emphasise and often denigrate unassisted cessation as failure-ridden folly (see Chapter 5).

2
How we study quitting smoking: a critical look

There is a vast amount of research about smoking cessation that's been published with increasing frequency since the 1970s. Those who have been trained in critical appraisal of evidence in public health develop skills in being able to assess the strengths and weaknesses of research designs, and the ways in which authors of research papers and those who publicise them both select and highlight aspects of studies. In this chapter, I'll look critically at the types of evidence that are used in debates about particular ways of quitting and discuss some of their implications for the overarching question of how to maximise successful, permanent smoking cessation across whole populations. Many of the limitations of different sorts of evidence need to be kept closely in mind when appraising arguments put forward for various approaches to quitting.

Evidence is not the plural of anecdote

In the early 1990s on a World No Tobacco Day in March, I was the guest of the local health service in Broken Hill, a mining town in the far west of New South Wales. The staff had arranged for me to be interviewed by the local radio station that had a massive footprint across the extensive far west of the state. The host invited former smokers to call in and talk

2 How we study quitting smoking: a critical look

about *how* they had quit. Consistent with everything we know about the method most ex-smokers use at their final successful attempt to quit, many callers wanted to talk about *why* they had quit (see Chapter 3). As had occurred many times before during similar interviews, I mostly had to probe them to talk about *how* they had quit. Nearly all had quit unassisted, going cold turkey.

However, I recall the last caller wanting to tell all listening across the far west of NSW that the various ways of quitting earlier callers had named were all very well. But no one had mentioned the very best method. Could our expert up from Sydney guess it? No, you tell us all, I suggested. Our caller then extolled the importance of letting Jesus Christ into your life. Jesus had stopped him smoking and could stop anyone smoking. Everyone needed to know this, he said. His own experience was all the evidence we needed.

Doubtless there are many people around the world who would make similar claims that their religious faith helped them quit. And those imbued with religious faith often don't hold back about it. They make these claims sincerely and often passionately, wanting to share their experience with others to inspire them. But how effective is faith in Jesus in helping any random smoker, even one with strong faith, to quit smoking? How many who pray to quit succeed and how many fail?

Lo and behold, we have some information on this! A 2017 paper studied 2,839 people in a US national survey who smoked in the year prior to interview and attempted to quit during that year. It found the odds of reporting no longer smoking at the time of interview "were no greater for those who used prayer, any mind–body therapy, or both, than in those using neither" (Gillum, Santibanez et al. 2009). But such evidence is unlikely to deter those who found prayer successful in stopping smoking from proselytising about their "way".

If you have quit smoking by taking a particular approach, and know others who have also succeeded that way, it can be hard to understand why there could ever be any debate that your method should not therefore be regarded as a self-evidently successful way to quit. And that anyone wanting to help others to quit too, would not want to shout about their way from the rooftops.

In the 2020 Australian Senate inquiry into vaping, the chair of the Select Committee on Tobacco Harm Reduction conservative Senator

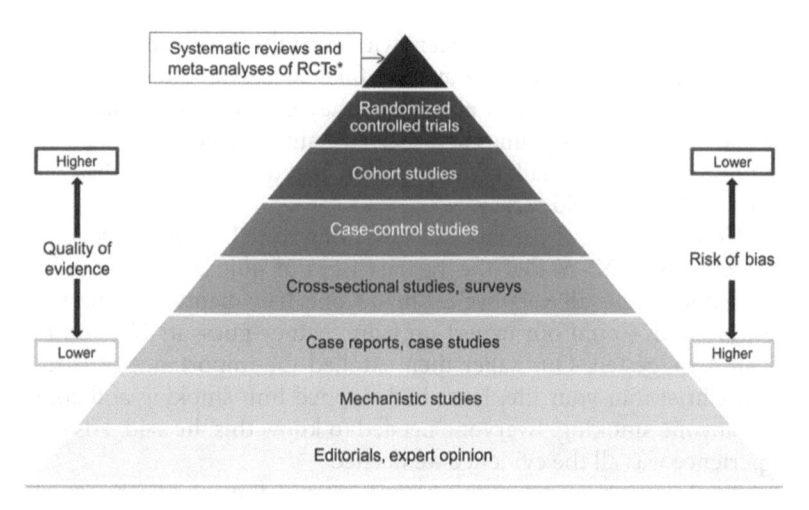

Figure 2.1 The quality of evidence pyramid.

Hollie Hughes, declared in an evidence session that she had herself recently quit smoking by taking up vaping. She put this question to two vapers who had been selected to give evidence to the Committee:

> One of the things that we keep hearing from experts is that stories like yours and, increasingly, stories like mine – I am 60 days without a cigarette – are nothing but anecdotes and that we are individuals and irrelevant to the broader study. We've had a significant number of submissions and I've had the privilege of speaking to an awful lot of people who have quit smoking using this method. Could you maybe tell me how it makes you feel when you're referred to as "nothing but an anecdote"? (H. Hughes 2020).

So let's consider why anecdotal evidence about quitting is always placed low in quality and importance when compared with all other forms of evidence (see Figure 2.1).

Self-selection bias

While sometimes compelling, personal anecdotes about how people quit smoking all wear the evidence-constricting crown of self-selection bias. People are far more at ease relating their success stories than failures. Those who have tried and failed to quit using any given method are understandably far less likely to be enthusiastic and evangelical than those who succeeded in stopping. Just as someone who tried to lose weight and failed is highly unlikely to want to take the time to write a political submission about their failure or call up a radio program discussing failed weight-loss methods, so too is it less likely that smokers who tried and failed would bother to spread their stories on every opportune soapbox.

In the opening statement of my evidence to the same 2020 Australian Senate inquiry on tobacco harm reduction I said:

> There are two broad claims made about vaping. One is that it's far superior to all other ways of quitting smoking, and many vapers, of course, have made submissions emphasising this. But there are no submissions from people who vaped and failed to quit and kept smoking or took it up again, and yet we know that this is by far the most common trajectory for vaping. We don't assess the effectiveness of anything by considering only those who had a positive outcome. That's why people who swear, for example, that they can drive perfectly well after drinking is not strong evidence that they actually can. Nor is it strong evidence for effective smoking cessation to point to online testimonials about the effectiveness of someone who might, for example, point a laser beam at your meridians, whisper reassurance and then take $500 from your wallet (Chapman 2020a).

Those who have not succeeded in quitting may feel that part of the problem lay with them, not with the method they used. They may feel they did not persevere as much as they should have, did not use a quit-smoking drug strictly as advised or complete the recommended course of the drug or procedure. They may feel awkward that others might draw that conclusion too, even if they did not mention these things themselves. Therefore we are likely to hear about failures less often.

So when we read the comment sections under online news articles, or hear smokers calling into radio programs with stories of their success, it's likely that there is considerable self-selection bias at play. Uncritical readers or listeners may get the impression that the drug being talked about is far more useful than it actually is: "Wow, almost everyone who called in was praising this method of quitting."

Such positive personal testimonies represent self-selection bias (Wikipedia 2020) about success and, while true for the individuals concerned, cannot be given credibility when it comes to making generalisations about the success or otherwise of any cessation method.

However, some find it self-evident that if someone swears by a method of quitting, that's 95% of all we need to know. If it worked for this person, it will probably work for many others. But pointing out that anecdotal evidence is the lowest level of evidence often raises hackles, as we saw earlier in Senator Hollie Hughes' attempt to provoke witnesses to the 2020 Senate Committee. I have often seen indignant comments on social media, particularly from vapers, saying, "Apparently I'm not a person with a lived personal experience of quitting smoking through vaping. I'm only an anecdote, understand. You need to speak to real people!"

Across a 45-year career in public health, I've heard and read countless testimonies supporting miracle smoking cures. These range from fairground hypnotism, acupuncture, herbal remedies, dipping your cigarettes in unpleasant-tasting potions before you smoke them (Chiang and Chapman 2006), paying someone to point a "laser" at special parts of your body while they charge you hundreds of dollars for the privilege, Alcoholics Anonymous–style smoking temptation story-sharing, thinly disguised religious pitches from church-based health groups talking about "higher powers", mantras to recite when tempted to smoke, and various offerings from the pharmaceutical industry.

Glowing testimonies can be found from those who've tried every imaginable quitting strategy. Take "laser acupuncture", for example. A very grateful "Crystal" (Crystal 2020) has this to say:

> I had gone in to LaZer iZ to help me quit smoking after smoking 1–2 packs a day walked in there stressed, nervous, moody and more but

after treatment I walked out calm, happy and so much more I was so happy it worked and now 5.5 years later I'm still smoke free: staff were great and I recommend them to everyone I know and even people that I don't. THANK YOU for helping me kick the smokes.

Acuquit, an Australian chain of 11 laser clinics, charges its customers $495 for an "overall treatment time [of] 30–45 minutes". If required, a follow-up session is available for the knock-down price of $195. Its website states, "Laser Acupuncture had an 84% success rate in recent research (Lim 2018) with many participants reporting they no longer had the urge to smoke." That claim is based on self-reports of those after they had completed seven sessions of laser therapy ("there was no long-term follow-up"). This is what is known as "end-of-treatment" results: the smoking status of participants as they finish a course of treatment and complete a questionnaire before leaving.

Because of the endemic problem of relapse into smoking (see later in this chapter), end-of-treatment quit outcomes are a highly inflated way of describing success rates in quitting. And when they are self-reports which are not verified by any biochemical testing, their status sinks even lower. This is particularly so when the record of the self-report is given to someone connected with the delivery of treatment. Smokers "get" that those trying to help them quit are very hopeful that they succeed, and so a "pleasing the therapist" phenomenon can occur where smokers say they have quit, even when they may have not.

The Instant Laser Clinic in Melbourne provides three 15-minute laser sessions for people wishing to quit smoking. Its website says:

Our professional laser consultants will apply a specialised laser handpiece on specific locations on the body, called "Meridian Points", such as the ears, face, hands and wrists – the areas of your body responsible for nicotine addiction. The light energy triggers the release of endorphins to help your body detox and eliminate any possible withdrawal symptoms.* In as little as 3–4 days after laser treatment to stop smoking, your body will be free of nicotine, and craving symptoms will disappear . . . amazingly!*
*Individual results may vary

Yes, these claims are indeed quite *amazing*, because few visitors to this website would be aware that the evidence for acupuncture and related methods (which include laser procedures) is "not shown to be more effective than a waiting list control for long-term abstinence". In other words, the long-term impact of acupuncture or laser treatment on smoking cessation is no different to the effect of placing your name on a waiting list for such treatments but not ever actually having them (White, Rampes et al. 2014). Few would also be aware that detectable nicotine remains in the bloodstream for only one to three days, with its metabolite cotinine able to be detected for up to 10 days. So having a body free of nicotine if you fully stopped smoking using *any* method would result in exactly the same lack of nicotine as the claim made by Instant Laser Clinic.

Randomised controlled trials

The 2020–21 COVID-19 pandemic has seen two words, efficacy and effectiveness, given perhaps their most intense ever public workout as debate rages about vaccines. Often the two words are used interchangeably by journalists and the public. But in public health and epidemiology their meaning is quite different (Streiner 2002).

Efficacy refers to the performance of an intervention (such as a drug) under the near-to-ideal conditions that can be organised when conducting carefully controlled and monitored trials. Effectiveness refers to performance in uncontrolled real-world use: how well a drug works in the circumstances of its actual use, away from regular monitoring or oversight from researchers. As I'll now explain, these differences are critically important for any understanding of what research tells us about how useful any quit-smoking method is or is likely to be throughout a population.

Randomised controlled trials (RCTs) have often been used to assess the efficacy of smoking cessation interventions. RCTs are revered in experimental and clinical science as being "gold standard" evidence about whether an intervention (often a drug) makes a difference to outcomes of interest, such as smoking cessation.

In the world of evidence-based medicine and public health, RCTs sit just below the apex of what is known as the quality of evidence pyramid (see Figure 2.1 earlier). The only evidence sitting above them in importance are studies that pool all quality RCTs on the same issues, weight results from the higher standard RCTs and draw conclusions about outcomes across all studies which reach high standards of evidence. RCTs are venerated because randomisation should ensure equal probability to any conceivable confounding variable that might bias the probability of any outcome being equally distributed between those in a trial allocated to the active and control arms of a trial.

Ideally, RCTs should also be double blinded: when the effects of a drug and a placebo are being compared, it is ideal if both those taking the drugs and placebos and those conducting the analysis of the results do not know who is in the control (often placebo) group and who is in the active drug group. Only after analysis is complete should the status of those in the placebo and active drug allocations be unmasked to those in the trial and to those who conducted the analysis.

If trial participants know they are taking the active drug or placebo, their expectations of effect will be different. If trial staff know who is in what group, they may inadvertently let slip body language or hints to the participants about the group they are in, compromising the integrity of blindness.

But as we will see below, there is a problem in preserving the blindness integrity of nicotine replacement drugs (including e-cigarettes which deliver nicotine) when all trial subjects are people who often have many years experience of negative biofeedback when they are being deprived of nicotine. If they are allocated to the placebo (no nicotine) arm of a trial, they tend to work that out very quickly.

And when RCTs exclude many subjects who in the real world would be considered high-priority candidates for an effective treatment, we have to ask questions about whether the results from such RCTs can be seamlessly generalised to real-world use. As we will see, this is another huge problem for RCTs in smoking cessation.

The Cochrane Collaboration is a global project founded in 1993 to assess evidence of safety and efficacy of therapeutics, interventions and diagnostics. Its tobacco addiction site (Cochrane Collaboration 2020) lists 78 reviews, including RCTs with bupropion, varenicline, various forms of nicotine replacement therapy, antidepressants, anxiolytics, e-cigarettes, and many other drugs and interventions to stop and reduce smoking. It never includes anecdotes in its assessments.

RCTs can compare a drug with another drug used for a similar purpose, with a placebo, or with "usual care". Usual care in smoking cessation RCTs can be the sort of advice that a doctor or other health professional might ordinarily offer to a smoker when they were not participating in a study. As such advice is often provided as part of responsible clinical practice, especially when a medication is involved, it is important to assess whether the medication has any additional cessation effect on top of the advice or routines to which smokers would normally be exposed in their interactions with a healthcare provider or service.

But when smokers access drugs in real-world circumstances, they are most likely to receive no support or advice (for example, when buying NRT from a supermarket) or only brief, sometimes perfunctory advice when a healthcare provider or pharmacist is too busy to spend much time with a customer. A NSW survey of 700 pharmacies (Paul, Tzelepis et al. 2007) reported that pharmacists claimed to spend an average of five minutes discussing stop smoking medications with smokers, which means that many would spend less time than that.

Smoking cessation medications do not act rapidly like an analgesic, a sleeping tablet, a topical mild local anaesthetic for an insect bite or a decongestant. Their pharmacological effect is far more subtle; often it is "slow release" and imperceptible. If smokers are not given support or detailed instructions about what to expect, it's understandable that many might quickly discontinue use, thinking that the drug is not working.

Those conducting RCTs can recruit their participants in a variety of ways, some of which introduce important biases into the population being studied. In the smoking cessation field, we often see subjects recruited from sources like quit-smoking clinics, telephone quitline callers, general practitioner and other primary healthcare patients, smoking cessation or vaping website and chat room visitors. Vaping studies sometimes recruit from vaping online chat rooms populated by deeply committed vapers embracing a "vaping lifestyle". With each of these, we need to ask whether smokers or vapers recruited in such ways are different in important ways to randomly selected smokers or vapers in the population at large. Self-selection bias is very relevant here. We are likely to be dealing with those who are more help-seeking. This may mean they are more motivated to quit than smokers in the general population, and it may also mean they are people with lower self-efficacy (lower confidence in their ability to quit unaided).

Often researchers attempt to address this concern by demonstrating that those who have been recruited into trials are comparable to smokers in the whole population on a range of variables like demographics, smoking history, level of nicotine dependency, intention to quit and so on. But, beyond all these characteristics in a very important respect they *are* different: they have often taken steps at help-seeking in their hopes to stop smoking. As we will see in Chapter 3, the great majority of smokers who quit don't seek help to do so when they finally succeed. So those who volunteer to take part in trials recruited in these ways are help-seeking volunteers.

Trial exclusion criteria

For a large variety of reasons, trialists are often unrepresentative of the general population (Schulz and Grimes 2002, Rothwell 2005). This can reflect characteristics of those who are willing to volunteer or consent compared to those who are not. Those running trials will often exclude people from trial participation for a variety of reasons. Those who have language problems are often excluded as interpreters are expensive to add to constrained research budgets. Those with drug or alcohol dependency, serious mental health problems like depression, psychosis or bipolar disorder can also be excluded, as can those with no fixed address, or who move addresses often, are in prison or who have a serious illness which might reduce their life expectancy (and so participation in the study down the track). Those with low motivation to quit can also be excluded.

One study (Le Strat, Rehm et al. 2011) reviewed 54 smoking cessation RCTs for criteria for exclusion and found 25 separate criteria being used across these trials. They then applied 12 of the most commonly used criteria to 4,962 adults with nicotine dependence in the past 12 months from a US national survey on alcohol use (National Epidemiologic Survey on Alcohol and Related Conditions – NESARC) and to a subgroup of participants motivated to quit (See Table 2.1).

Table 2.1 Estimated (rounded) percentages of adults with nicotine dependence in NESARC excluded from typical trials of treatments for nicotine dependence by traditional ineligibility criteria. NA = information not available in NESARC. Source: Le Strat, Rehm et al. 2011.

Exclusion variable	Current nicotine dependence (n=4962) %	Motivated to quit smoking (n=4121) %
Pregnancy	3	3
Cardiovascular disease	7	7
Smoking <10 cigarettes/day	32	34
Current/past 6m use of any psychotropic medication	NA	NA
High alcohol consumption	14	13
Not motivated to quit	18	0
Use of other drugs	3	3
Current depression	17	16
Current/past 6m use of bupropion and/or NRT	NA	NA
Eating disorder	NA	NA
History of psychosis	2	2
History of bipolar disorder	10	10
Exclusion by any criterion	66	59

They found two-thirds of participants with nicotine dependence would have been excluded from clinical trials by at least one criterion, with 59% of the subgroup of motivated-to-quit smokers also being excluded. Those in such trials are thus very unrepresentative of all smokers wanting to quit. This may result in important participation biases which reduce the applicability of the results to smokers at large, or even smokers at large who want to quit.

Of note in Table 2.1 above is the exclusion from trials of those who have mental health problems (depression, psychosis, bipolar disorder, eating disorders). A 2000 paper in the *Journal of the American Medical Association* reporting on smoking rates in the 1991-92 US National Comorbidity Survey found that current smoking rates for those with mental illness were 41% (past-month mental illness), 34.8% (any lifetime mental illness) and 22.5% for those with no mental illness. Those with any mental disorder in the past month consumed approximately 44.3% of all cigarettes smoked by this nationally representative sample (Lasser, Boyd et al. 2000). By excluding those with mental illness from smoking cessation trials, RCTs shut out a hugely significant proportion of smokers in the USA.

In an analysis of data from the 2007 Australian National Survey of Mental Health and Wellbeing, having a mental illness in the past 12 months was the most prevalent factor strongly associated with smoking, and associated with both increased current smoking and reduced likelihood of smoking cessation (Lawrence, Hafekost et al. 2013). The situation is likely to be similar in many other countries.

Hawthorne, attention and social desirability effects in RCTs

The Hawthorne effect refers to behavioural change attributable to awareness of being observed or monitored. While the originally described Hawthorne effect has been challenged and debated (Wickstrom and Bendix 2000, Kompier 2006, Berthelot, Le Goff et al. 2011), there is little dispute that participation in a study or trial *in itself* can cause changes in outcomes that would not occur in people's lives had they not been involved in a study where awareness of the observations and judgements of others may influence changes in behaviour or response. One of these participation effects is the social desirability effect where some study participants answer in particular ways that they are aware would be considered more socially desirable than others (Persoskie and Nelson 2013). By offering these responses, interviewees might anticipate being thought of more positively by researchers who they might not have ever met before or are unlikely to ever again.

In smoking cessation trials, subjects understand that quitting smoking is the key outcome of interest to the researchers and are likely to assume that the personnel associated with the conduct of the trial have their hopes up that many trial participants who have been allocated to the active drug arm of the trial will quit smoking. In my long experience in the tobacco control field, this is highly likely to be the case. While trial staff will have been instructed to say or do nothing when interacting with participants that would indicate any predictions or hopes for outcomes, it is highly likely that this neutrality is often breached in conversational asides and other often unintentional ways.

When you are involved in a smoking cessation study, lots of attention is often paid to you. You get screened to ensure you are eligible to be in the study. You consent to be contacted, sometimes quite often, by the research team. For example, in the Jorenby et al. varenicline trial, subjects were contacted by study staff 28 times (eight by telephone, 20 in person), of which 18 involved some counselling (Jorenby, Hays et al. 2006). The Niaura et al. trial (Niaura, Hays et al. 2008) involved 24 contacts including counselling on 13 occasions. Walsh's 2008 review of 12 studies of over-the-counter (OTC), non-prescribed NRT use for their generalisability to real-world conditions of use found study subjects had an average of 7.6 interactions with research staff (range 4–11) (Walsh 2008).

Trialists sometimes attend a pre-trial information session with other study participants, where a sense of teamwork to help science can be fostered. This, and the frequent contact with the research staff who are doing their best to ensure low rates of trial dropout, can combine to create an influential backdrop to using a quit-smoking medication or approach which is very different to the way people will use the same drugs or approach in "real-world" conditions outside a trial.

Trial participant retention strategies

Those running trials routinely put a lot of effort into maximising trial cohort retention rates. If lots of people drop out of the groups being

2 How we study quitting smoking: a critical look

studied, this can greatly compromise the integrity of trials, as important questions can be asked about whether those who pulled out or were lost to follow-up differed in important ways to those who remained in a study across its entire course.

Importantly, real-world studies have found high levels of premature discontinuation of medication use. A four-nation study of 1,219 smokers and recent quitters who had used medication in the last year found most (69.1%) discontinued medication use prematurely (71.4% of NRT users and 59.6% of bupropion and varenicline). NRT users who obtained their patches or gum OTC without prescription were particularly likely to discontinue (76.3%) (Balmford, Borland et al. 2011). A small national cross-sectional 2021 Australian study found 28% of those using cessation medications adhered to the recommended regimens (Mersha, Kennedy et al. 2021).

Evidence from Australia's Pharmaceutical Benefits Scheme (PBS) which subsidises the cost of drugs to patients, including smoking cessation drugs, shows that many who are prescribed smoking cessation drugs do not take them as directed. Data on the real-world experiences of bupropion and varenicline use indicate stark differences from experiences under research conditions. A 2002 New South Wales study of 151 smokers recruited from 11 general practices who were prescribed bupropion found 84% were taking the drug for a range of 1–12 weeks, with only 19% taking it for or beyond the minimum recommended duration of seven weeks (Zwar, Nasser et al. 2002). Forty-four to fifty percent of patients who received subsidised prescriptions for varenicline failed to commence the last eight weeks of treatment (no data were available to indicate what proportion of the remainder completed the last eight weeks of treatment), in contrast to 12-week completion rates of 68–76% in clinical trials (Walsh 2011). An unknown proportion complete even the first eight weeks after collecting their drugs from a pharmacy. Compliance is much higher in trials: for example, 69% (Niaura, Hays et al. 2008) and 76% of trialists (Jorenby, Hays et al. 2006) completed 12 weeks of treatment.

Yet between January 2008 and October 2009, the Australian government spent $93 million on varenicline prescriptions. This compares with $59 million allocated over four years to social marketing campaigns designed to promote quit attempts in Australia. Given this relatively high spending on pharmacotherapy, it is essential that we are realistic about its potential impact on population smoking prevalence, and whether attention would be better focused on boosting the campaigns known to stimulate mass cessation (see Chapter 8).

Much wisdom has accumulated in professional trial communities about cohort retention. Strategies include reducing any barriers to participation, efforts to build a sense of community and belonging among trialists, follow-up and reminder strategies, and tracing techniques (Teague, Youssef et al. 2018). Community-building strategies can be particularly important, as well as trial staff who have good "people" skills. This often fosters positive attitudes and a sense of responsibility among participants about helping the trial maintain low levels of dropout. They can be made to feel important that they are contributing to the advance of science and the health of communities.

Trial staff often include young investigators whose PhD or research work is focused on a trial. These people have particularly strong motivation to develop good personal relationships with trialists as the work they do will be assessed by their thesis and publication reviewers, and major problems like high dropout rates can be fatal to publication. Someone mildly irritated with the ongoing demands of a study to complete questionnaires, provide biological samples and keep personal data records may feel a sense of "that nice young researcher who contacts me every few months would be very unhappy if I pulled out". Strategies like sending thank-you, birthday and holiday cards, trial newsletters, supplying trial logo material like caps and T-shirts are also often used.

Trialists are often paid and drugs are free

The drugs used in trials are given free of charge to trialists. Even where governments subsidise the cost of approved prescribed medications, the drugs are only seldom handed out free, such as during special quit-smoking promotions (Miller, Frieden et al. 2005), and to those on very low incomes. Even subsidised drugs can still constitute a significant outlay to those on low incomes. This may inhibit them being used into the medium or longer term by those who feel they need to continue using them.

It is also increasingly common for trialists to be paid for their participation in trials (National Health and Medical Research Council 2019). This is intended to act as both fair compensation for their time and cover any out-of-pocket expenses like travel to the research centre, but may also act as an incentive to continue participation, particularly for those on low incomes or who are unemployed. In real-world, unmonitored or unsupervised quit attempts, smokers are never paid to use quitting aids. These differences may give an extra boost to high compliance across the recommended course of smoking cessation aid use, something that is often far from the case in real-world use.

Blindness integrity problems

In most RCTs, as mentioned above, participants are not told whether they have been randomised to receive the active or placebo (control) drug. This is called subject "blinding": they are blind to whether they are getting the active drug or the dummy, inert, control drug. Research team members are also often blinded to which treatment or control arm each study participant has been allocated. This is called double blinding and is undertaken to remove the possibility of researchers actively or inadvertently communicating expectations of effects to study participants. A researcher who might have hopes that a particular treatment is efficacious and who knows that certain study participants have been allocated to the active drug may make comments to these patients that suggest to them it is likely that they are on the active drug. Researchers with expectations that successful outcomes of a trial (i.e. where the active drug is shown to be far better than a placebo) might lead to valuable, career-enhancing opportunities may sometimes be tempted to compromise the integrity of the blinding of a trial.

NRT is a strong candidate for a failure in blindness integrity. Nearly all smokers have often experienced interoceptive cues when they are craving nicotine. Here, we need only think of the speed with which many smokers light up a cigarette soon after waking each morning, the once-common sight of smokers rushing to light up after alighting from non-smoking public transport, and standing outside office blocks and restaurants. These sights tell us that smokers are very familiar with sensations that remind them of their need to re-dose with nicotine and the relief and pleasant sensations they experience shortly after doing this. Let's stay with this pleasure issue for a moment.

The pleasures of smoking?

We sometimes hear smokers talking about the "pleasures" they get from smoking. The picture being painted here is that if you smoke, your days will be filled with particular sensual delights inaccessible to non-smokers. With cigarettes, not only do smokers have the accoutrements for the full public smoking performance (the elegant cigarette, a tasteful lighter, the full hand gesturing and exhaling repertoire catalogued in Richard Klein's *Cigarettes are sublime* (Klein 1993), but they are constantly pleasuring themselves around the clock in a way denied to non-smokers who have not woken up to the joys of nicotine.

But what is it that nicotine-dependent people "like" about pulling smoke and nicotine deep into their lungs 87,660 times a year (12 puffs per cigarette x 20 cigarettes a day x 365.25 days)?

In 1994, the *New York Times* published the ratings of two of the USA's most renowned addiction specialists, Neil Benowitz and Jack Henningfield, on the relative addictiveness of nicotine, caffeine, heroin, cocaine, alcohol and marijuana (cannabis) (Hilts 1994). They rated each of these on a scale of 1 (most serious) to 6 (least serious) – see Table 2.2.

Both rated nicotine higher on the dependence criterion than all the other drugs. By "dependence" they meant "how difficult it is for the user to quit, the relapse rate, the percentage of people who eventually become dependent". Nicotine withdrawal also rated high (third behind the often-depicted agonies of alcohol delirium tremens and heroin withdrawal). Both experts rated nicotine fourth behind cocaine, heroin and alcohol when it came to reinforcement (essentially the pleasure given by the drug). But both rated nicotine last on intoxication, behind even caffeine.

Taking all this together, a picture emerges of nicotine-dependent people living in full knowledge of their high dependency, experiencing often unpleasant and insistent withdrawal symptoms when they have

Table 2.2 Henningfield and Benowitz ratings of drug dependency components. Source: Hilts 1994.

HENNINGFIELD RATINGS

Substance	Withdrawal	Reinforcement	Tolerance	Dependence	Intoxication
Nicotine	3	4	2	1	5
Heroin	2	2	1	2	2
Cocaine	4	1	4	3	3
Alcohol	1	3	3	4	1
Caffeine	5	6	5	5	6
Marijuana	6	5	6	6	4

BENOWITZ RATINGS

Substance	Withdrawal	Reinforcement	Tolerance	Dependence	Intoxication
Nicotine	3*	4	4	1	6
Heroin	2	2	2	2	2
Cocaine	3*	1	1	3	3
Alcohol	1	3	4	4	1
Caffeine	4	5	3	5	5
Marijuana	5	6	5	6	4

not been able to smoke for a while, and being quickly relieved of this unpleasantness when lighting up another cigarette.

Nicotine withdrawal symptoms can include headache, nausea, constipation or diarrhoea, fatigue, drowsiness and insomnia, irritability, difficulty concentrating, anxiety, depressed mood, increased hunger and caloric intake, and, of course, constant tobacco cravings.

Smokers know from the earliest days of their addiction that these feelings can disappear within seconds as nicotine is rapidly transported from their lungs to their brains where dopamine is released and experienced as pleasurable.

Smokers and vapers insist that the pleasure from this release can somehow be experienced independently of the pleasures of the nicotine withdrawal symptoms rapidly dissipating: they keep smoking to pleasure themselves, not to relieve withdrawal symptoms.

So what is the "pleasure" being experienced here? When you have a bad toothache and this is relieved by a strong analgesic, your mood can elevate by the minute as the codeine begins to kick in. We've all sat through an execrable movie in a cinema and decided we will endure it rather than disturbing all those between where we are sitting trapped and the end of the row. The agony of watching piles higher and higher, and the eventual escape outside is experienced as pure bliss. But few of us would disagree that while escape from a bad movie or concert is pleasurable, we don't seek out awful movies or music to experience the pleasure of escaping from them.

The argument that smoking and inhaling nicotine is "pleasurable" is a bit like saying that being beaten up several times every day when you haven't been able to smoke is something you want to continue with, because it feels so good when the beating stops for a while.

When a smoker is randomly allocated to receive a placebo in an NRT-placebo blinded trial, it seems highly likely that those allocated to placebo will quickly feel very confident that they are not in the active NRT arm. Their body will be telling this to them as it has every day when they knew that they badly needed more nicotine. All this suggests that those in NRT trials who are allocated to placebos (gum, patch, inhaler or lozenge not containing nicotine) will be able to guess this very quickly.

Can smokers guess if they have been allocated to the placebo arm?

In a very important way, RCTs of smoking cessation drugs differ from those involving many other drugs. If you are involved in a trial assessing the efficacy of a drug for a condition which has few if any obvious symptoms, and where the outcome must be assessed by some test, this is very different to a situation where the trialists experience symptoms or sensations which make it very clear to them that they have been allocated to the active drug in the trial, and not to the placebo arm. Trials of blood pressure or cholesterol reducing drugs are good examples of where trialists may not be able to accurately guess their allocation, with the changes only being detectable by a sphygmomanometer (blood pressure) or blood test (cholesterol).

Smokers who are nicotine dependent are very aware of when they feel compelled to light up their next cigarette. They have become thoroughly attuned across sometimes decades of smoking to recognising when they feel nicotine-deprived and to the relief and pleasure they experience when they inhale the first puff of nicotine from a new cigarette. For this reason, there is an obvious cause for concern that smokers participating in RCTs where they are not told whether they have been allocated to the active (NRT) arm of the trial or to the control (placebo) arm can accurately guess to which arm they have in fact (Schnoll, Epstein et al. 2008) been allocated.

In 2004, Mooney, White and Hatsukami published a review of blinding integrity in 73 NRT trials (Mooney, White et al. 2004). Remarkably, they found that only 17 (23%) reported any assessment of blindness integrity, and of these 12 (71%) found that subjects accurately judged treatment assignment at a rate significantly above chance. Of those allocated to placebo, 63.6% accurately guessed they were in the placebo arm, and 57% of those using NRT correctly guessed they were getting nicotine. Only three of the 17 trials which assessed blindness integrity adjusted for it in reporting their results.

A similar concern may apply to other smoking cessation medications. In another study of smokers randomised to take bupropion or placebo (Schnoll, Epstein et al. 2008), participants were asked to guess which they were on (or were not sure). Overall, 55% of subjects guessed their allocation correctly. Compared to guessing "not sure", those who guessed they were taking bupropion were more than twice as likely to have been randomised to bupropion. Equally, those who guessed placebo were twice as likely to have been randomised to placebo. Importantly, when the authors included treatment arm guess with actual treatment arm allocation in their modelling, the odds ratio of bupropion being more successful than placebo significantly reduced when measured at end of treatment, at both 6 months and 12 months.

It is not difficult to place yourselves in the shoes of a trialist who believes they had been allocated to the placebo arm of a smoking cessation trial. Such a belief would evaporate expectations that what you were taking was likely to have any benefit. This would likely reduce the probability of quitting. Equally, if you believed you had been allocated to the active arm of a trial, this would likely give you faith that what you were using might help you stop smoking.

These considerations add another layer of important difference to what happens when you try to quit smoking with a drug in an RCT with what happens when you use the drug in real-world conditions.

Competing interest bias

There is another important source of bias in smoking cessation studies: the presence of research or researcher funding by industries which have a financial interest in the outcome of the research. The adage that "those who pay the piper, call the tune" is familiar to all. We understand from it that when you are being paid by someone – particularly on a continuing basis – there are expectations that what you produce will be pleasing to those paying you. If you are in the habit of producing information that creates serious problems for your benefactor's business, it is likely that such funders will stop funding your work.

Cochrane has very strong rules about researchers with competing interests authoring reviews for Cochrane (Cochrane Community 2020). Taking effect from 2020, it now requires that:

- Authors without conflicts of interest must make up at least two-thirds of the author team.
- Both last-listed as well as first-listed authors must be entirely free of conflicts of interest (the first and last authors on papers are commonly those who have most influence on the planning, conduct and reporting of studies).
- Authors of clinical studies that are funded by industry and are relevant to the topic of a review may not be the first or last author of a Cochrane Review.

In biomedical research, it has long been known that studies with authors who have competing interests are more likely to report outcomes which are helpful to the interests funding the research. This has been documented across a wide range of research areas (Dunn, Coiera et al. 2016) that includes pharmaceuticals, asbestos, gambling, food additives, sugary drinks, alcohol, tobacco and e-cigarettes (Pisinger, Godtfredsen et al. 2019). Biases associated with receipt of funding include selective reporting of outcomes, poorer study quality and reliability, and an increased likelihood that funded authors will interpret evidence as supporting an intervention and megaphone this in publicity surrounding the publication of their research, all to the delight of their funders.

Positive outcome bias

Further, "positive outcome bias" – the tendency for studies reporting positive outcomes to be published and accepted for presentation at scientific conferences – is a recognised phenomenon, with a recent systematic review concluding:

> There is strong evidence of an association between significant results and publication; studies that report positive or significant results are more likely to be published and outcomes that are statistically significant have higher odds of being fully reported. Trials which show drugs have mediocre effects may have more difficulty in being published than those which have clear and obvious positive impacts (Dwan, Gamble et al. 2013).

Trial registration (De Angelis, Drazen et al. 2004) and journals making it mandatory that all studies submitted for publication must supply details of that registration are a major step in the direction of allowing greater transparency to others about the protocols and methods used in trials. But it may be that reviewers and especially editors working to publishers' space limit budgets may be less inclined to publish trials with negative or unclear findings about efficacy (Hopewell, Loudon et al. 2009, Bala, Akl et al. 2013). Rejected papers are often "moved down the food chain" to journals less preferred by authors where they are still published (Nguyen and Chapman 2005).

Many studies on smoking cessation drugs are funded by pharmaceutical companies which plainly have strong interests and hopes that their new drugs, formulations or delivery systems will be found to be useful to smokers. Armed with such evidence, many opportunities open up for marketing and promoting these drugs. Huge increases in sales and profits can follow. The same is obviously true with tobacco and vaping industry-funded research about putative harm-reduction products. Researchers who seek and accept pharmaceutical, tobacco or vaping industry funding also have competing interests in that successful outcomes with treatments manufactured by these sources are more likely to see further funding sent their way than would be the case if the treatment outcome was unsatisfactory. Pharmaceutical companies invest heavily in promoting the findings of favourable trials to both smokers and doctors.

In 2021, a study that received extensive global media publicity, was retracted by the *European Respiratory Journal*, which had accepted it for publication and published it online before the editors realised that authors on the paper with tobacco industry financial support had not declared these interests at the time of the paper's submission, as they were required to do. The paper had concluded that smokers had a lower incidence of COVID-19 infection and severity than non-smokers in Mexico (Editors of *Eur Respir J* 2021), a finding that would have been very pleasing to those in the tobacco industry.

Etter and colleagues (Etter, Burri et al. 2007) assessed whether source of funding affected the results of trials of NRT for smoking cessation. They reviewed 90 trials of gum which were included in a Cochrane Review (52 with nicotine gum and 38 with nicotine patch. Forty-nine studies had received industry support). They found 51% of industry-supported trials reported statistically significant results, compared with nine (22%) trials not supported by NRT manufacturers. They concluded that "compared with independent trials, industry-supported trials were more likely to produce statistically significant results and larger odds ratios." They also speculated that,

Although we had no data on the amount of funding for each trial, it is possible that more resources led to higher treatment compliance and therefore greater efficacy in industry-supported trials. Differences can also possibly be explained by publication bias with several small, null-effect industry studies not having reached publication. After adjustment for this possible bias, results for industry trials were lower and similar to non-industry results. Similarly, the overall estimate of the net effect for these products reduces to about 5% attributable 1-year successes. This remains of considerable public health benefit.

Given all the preceding discussion about the important and varied differences between RCTs and real-world use, it is remarkable that the authors of this paper felt moved to describe a 5% success rate (i.e. a 95% failure rate) as a "considerable public health benefit" when the true real-world impact away from RCTs would have probably been far less.

Another 2010 examination of 107 smoking cessation trials (70 industry funded and 37 non-industry funded) sought to test anecdotal evidence that researchers might attempt to increase the likelihood of obtaining a statistically significant result in trials "by reducing the rate of placebo responding" (i.e. reducing quitting in placebo-allocated participants). They found that reduced placebo responses were responsible for greater than 70% of the variation in placebo arm quit rates and concluded: "These results suggest that there may be important differences in the design and conduct of industry-sponsored trials compared with non-industry trials, which impact specifically upon placebo response rates to increase the likelihood of observing a statistically significant treatment effect" (Greene, Taylor et al. 2010).

A 2019 review of 826 tobacco harm reduction (THR) publications published between 1992 and 2016 found only 23.9% disclosed industry associations. The authors reported that support from the e-cigarette, tobacco or pharmaceutical industries was significantly associated with supportive stance on THR in analyses, and emphasised that public health practitioners and researchers need to account for industry funding when interpreting evidence in THR debates (Hendlin, Vora et al. 2019).

Authors who are funded by industries with a strong commercial interest in particular outcomes are often deeply offended by any suggestion that their work ought to be viewed with heightened circumspection. They often demand of anyone suggesting this that they provide precise evidence of any scientific misconduct, problematic analysis or unwarranted interpretation. Such challenges can be difficult to meet because of the multitude of ways that researchers hoping to "produce" a conclusion can avoid full transparency of all the decisions taken during the course of their research.

"Intention to treat" analysis

When RCTs commence, it is almost inevitable that some recruits who consent to participate drop out of the trials before they conclude. People sometimes move from where they live, change their email addresses and phone numbers, and are lost to follow-up. Some die or become too ill to participate. Some withdraw from the study. This can be for a variety of reasons, some of which have little to do with the key outcomes. But we know that those who withdraw from RCTs on smoking cessation are more likely to be smokers who have relapsed back to smoking. Some of these people may feel embarrassed about their lack of resolve or failure to quit and anticipate awkwardness when interacting with the researchers, even when these researchers may be contracted survey company staff with no personal interest or investment in a cessation intervention succeeding.

If we see RCTs as being a reasonable guide to how a smoking cessation drug performs, and believe they have high relevance for real-world policy and practice, we need to express final outcome measures in terms of the number of participants who *started* the trial intending to quit smoking. This is known as "intention to treat" analysis. It is highly misleading to conveniently remove all those who dropped out or were lost to follow-up from study participant denominators, because this would artificially flatter success rates by setting aside a subgroup of participants that is likely to include many non-successes.

Most journals insist on data being reported in intention to treat analysis. But some do not. It is wise to carefully look to see whether authors have avoided this and presented flattering data.

Citation bias

Large, attention-grabbing numbers are almost by definition more memorable and repeatable than those not waving look-at-me flags and blowing loud public relations sirens. So when journalists report research findings, it's perhaps predictable that a big bold number in a report is likely to draw both their and the readers or audiences' attention more than numbers less startling. This can have important implications for smoking cessation statistics being thrown about in policy debates.

In 2008, I had noticed in the introductory and discussion sections of research papers and in press reports and websites that smoking prevalence among people with schizophrenia was often reported as being much higher than that in the general population. It was frequently described as being "around", "up to" or "about" 90%, when smoking in the general population in nations like the US, the UK and Australia at the time were in the early 20% region.

At the time, the most recent review of studies reporting on smoking and schizophrenia showed that the pooled prevalence of smoking in people with schizophrenia in published studies across 20 nations was 62%, with a range of 14–88% (de Leon and Diaz 2005). Smoking prevalence of over 80% was found in just 6 out of 42 (14.3%) of the studies, with the numbers of smoking patients in these six studies totalling 484 out of 4686 (10.3%) of all smokers across all of the studies in the review. A widely publicised report on smoking by people with mental illness in Australia recycled the same statement ("People with schizophrenia in particular have extremely high rates of smoking, with most studies finding a prevalence rate of about 90%") (Chapman 2008b).

This looked to us like a classic case of citation bias playing out. Citation bias is the selective citation of published results to support the findings, arguments or interests of authors and those funding their work (Egger and Smith 1998). Those wanting to draw the attention of journalists, the public and policymakers to the far greater rates of smoking in people with psychosis probably thought, "Let's find a study with a very high smoking prevalence number in it."

So where did this "90%" come from? It is likely that it originated from a small but highly influential early paper by Hughes and others, which showed the prevalence of smoking in a sample of people with schizophrenia to be 88% (Hughes, Hatsukami et al. 1986). This finding derived from a sample of just 24 people with schizophrenia living in one US city and attending a hospital outpatient service in 1981–82. As of March 2022, researchers have since cited the paper an amazing 1,433 times, despite its age and very small sample size. One example of how it was cited was in 2008 (27 years after the data collection) in *Physiological Reviews* where the authors wrote, "it has been shown that people with schizophrenia smoke cigarettes at a very high rate, ~80–90% compared with the 45–70% of patients with other psychiatric disorders and 30% of the general population" (Lendvai and Vizi 2008).

Numbers like this, while not being wrong, are nonetheless very misleading when seen in the context of all other relevant studies. Erroneous assumptions about the near inevitability of smoking in people with schizophrenia may reinforce institutional and clinical neglect of this stigmatised group of people and stultify innovation in targeted support to help this group. While it is possible that the decades-long repetition of the "around 90%" factoid may be motivated by a well-meaning concern to magnify the severity of the issue to attract support or funding, uncritical recitation of statements about misleadingly high smoking rates in schizophrenic patients is often inaccurate and should be challenged.

When critically assessing claims about smoking cessation, it is therefore important to ask whether commonly quoted numbers might reflect citation bias. Big and bold numbers repeatedly used to demonstrate the success of a way of quitting should be traced to the source and compared with estimates in meta-analyses and reviews.

I'll now turn to two other very common ways of studying cessation: real-world observational studies. We'll first look at cross-sectional surveys (including time-series studies) and then at longitudinal cohort studies.

Real-world observational studies 1: Cross-sectional surveys

Cross-sectional studies reporting on smoking cessation are those where researchers select participants from the general or particular subpopulations (for example, armed forces, Indigenous populations, school students), and ask them questions about their smoking. These studies can be single "snapshot" surveys or part of a time-series where the same questions are put to different samples selected in the same way annually or every third year, for example. With time-series reports, differences between data collected in different years can be compared, trend lines constructed and statistical tests of significance for differences calculated to provide descriptive accounts of "changes".

Such repeated, time-series cross-sectional series can be very useful in illuminating some questions about cessation, but have inherent limitations when addressing others. Snapshot and time-series surveys allow us to measure changes in the prevalence of smoking overall or in the prevalence of measurements like the proportion of a population who smoke over time, including changes happening in different groups, but they do not allow any causal inferences to be drawn on what factors are responsible for the changes noted. Other weaknesses include:

- Inability to determine whether an outcome has followed exposure in time or whether exposure resulted from the outcome (reverse causality).
- Inability to measure incidence (new cases of a disease or behaviour like smoking across a specified period).
- Susceptibility to bias due to low response and misclassification due to recall bias when subjects are asked to provide information from the past.

Low response rates in cross-sectional surveys

In recent decades, survey research has been deeply impacted by declines in response rates to surveys, particularly when conducted by telephone. Technological advances (increased use of unlisted mobile phones, use of answering machines and voicemail to screen unwanted calls and caller identification, screening and blocking) have caused increases in under-reporting. According to the California Tobacco

Surveys, response rates fell from 70% in 1992–93 to 51.1% in 1998–99 (Biener, Garrett et al. 2004). However, one study comparing estimates obtained from the US Current Population Survey, which used expensive door-to-door interviewing and obtained significantly higher response rates than phone surveys, showed that "under or over-representation of population sub-groups has not changed as response rates have declined". In 2003 the Canadian Marketing Research and Intelligence Association reported that refusal rates to one-off telephone surveys increased from 66% in 1995 to 78% in 2003 (Allen, Ambrose et al. 2003). By 2018, the US Pew Research Center reported that telephone survey response rates had fallen to a truly dismal 6% (Kennedy and Hartig 2019).

Online surveys can perform better. The popular platform Survey Monkey reports response rates "as high as 20 to 30 percent", meaning that 70 to 80 percent of those contacted decline (Porter 2021). Incentives can boost responses. A University of Michigan series of experiments in increasing web-mailed survey completion rates between 2011 and 2012 found "fresh" first-time requests to do an online survey saw 17.4% completed compared with 34.5% when offered a US$5 incentive. Recontacting people saw 50.3% respond with no incentive, rising to 70.1% with an incentive (Suzer-Gurtekin, McBee et al. 2016).

Self-selecting, motivated samples vs. whole population randomly selected samples

It is always important to look at studies of smoking cessation for details of the study population involved and how they have been recruited. Those promoting particular methods of quitting will often gloss over such details in the rush to highlight headline results. But results from surveys of clearly biased populations of smokers are of almost no value in extrapolating findings to all smokers. An online survey of over 19,000 people who completed a questionnaire on an electronic cigarette advocacy website reported that 81% of smokers had completely abandoned smoking (Farsalinos, Romagna et al. 2014). This finding was lauded by vaping advocates on social media who seemed to believe that a survey completed by like-minded dedicated pro-vaping advocates had any relevance for what was happening with vaping in the wider population. It was rather like a survey of members of a whisky appreciation club on their drinking habits being seen by some as a reasonable guide to whisky drinking in the whole population.

Many studies of smoking cessation are conducted with study populations of smokers who have come forward to participate in a clinical service providing smoking cessation interventions. Others involve outreach efforts to attract smokers by advertising the availability of self-help materials or minimal, low-intensity support like supportive phone calls, booklets, online quit-buddy support networks, or quit apps. In all these cases, those being researched are smokers who have an intention to quit which has motivated them to seek help or enquire about self-help materials that are unlikely to require them to attend a sometimes time-consuming quit-smoking service. An early review of 10 prospective trials of smokers intending to quit who had responded to advertisements offering self-help materials or seeking intending quitters who wanted to try to quit without assistance, found a 13.9% quit rate at 12 months (Cohen, Lichtenstein et al. 1989).

By contrast, Australian researchers Baillie, Mattick and Hall in 1995 published a meta-analysis of the available literature on the rate of smoking cessation in randomised controlled trials which involved control groups who were deliberately given no smoking cessation treatment or given only "usual care" by staff at health facilities where they were recruited into the studies. Fourteen such studies were found and results pooled in the meta-analysis. Across the studies they found a 7.3% quit rate over a 10-month period, nearly half that found in the analysis of smokers who were *intending* to quit, described above (Baillie, Mattick et al. 1995). The Australian authors' finding was based on the longest follow-up period reported in each of the 14 papers they reviewed, which varied. However, this 7.3% figure was not a finding of continuous abstinence across that period. Some smokers may have been continually abstinent, while others may have relapsed during the follow-up periods but may have quit again and were not smoking when the final, longest follow-up was conducted.

Comparisons of quit rates between those given assistance to quit and matched smoking controls not given any special assistance allow us to consider the size of any additional quit rate above and beyond that which might have been expected to occur among a group of smokers not offered assistance. So, taking the two studies just described, 13.9% less 7.3% gives an increased absolute quit rate of 6.6%, some 90% above the background unassisted quit rate. For decades, those promoting assisted cessation have spun this difference via the highly memorable claim that research shows that assisted cessation "doubles your chances of quitting".

But for the many reasons discussed so far, there are strong caveats that should be applied to this glib comparison.

A 2016 paper in *Addiction* reporting on a cross-sectional survey of 27,460 Europeans aged 15 and over in all 28 EU nations concluded that an estimated 6.1 million citizens had quit smoking with the help of e-cigarettes (Farsalinos, Poulas et al. 2016). The take-home message highlighted in publicity about this study was that there were over 6 million people in Europe who used to smoke and reported that they now no longer did on the day they answered the questionnaire, thanks to taking up vaping. But this paper was savaged in a response which made the following criticisms (Maziak and Ben Taleb 2017):

1. It is impossible to know how many of those who claim that they have stopped with the aid of e-cigarettes would have stopped anyway, and how many of those who used an e-cigarette but failed to stop would have stopped had they used another method.
2. With smoking status being highly unstable (smokers quitting, then relapsing, then quitting again) the cross-sectional design could never account for known high levels of relapse in those who make quit attempts.
3. The study's key question ("Did the use of electronic cigarettes or any similar device help you to stop or reduce your tobacco consumption?") can result in the misclassification of short cessation periods as full cessation.

Real-world observational studies 2. Longitudinal cohorts

Longitudinal cohort studies involve a group of people being studied across successive time intervals to measure changes or transitions in outcomes of interest. In smoking cohort studies, we find studies looking at uptake of smoking and vaping, relapse back to smoking, attempts at quitting

2 How we study quitting smoking: a critical look

and how long these last, further attempts at quitting after failed attempts and dual use (smoking as well as vaping by individuals). Like snapshot cross-sectional studies, cohorts can recruit randomly drawn samples from the general population, or focus only on special populations.

The important difference between cross-sectional "snapshot" studies and longitudinal cohort studies is that with the latter, the *same individuals* are followed, repeatedly questioned at several points in time and often biochemically tested for signs of smoking (typically, exhaled carbon monoxide levels or salivary or urine cotinine, a metabolite of nicotine). Enduring cohorts can thus have many data points across the duration of the study. While snapshot prevalence studies often include questions about past quit attempts and their duration, longitudinal data for the same individuals allow direct analysis of stability or transitions in self-reported smoking and quitting attempts. As will be discussed, serious problems with accurate recall of quit attempts and number of cigarettes smoked are far more common in snapshot cross-sectional studies that ask about past smoking than in cohort studies where current status is typically recorded for recent periods.

Moreover, Hughes et al. note that, unlike RCTs, most cohort samples of smokers "have few inclusion criteria and most are of smokers not enrolled in any formal treatment program" (Hughes, Peters et al. 2011). They are therefore important data sets for considering real-world quitting transitions.

Because it is critical to the very core of cohort studies' value that they have high respondent retention rates, those managing these studies generally invest in ensuring that loss to follow-up is as low as possible. Cohort studies invariably experience attrition or loss to follow-up problems where those in the study either cannot be located at later phases of the study, or decline to continue to be involved. There are statistical methods that can be used to adjust for attrition but these are often not undertaken, and attrition rates of greater than 20% pose serious threats to validity (Bankhead, Aronson et al. 2017).

Relapse

When we learn that someone has quit smoking, this can mean many different things. At one end of the spectrum, it can mean that a person has made an effort to stop either alone or with assistance and a very short time later (for example, at the end of the last session of a multi-session stop-smoking course) declares that right now, they are not smoking. It might mean that the day after their planned quit day, they have not had a cigarette for a day. This is often referred to as an "end-of-treatment" result and can often be found on commercial quit-smoking-quick websites. Today such information would struggle to find publication in anything but a pay-to-publish junk journal, because of decades of knowledge about relapse or remission back to smoking.

While there are some people who try to quit smoking and succeed permanently on their very first attempt, this is unusual. By far the most common pathway to permanent quitting is for smokers to have several and sometimes many attempts at quitting, only to relapse back to smoking for weeks, months or years and then repeat that cycle until their final, successful quit attempt. This has enormous implications for any critical appraisal of data in research reports on quit rates.

Relapse has been much studied across several decades. A 1994 Californian study found 71.1% of quit attempts lasted just two days before smokers lit up again; 58.5% last at least three days; 39.2% for a week or more; 19.6% for one month; and 14.1%, for three months (Gilpin and Pierce 1994). One of the most cited papers looking at this phenomenon is by US researcher John Hughes and colleagues from 2004, "The shape of the relapse curve and long-term abstinence in unaided quitters" (Hughes, Keely et al. 2004). This paper reviewed the paucity of prospective studies of people trying to quit without assistance (just two studies), and studies which had no-treatment control groups (five studies) available at that time. Summarising earlier work, the authors stated that "3–5% of self-quitters achieve prolonged abstinence for 6–12 months after a given quit attempt" (See Figure 2.2).

The data used in Figure 2.2 date from studies published in the late 1980s and the 1990s, and so could not reflect the more recent experiences of people trying to quit smoking in eras when modern tobacco control policies like smoke-free laws, significant tobacco tax

2 How we study quitting smoking: a critical look

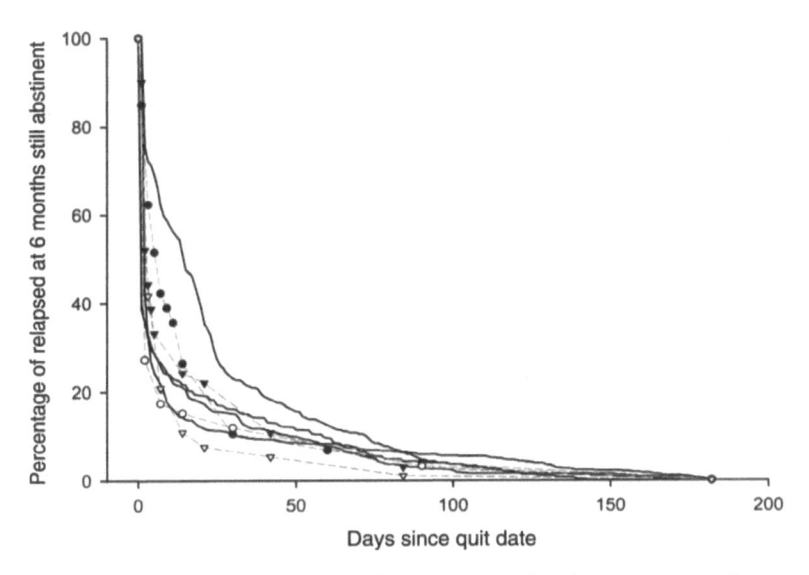

Figure 2.2 Among those who relapsed within six months, the proportion still abstinent over time in studies in Table 1 (Hughes, Keely et al. 2004). True survival curves (solid lines) and line-graph curves (dotted lines) in self-quitters (open circles and triangles) and those in control groups (solid circles and triangles).

increases, total advertising bans, graphic health warnings, extensive public awareness campaigns, plain packaging and the growing denormalisation of smoking combined to create an environment that is very different to that typical of earlier decades.

So what do more recent data show? A 2012 paper analysing seven years of data from 21,613 smokers recruited into the International Tobacco Control (ITC) four-country study (Australia, Canada, UK, USA) found that 40.1% of smokers reported quit attempts in the past year, with an average of 2.1 attempts. When the authors adjusted for recall bias (see below) and only included quit attempts made in the last month, the average fell to one per year (Borland, Partos et al. 2012a). This seems a peculiarly narrow, stringent window. Intuitively, it's hard to imagine that anything deserving to be seriously called a quit attempt would decay from memory after just one month. Another paper from the same study estimated that by the time the average smoker reaches 40 years, they will have made 40 attempts to quit (Borland, Partos et al. 2012b).

A British study of 1,578 former smokers who had quit for at least a year between 1991 and 2006 participating in the annual British Household Panel Survey, and followed up for a mean of 5.2 years after their initial one-year smoking abstinence had the authors estimate that 37% would relapse within 10 years. Increased length of abstinence, increased age, being married, being educated to degree level, and having a high frequency of general practitioner visits were significantly associated with a lower risk of relapse, while higher relapse rates were significantly associated with mental health problems and having a partner who started smoking (Hawkins, Hollingworth et al. 2010).

Most estimates of the average number of quit attempts made before final, long-term success derive from cross-sectional studies where smokers are asked to state how many lifetime attempts they have made, or how many in a more recent period, such as the past 12 months. As I will discuss below, recall of quit attempts and indeed agreement about what a "quit attempt" actually means are problematic. To reduce this problem, in 2016 Chaiton and colleagues looked at how many quit attempts smokers make by questioning the same 1,277 Ontario smokers who had reported a subjectively "serious" quit attempt during the last year. They re-interviewed these smokers every six months for up to three years. This enabled the researchers to validate more recent answers with those supplied by respondents in former years.

In a complex paper befitting an apparently simple but in fact very challenging question, they used four different approaches in their estimations, ranging from those which assumed that quit attempts reported in recent years would have also applied in more distant years to those which adjusted for various expected reporting biases and concluded, "The estimated average number of quit attempts expected before quitting successfully ranged from 6.1 under the assumptions consistent with prior research, 19.6 using a constant rate approach, 29.6 using the method with the expected lowest bias, to 142 using an approach including previous recall history" (Chaiton, Diemert et al. 2016).

Their open-access paper explains in great detail the strengths and limitations of each method, and their reasons for settling for the "Life Table, Observed Quit Rates" method which suggests that a smoker tries to quit on average 30 times or more before successfully quitting for one year or longer.

Finally, no discussion of relapse in a book looking at unassisted cessation could avoid considering a letter published in *Addiction* in 2012, authored by five giants of smoking cessation research (Hughes, Cummings et al. 2012). They were writing to criticise a press release about a case-control study in *Tobacco Control* where the authors concluded that "NRT is no more effective in helping people stop smoking in the long term than trying to quit on one's own" (Alpert, Connolly et al. 2012).

The Alpert et al. paper was important because it provided data on a question that is probably front of mind in most smokers wanting to quit and considering using NRT or a medication to do so: "How successful will this treatment be in getting me to stop smoking permanently?" I doubt that there would be many smokers who, in considering any given smoking cessation treatment, would ask, "How successful will this treatment be in getting me to stop smoking for a few days, a few weeks, a few months or even for a year?" Most would be thinking that, as they were making the effort to quit, those recommending a treatment would understand that most smokers would be interested in what the evidence showed about permanent quitting, not just temporary cessation.

The five authors wrote, "the [Alpert et al.] study tests whether the use of NRT in the distant past (up to 2 years prior to the survey) prevents relapse during the subsequent period [of] years after use of NRT. *Studies have found that the therapeutic effect of NRT is concentrated during the weeks it is being used, and after this the rate of relapse is similar between NRT and control conditions.* Thus, NRT does increase long-term abstinence, primarily by increasing the initial number of quitters" [my emphasis] (Hughes, Cummings et al. 2012). Here, they referenced a 2006 meta-analysis of 12 RCTs (Etter and Stapleton 2006) in support of their claim about the superiority of NRT to no-treatment in both short- and long-term success.

For all the reasons discussed in Chapter 2, we need to be very cautious in extrapolating NRT results to real-world results. And the Hughes et al. letter omitted to mention that the Etter and Stapleton meta-analysis stated "initial relapse after one year has the effect of diminishing the number of ex-smokers that can be ultimately attributed to NRT". They wrote that the frequent use of 6–12 month cessation data in reviews and treatment guidelines "will overestimate the lifetime benefit and cost-efficacy of NRT by about 30% ... the long-term benefit of NRT is modest".

So from this exchange, the best complexion we can put on the question of how good NRT is in keeping smokers abstinent into the longer term (here two years), is to say that NRT fares better than unassisted quitting while it is being used, but that both strongly fade as the months and years go by, to the point that there is no difference at two years. Smokers' curiosity about whether they will fare better in the long-term with a course of NRT than with unassisted cessation therefore looks like a "no".

Recall bias

A 2012 International Tobacco Control (ITC) Four Country study paper discussed earlier by Borland and others about systematic biases in cross-sectional studies of smoking cessation argued that these types of study are likely to underestimate the effectiveness of smoking cessation aids because of recall bias (Borland, Partos et al. 2012a).

The paper reported that those using stop smoking medications (SSMs) remembered quit attempts from further back than those attempting to quit unassisted. This finding was surely highly predictable. When you take SSMs (depending on the drug), you sometimes have to go and see a doctor to get a prescription. You then have to go and buy the drug, sometimes carry them around (as with nicotine gum or inhalers), and are meant to take them each day over a sustained period. There are therefore many cues to remembering that you took them compared to trying to quit without using any of these products. Unassisted "attempts" are often little more than an empty ritual in the style of "This weekend, I'm really going to stop". So when relapse occurs hours or days later, all rationalisations about "Well, I wasn't really serious" probably dissipate quickly, never to be recalled.

I certainly don't recall how many times in the last two years that I decided to lose five kilograms and so I just avoided alcohol during the week, tried smaller meal portions, walked to the shops a little quicker and walked 30 minutes to and from my regular tennis instead of driving, and then went back to my usual lower level of daily activity. But I certainly remember my "assisted" attempts: going on the 5:2 diet for three months, signing up for a gym, increasing my tennis to several times a week, and buying an indoor exercise bike and a rowing machine. If a researcher had called me, I would have recalled that the bike sat in a corner of the TV room unused after about 10 uses – I would have recalled the *failed* "assisted" attempt but probably not all the half-hearted unassisted ones.

But if your primary interest is in what approaches across whole populations produce the most permanent ex-smokers, *failed* attempts are not what is most important. The key question is what method was used at the final *permanently successful* attempt when ex-smokers are questioned: it's not about *quitting attempts*, but about the method used when a smoker *actually* finally quits. I cannot imagine any smoker who quit assisted or unassisted failing to recall how they quit, particularly when the final attempt was recent.

This 2012 Borland, Parthos et al. paper framed its research question against a background of questioning from some (a paper by me was referenced) about usefulness of SSMs in quitting when the real-world cohort data have often shown disappointing SSM effectiveness. The data used in their argument were on *recalled* quit attempts, not quit attempts that *actually succeeded* into the long-term. So I think the authors used a sleight of hand here: they drew attention to something that is not being disputed (that smokers make many attempts to quit). They thereby hoped to provide evidence about the question of the comparative head-to-head quit rates obtained from assisted vs. unassisted cessation attempts when these attempts were successful.

Given the variable reliability of recall of quit attempts, and indeed questions about what ought to be even described as a quit attempt, it seems sensible to approach the issue from a different direction. Instead of asking, "Are smokers more likely to quit by using assistance than by trying to quit unassisted?" we ask, "What if we take 1,000 former smokers who have not smoked for 12 months, and ask them what method they used in their final, successful attempt?"; we move from an individual to a population perspective in answering the question about what approach to quitting yields most long-term ex-smokers. And the answer has always been unassisted cessation.

Indication bias

When we see data that show real-world use of quit-smoking aids not performing as well as they did in many often highly publicised clinical trials, we tend to see authors and commentators arguing that this is unsurprising because of what is termed "indication bias". Saul Shiffman described it this way:

> Another important bias in uncontrolled population studies of cessation methods is that smokers self-select which method they use for quitting ... more dependent smokers – who have a lower probability of success in the first place – gravitate towards treatment (Shiffman 2007).

So if this assumption is correct, it would follow that in a large sample of smokers trying to quit who are recruited into a study from the community, there will be a higher concentration of heavily dependent smokers in those using NRT, a prescribed drug or by vaping than there will be in those who are trying to quit without any aids or professional assistance.

Being a more dependent or addicted smoker has long been known to predict relapse compared with less addicted smokers who try to quit. So when the proportions of successful quitters in both groups (aided vs. unaided) are compared, no one should be surprised if, at first blush, it looks like unassisted quitters did as well as or even better than those who were using assistance.

Appreciating the impact of this confounder, some studies take care to control for this form of bias. Here, researchers can include questions designed to measure the degree of addiction or heaviness of smoking (Chaiton, Cohen et al. 2007) in their battery of questions. If it emerges that, in fact, there are indeed significant differences in these variables between the assisted and unassisted groups (Borland, Partos et al. 2012a), weighting can be introduced into the statistical analysis of the outcomes for the two groups to produce an adjusted "apples with apples" comparison.

What we see happening here is a quiet refinement of expectations for assisted cessation methods. Starting from an argument that *all* smokers would benefit from pharmaceutical and professional assistance, and explicit warnings to not try to quit cold turkey (see Chapter 5), we then see statistical techniques applied in cessation studies to mask the fact that more heavily nicotine-dependent smokers will likely have poorer quit outcomes than less dependent smokers; often worse than control-group comparators who are commonly those who attempt to quit unassisted.

Despite these heavily qualified outcomes, bald public statements about the performance of various forms of assisted smoking cessation being superior to unassisted quitting remain very common. Part of the explanation for this is the sheer brevity of most health communication. Public messaging about smoking cessation is often highly constrained by cost factors in paid advertising (15 or 30 seconds being the most common duration) and in sound bites used by news bulletins. My work on the parameters of Sydney television news items found the average duration of comment by a person appearing in a news item is just 7.2 seconds (Chapman, Holding et al. 2009).

Much discussion of quitting has long been infected with commercial agendas. Clinical and research consultants to the pharmaceutical industry are often given media training with product-friendly talking points. So when a smoker sees an advertisement for a quit smoking drug or hears an expert being interviewed on television, what survives are headline messages, slogans and sound bites like "twice as effective" or "double your chances of quitting". Smokers won't be told that hidden behind such breezy claims are the sort of caveats I discuss throughout this book. "Doubles your chance of quitting" is a sales pitch, not a relative risk statement.

Ways of quitting smoking

I refer in this book to both assisted and unassisted cessation. It's important that this distinction is clarified. In a 2015 review I conducted with Andrea Smith and others of unassisted smoking cessation in Australian research literature, we defined assisted smoking cessation as:

quitting methods that have been "opted in" by the smoker and that provide assistance on more than a one-off basis. All of the included studies [re-reviewed] agreed that use of NRT or stop-smoking medications constituted assistance; however, studies differed in whether or not they classified brief advice from a health professional, use of self-help materials, ever calling a quitline service, or seeking information on the internet as assistance. In addition, several studies used "cold turkey" to refer to quitting abruptly without professionally or pharmacologically mediated assistance, but the term was also used to refer to quitting abruptly with professionally or pharmacologically mediated assistance. A standard definition of unassisted cessation was required with which we could assess every study for eligibility. The rationale for the definitions adopted for assisted and unassisted cessation was that it reflected the stance taken by the Cochrane Collaboration, whose reviews of smoking cessation interventions differentiate between quit attempts that are formally supported by the ongoing help of a health professional or counsellor and those that are not. Our definition of "unassisted" cessation therefore included, for example, smokers who received brief advice [from a primary healthcare worker] or who called a quitline but who did not receive ongoing support from a GP or counsellor (Smith, Chapman et al. 2015).

This is the approach I have again adopted in this book. It means that by "assisted cessation", I'm including the following ways of attempting to quit: pharmacotherapy (NRT, bupropion, varenicline or other prescribed drugs); vapourised nicotine products; behavioural individual or group counselling whether delivered through a dedicated smoking cessation service, by a HCP in formal sessions, the use of a telephone quitline, an online website or phone app over several sessions; the use of a guided book such as the Allan Carr program; and complementary and alternative therapies (e.g. hypnosis and acupuncture).

What, in my view, cannot reasonably be considered formal assistance is the brief mention of the desirability of quitting by a healthcare practitioner during the course of consultation for another purpose; a one-off curiosity call to a quitline; reading an article every now and then about quitting smoking online, in a magazine or newspaper; talking with an ex-smoking friend or acquaintance about how they quit; seeing smoking cessation advertisements on television, noticing graphic health warnings on cigarette packs or many other encounters with routinely "smoking denormalised" signage, customs or policies (such as working in a non-smoking building).

This is because all these activities are extremely commonplace, unavoidable, often only crudely quantifiable and rarely researched in any detail. Collectively, they are all part of what we might call the "background environment" of factors that together, acting synergistically, bring smokers to points in their smoking careers when they decide to try to quit (see Chapter 8). To sweep them all into a very broad definition of "assisted" cessation would mean that *all* quit attempts would have to be regarded as assisted. There is no smoker in any country with graphic cigarette pack warnings, who has never seen one of these. There are possibly smokers who have never been in a conversation with a friend, family member or workmate who has quit and wanted to talk about it, but they would be very rare.

A very recent paper from the International Tobacco Control (ITC) Four Country Smoking and Vaping Survey looked at the different quit methods used at the most recent quit attempt in samples from the USA, UK, Canada and Australia in the last 24 months (Gravely, Cummings et al. 2021). The most common method used was "no aid" (i.e. unassisted cessation) named by 38.6%, followed by NRT (28.8%) and NVP (nicotine vaping products) at 28%. Many used different methods in combination at their latest quit attempt. In total, the authors stated that 61.4% made an aided quit attempt.

However, a footnote in the paper unpacks a residual category named "other support" which a substantial 16.5% of respondents reported using. This category included "mobile apps, cessation website, pamphlets/brochures, books, acupuncture, laser therapy, hypnosis, support groups, social media, cognitive behavioural therapy, meditation/mindfulness." Some of these (cessation websites, pamphlets/brochures, books and social media) may well have involved quite superficial and fleeting engagement. A person who responded "cessation website" or "social media" for example, could have just briefly browsed such sites or could have fully engaged with them over a sustained period. The paper provides no way of knowing. So it seems reasonable to be sceptical that all 16.5% of the sample were indeed meaningfully being seriously "aided" in their most recent quit attempt, rather than casually browsing material related to quitting smoking.

Success rates versus intervention and policy reach

When we look at research evaluating smoking cessation policies and interventions through a population-wide focused lens, the two most elementary questions we need to ask concern the long-term success rate of an intervention or policy and their "reach" into the population at large, here meaning all smokers. In this chapter I've looked at most of the caveats and qualifiers that need to be borne in mind when critically appraising claims about success. But so often claims about the great promise shown by a quit-smoking method or a policy initiative which might stimulate lots of quitting activity fail to look openly at the considerations of how many smokers are ever likely to actually use a method or be exposed to a policy.

A method of quitting shown experimentally to be spectacularly successful but which would be hugely expensive to manufacture or require a large professional workforce to deliver it (where such a workforce would often not even exist) would invariably have inconsequential uptake in the real world, regardless of how efficacious it might be. For example, if it could be shown experimentally that paying smokers several thousands of dollars to quit resulted in pleasingly high rates of permanent quitting, the very first questions needing to be asked are, "How many employers would ever be willing to implement such a policy?" and "Would any government ever adopt such a policy?". Also, many non-smokers might reasonably ask, "So, do I also get a few thousand dollars for never taking up smoking? This seems very unfair". I look at paid incentives further in Chapter 4, along with perhaps the world's largest experiment in government funding of labour and pharmacological intensive smoking cessation, the decade long English embrace of quit-smoking centres.

Flipping this the other way, we can also see that an intervention with very low rates of success which becomes part of the day-to-day world of every smoker might nonetheless have an important public health impact across the whole population of smokers. Policies like graphic health warnings on cigarette packs, tobacco tax rises which impact on retail prices, and the introduction of policies which prevent smoking in workplaces and public places where smokers might otherwise be smoking lots of cigarettes each day reach *every* smoker.

Consider a hypothetical stop-smoking intervention which has been shown in trials or pilot studies to cause 20% of smokers to permanently quit. Imagine it was taken up by a national company employing 10,000 smokers, of which 20% participated in the intervention offered at work. This means that 400 smokers would quit.

But then consider the rollout of a rotated set of see-and-never-forget graphic pack warnings. Imagine a post-rollout evaluation of randomly selected smokers in a national population of 3 million smokers being interviewed about possible impacts of the warnings on their intentions to quit. Imagine that only 5% of smokers interviewed reported that the warnings had stimulated them to make a serious quit attempt, and that a derisory 2% of those had succeeded and were comfortable in attributing their decision to quit as being a response to the warnings – a straw that had broken the camel's back.

So with all smokers seeing the graphic warnings every time they notice or reach for their pack, here we have 3 million x 5% being stimulated to make a quit attempt (150,000) x 2% who quit (3,000 ex-smokers), far more than our hypothetical stop-smoking intervention described above.

Moreover, in Chapter 4, I'll look at how common it is for researched interventions like trials of workplace quit-smoking programs to be "upscaled" to a situation where they proliferate in wholesale ways throughout communities. Spoiler: they very rarely do.

All this also assumes huge faith in reductionism – the belief that, when it comes to explaining population-wide changes in complex health behaviours like diet, physical activity and smoking, it is possible to forensically and neatly reduce explanations of causal factors to individual influences. In Chapter 8, I'll take this up again.

3
Quitting unassisted: before and after "evidence-based" methods

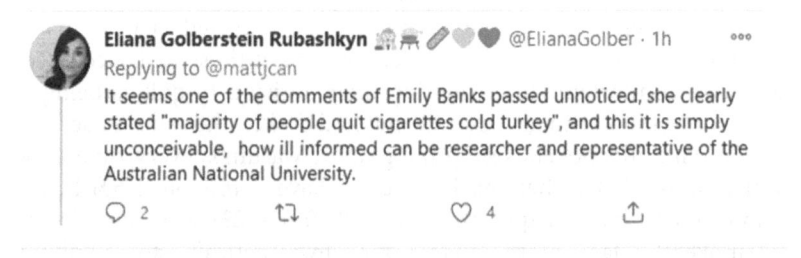

> **Eliana Golberstein Rubashkyn** @ElianaGolber · 1h
> Replying to @mattjcan
> It seems one of the comments of Emily Banks passed unnoticed, she clearly stated "majority of people quit cigarettes cold turkey", and this it is simply unconceivable, how ill informed can be researcher and representative of the Australian National University.
> ♡ 2   ⇄   ♥ 4   ⬆

Tweet from New Zealand vaping activist to Australian Senator Matt Canavan (pro-vaping member of the 2020 Senate Select Committee on Tobacco Harm Reduction), 13 November 2020. Source: https://twitter.com/ElianaRubashkyn/status/1327047735586021380

Most of the 20th century saw astronomical growth in smoking in many nations. This was almost entirely ignited by the mechanisation of cigarette production, which commenced from 1880. This dramatically reduced labour costs in what had hitherto been a highly labour-intensive industry involving the hand-rolling of cigarettes. Prior to mechanisation, an experienced worker in a factory could make about 240 cigarettes per hour. The first mechanised cigarette-rolling machine could make 12,000 an hour. Today's Philip Morris International machines churn out 1.2 million cigarettes an hour (Philip Morris

3 Quitting unassisted: before and after "evidence-based" methods

International 2021). Mechanisation saw the price of cigarettes fall rapidly, making them affordable to even those on meagre incomes. The rise of the advertising industry in the 1920s (Ewen 1976) enabled smoking to be invested with a host of meanings that saw the wholesale normalisation and glamourisation of smoking, first among men and later among women (Amos and Haglund 2000).

In these early decades of the 20th century, fragmentary references to advice and efforts to help people stop smoking can be found. But overwhelmingly, this period was a story of unstoppable smoking uptake, and the untrammelled promotion of smoking. On my bookshelves are numerous historical books about smoking, often given to me as gifts by graduating students who found them in second-hand bookshops and knew my love of history. These extol the delights of smoking (MacKenzie 1957), fulminate about the smoking "scourge", provide advice about how to rid oneself of this vice and mention early "cures".

Arthur King published a small book in 1913, *The cigarette habit: a scientific cure* (King 1913). The book commences with case studies on those who found quitting smoking agonisingly difficult. King openly declares smoking is an addiction for many, after having come to this realisation about himself ("If I couldn't quit smoking, maybe I was addicted to smoking, just as much as the morphine user is addicted, or the chronic alcoholic"). Most of the book is then devoted to explaining his cure, which he explains is based on "a classic axiom in drug-addiction treatment that it takes exactly *twenty-one* days to get the patient 'off the hook'".

His "cure" involved many of the standard folk wisdoms that have persisted for over a hundred years in tips that are still often passed to smokers about how to overcome cravings when quitting. King gave lots of advice about drinking fruit juice and water, cleaning the teeth, deliberately banishing thoughts about smoking, going for walks, writing out long lists about all the pluses of quitting and so on. But there are also early examples of self-medication, with smokers advised to stock up on caffeine tablets, antihistamines, and Boots' (the British pharmacy chain) "Anti-Smoking Tablets". Addicted smokers were urged to obtain five 5 mg dexedrine (amphetamine) tablets, and 10 half-gram phenobarbitone tablets (used to control epilepsy) to assist them with quitting.

Allan Brandt's epic history of the rise and decline of smoking in the 20th century, *The cigarette century* (Brandt 2007) notes that in the first decades, anti-smoking views were found among those who saw smoking as a vice and "a profound moral failing and a sign of other social and characterological flaws". Youths who smoked were commonly believed to be "stunted in growth and under-developed in mind", generating much tut-tutting and parliamentary activity designed to keep youth away from tobacco. But there are few accounts of efforts to promote quitting. Brandt describes (Brandt 2007, 48–9) the establishment of stop-smoking clinics in Los Angeles, Chicago, Hoboken and "many cities" that drew "a veritable mob" of smokers looking for treatments. These treatments included mouthwashes and swabs sometimes using silver nitrate designed to make the taste of smoking unpalatable.

A 1923 book published in Melbourne, *Secret recipes* (Holmes 1923), believed to be written by World War I medical officer Thomas J. Holmes, described an "anti-smoking mixture" where 36 grains of silver nitrate were mixed with 475 ml of water for use as an aversive mouthwash after meals. The book cautioned, "Do not swallow any of the mixture. It is almost tasteless, but is instantaneous in removing the desire to smoke". A medical advice column in the *Detroit News* from 1949 also recommended the same path, cautioning that silver nitrate "is sometimes used to mark the skin". It had often been used as a wart corrosive. The column continued, "One trying to quit smoking should exclude from his diet meat soups, broths or extracts, highly seasoned sauces or dishes. He or she should eat freely of apples, baked with meals or raw the first thing for breakfast and the last thing at night" (Brady 1949).

Such folksy hokum persisted for decades in leaflets and how-to-quit tip sheets often provided by health departments. For example, this Ugandan advice from 2004 counselled: "Nature has the remedy. Stretch out your arm and pick up a carrot. Chew it and smile. Within a few hours, all your distress will be gone. This orange root has large amounts of charm that is appropriate for those who wish to give up smoking. It accelerates the elimination of nicotine and its content of carotene reconstructs the mucosal membrane of the respiratory system that might have been damaged by smoking" (Nadawula 2004).

3 Quitting unassisted: before and after "evidence-based" methods

As I'll discuss later in this chapter, the advent of nicotine replacement therapy (NRT) from the late 1980s and its 30 years of subsequent widespread use marked the first time that attempts at stopping smoking often involved large-scale efforts to promote using medication to assist quitting. Prior to NRT, those who "took something" to help them quit used preparations that made money for the patent medicine spruikers selling them, but as far as I can tell from the thin historical record, none of the snake oils touted by their commercial and moral evangelists ever saw them in widespread use. But as we will now see, very large numbers of smokers began quitting when news reports of the first serious case-control studies started being published from the early 1950s.

In the introduction to this book, I noted that the publication of the seminal British and US case-control studies on smoking and lung cancer in the early 1950s saw a rise in news and commentary about smoking. This was greatly amplified in the early 1960s with the publication of the summary reports on smoking and health by the Royal College of Physicians of London (1962) and the United States Surgeon General (1964).

In 1955, just five years after Wynder and Graham's historic study of smokers and lung cancer was published in *JAMA* (Wynder and Graham 1950) and received widespread news publicity, 7.7 million Americans aged 13 and over (6.4% of the population) were former smokers. Ten years later in 1965, following further widespread publicity surrounding the 1964 US Surgeon General's Report, *Smoking and Health*, the number of ex-smokers had ballooned to 19.2 million (13.5% of the population aged 13 and over were ex-smokers). At the Second World Conference on Smoking and Health held in London in 1971, Daniel Horn, the director of the US National Clearinghouse for Smoking and Health, presented results of a cohort of 2,000 US smokers interviewed in 1966 and then again in 1970. Twenty-six percent of men and 17% of women had stopped smoking for a year or more in this time. Horn noted that 99% had done so without any formal help: "The level of change in smoking habits in the United States has become quite massive and I regard it as a change in health behaviour that is largely dependent on individual decision" (Horn 1972).

By 1975, 32.6 million Americans (19.4%) had stopped smoking (Horn 1978). Quitting smoking had become a major phenomenon. In 1979, the then director of the US Office on Smoking and Health noted in a National Institute on Drug Abuse Monograph Series, "In the past 15 years, 30 million smokers have quit the habit, almost all of them on their own" (Krasnegor 1979). Many of these quitters had been very heavy smokers. The same monograph also stated that "longitudinal studies should be designed to investigate the natural history of spontaneous quitters ... We know virtually nothing about such people or their success at achieving and maintaining abstinence" (Krasnegor 1979). In 2022, we have much improved on that situation, but the overwhelming majority of research on cessation has always focused on the "tail" of assisted cessation, not on the "dog" of unassisted quitting.

This major and enduring social and public health phenomenon of quitting smoking largely escaped the interest of researchers. There were very few research papers published in the 1960s and early 1970s about quitting. An early example by Graham and Gibson (Graham and Gibson 1971) reported on 382 smokers who had given up for at least a week. One hundred and twelve were classified as "successes" and the rest "recidivists". Of the successes, 89% had apparently stopped completely on their first attempt, with the others having up to four attempts before succeeding.

How did they do it? The authors asked about aids used, which in those days appeared to consist of either eating sweets or chewing gum (the wisdom of the day seemed to be that smokers needed to have something going into their mouths instead of a cigarette), 48% of the successes had used such aids compared with 70% of the recidivists. The authors noted that "various authorities and bodies ... issued statements condemning smoking, and data were published in newspapers from additional studies of prospective design".

A 1972 US paper reported on a cohort of smokers interviewed in 1966 and again 1968 (Eisenger 1972). Fifteen percent reported having quit in the two years between the interviews. The author attributed this to "expanded efforts by the US Public Health Service, American Cancer Society and others to inform the public of the health hazards of smoking". Again, this paper contained no information on how ex-smokers had quit. This might suggest that in those days, the question

3 Quitting unassisted: before and after "evidence-based" methods

may have never occurred to researchers: it was obvious that if smokers were quitting in large numbers, they were doing it unaided.

Ken Warner's 1977 paper in the *American Journal of Public Health* (Warner 1977) was probably the first time a helicopter view had been taken of population trends in per capita cigarette consumption across an early era in tobacco control. Using US data, he estimated:

> While individual anti-smoking "events" such as the Surgeon General's Report, appear to have had a transitory and relatively small impact on cigarette smoking, the evidence from this study indicates that the cumulative effect of years of anti-smoking publicity has been substantial. The analysis suggests that per capita consumption would have been one-fifth to one-third larger than it actually is, had the years of anti-smoking publicity never materialized. Increases in per capita cigarette smoking from 1970 through 1973 have been cited as evidence that the campaign has been ineffective; yet those increases totalled only 40 percent of what might have been anticipated in the aftermath of the TV-radio ads had there been no continuing effects of the campaign. Furthermore, in 1973 through 1975, abstracting from the effects of the campaign, conditions were conducive to the largest increases in consumption during the post-Report years – relative cigarette prices were falling for the first time; predicted consumption increased 16 percent during those three years. Yet following a 2 percent increase in 1973, actual consumption levelled out in 1974 and declined slightly in 1975.

Warner focused on the impact of mandated anti-smoking advertising that was broadcast across the US following a ruling under the Fairness Doctrine between 1968 and 1974. Following advocacy by pioneering US tobacco control advocate John Banzhaf III, and the Federal Communications Commission, the broadcast Fairness Doctrine which required television and radio licensees to "operate in the public interest and to afford reasonable opportunity for the discussion of conflicting views on issues of public importance" was expanded from the discussion of political issues to also include the smoking and health debate. With the tobacco industry spending millions on broadcast advertising of tobacco products, the advocates succeeded in requiring anti-smoking advertisements to be broadcast between 1968 and 1970. Health groups received US$75 million each year to pay radio and television stations to run the ads. For example, the American Lung Association delivered 1,269 ads between 1969 and 1970 with this funding (Warner 1977).

Warner calculated that publicity arising from "the smoking-health scares of the early 1950s reduced consumption by about 3 percent in 1953 and about 8 percent the following year, with the effect trailing off throughout the 1950s. In 1964, the Surgeon General's Report decreased per capita consumption by almost 5 percent. The anti-smoking TV and radio ads reduced consumption an average of better than 4 percent each of the three years they were aired under the Fairness Doctrine".

So effective was the impact of this advertising that the tobacco industry agreed voluntarily to stop all tobacco advertising in broadcast media in a bargaining deal to end funding for the anti-smoking advertisements. This took effect from 1 January 1971. While the American Lung Association had paid via Fairness Doctrine funding for 1,269 TV ads from 1969 to 1970, between 1971 and 1974 it ran only 569 ads when it had to finance the cost itself after the Fairness Doctrine funding tap was turned off. Gideon Doron's 1979 book *The smoking paradox* documented this early episode in tobacco control history (Doron 1979).

Neither Warner's nor Doron's analyses made any mention of the reductions in smoking they reported as being in any way attributable to assisted smoking cessation activity, but to reductions stimulated by mass-reach anti-smoking messaging. The only tobacco control policy in place for around a decade from the mid-1960s in a tiny handful of vanguard nations was tepid, general and very small health warnings on cigarette packs. The main drivers of all the quitting described above had been news publicity about the dangers of smoking. This shaped public views about the wisdom of continuing to smoke, and the US 1969–74 period where mass-reach anti-smoking advertising was broadcast in the USA at an average of only 306 screened ads a year, a tiny amount by the levels of major campaigns in later years (Dunlop, Cotter et al. 2013).

Of huge importance is Warner's comment above that "individual anti-smoking 'events' such as the Surgeon General's Report, appear to have had a transitory and relatively small impact on cigarette smoking, the evidence from this study indicates that the cumulative effect of years of anti-smoking publicity has been substantial". It should counsel us to be wary of being what renowned Australian epidemiologist A.J (Tony) McMichael (1942–2014) described as "prisoners of the proximate" in our search for causal factors that are responsible for changing highly complex phenomena like smoking throughout a population. Rather, we need to understand by shifting to a more ecological understanding of the complexity of change that large-scale social, attitudinal and behavioural change percolates for years, reflecting the interplay of both proximal and distal factors (McMichael 1999) I will return to this issue in Chapter 8.

In 1990, Michael Fiore and colleagues published findings from the 1986 US national Adult Use of Tobacco Survey (Fiore, Novotny et al. 1990). They set their report against the dramatic fall in smoking prevalence from 40% in 1965 to 29% in 1987. Yet again, their central finding was that smokers who quit overwhelmingly did so unaided:

> About 90% of successful quitters and 80% of unsuccessful quitters used individual methods of smoking cessation rather than organized programs. Most of these smokers who quit on their own used a "cold turkey" approach … Daily cigarette consumption, however, did not predict whether persons would succeed or fail during their attempts to quit smoking. Rather, the cessation method used was the strongest predictor of success. Among smokers who had attempted cessation within the previous 10 years, 47.5% of persons who tried to quit on their own were successful whereas only 23.6% of persons who used cessation programs succeeded.

As I discussed in Chapter 2, in later years commentators noting the frequent finding in population surveys that smokers quitting unassisted in real-world conditions succeeded more than those using assistance explained this as "indication bias". They argued that those who were heavier, more nicotine-addicted smokers were going to find it harder to quit and would gravitate toward using aids and professional help. They were therefore biased as being a group who were likely to struggle more to quit than those who used aids. They argued that no one should be surprised that those who believed they could quit without help (because they were allegedly mostly less addicted, lighter smokers) were more likely to succeed in quitting than those who were more heavily addicted.

So the Fiore group's findings summarised above are rather awkward for this explanation: they found no difference in quitting when comparing higher with low daily consumption – a key marker of nicotine dependency. It was quitting unassisted – regardless of daily smoking rate – that predicted success.

A systematic review of 26 studies which had reported on rates of cessation attempts from nine nations published between 1986 and 2010 found that all but two reported that smokers attempting to quit unassisted were in the majority (Edwards, Bondy et al. 2014). Heterogeneity in the papers about key issues like the duration of quitting precluded any pooled estimate of how many of those attempting to quit try to do so unassisted, but the range across the 26 papers was between 40.6% and 95.3%. Only some of the 26 studies provided data on whether their final successful attempt was unassisted (many quitters try a variety of ways to quit across a given year).

Of four that reported success rates differentiating assisted from unassisted, for unassisted these ranged from 79.5% in 1990 (Fiore, Novotny et al. 1990), 45.4% in 1994 (Lennox and Taylor 1994), 72.1% in 2007 (Lee and Kahende 2007), 66.9% prior to 1983, 57.4% in 1984–95 and 43.9% in 1996–97 (Yeomans, Payne et al. 2011). Each of these rates would be regarded as highly impressive if reported for any method of smoking cessation, particularly if the cessation was long-term.

We are hugely amnesic in forgetting or ignoring what happened in the days when what are today routinely called "evidence-based" treatments were unavailable. In the 1960s to late 1980s, there was nothing remotely approximating today's suite of tobacco control policies that have slowly driven down smoking in countries like Australia from 41% of men and 29% of women in 1975 (Gray and Hill 1975) to only 11% of those aged 14 and over smoking daily today (Australian Institute of Health and Welfare 2020e). In those days, there were no complete tobacco advertising bans, cigarettes were dirt cheap, there were few sustained (Lee and Kahende 2007) mass-reach anti-smoking campaigns, smoking was allowed almost everywhere and pack warnings, where they even existed, were tiny and timid (Chapman

3 Quitting unassisted: before and after "evidence-based" methods

and Carter 2003). Yet hundreds of millions of smokers across the world were motivated to quit smoking without help, and a huge number did so permanently.

In looking to the future of smoking cessation we should not forget the often-repeated, important lessons from its past. But as we shall see in Chapter 5, drawing attention today to the enduring, heavy-lifting contribution of unassisted quitting to the ranks of ex-smokers has become something of a profanity in professional smoking-cessation circles, which are dominated by those determined to encourage smokers to do anything but try to quit on their own.

Enter Nicotine Replacement Therapy (NRT) and prescribed medications

A search of the PubMed database of health and medical research shows the first paper published on gum containing nicotine for use in controlling smoking was published in 1973 (Brantmark, Ohlin et al. 1973). By the end of the 1970s, 15 papers had been published on the topic, and during the 1980s, turbo-charged growth saw another 293. Growing understanding of the effects of nicotine on the central nervous system, its addictiveness and on the potential for NRT to ease withdrawal prompted the widespread belief that cushioning withdrawal reactions by replacing nicotine in cigarettes with that in NRT would facilitate increased quitting. By the early 1990s, interventionists who focused on individualistic clinical models of smoking cessation were excited about what they saw as the first potentially mass-reach effective approach to cessation and were writing obituaries for face-to-face therapies:

> What is required is a broader perspective and greater respect for the limited role of individual and even small group interventions. Over the past decade we have witnessed a sometimes grudging acknowledgement of and interest in the pharmacological aspects and addictive properties of tobacco (Lichtenstein and Glasgow 1992).

In Australia, NRT gum became prescribable by doctors from 1984, and patches from 1986. Both gum and patches were rescheduled by the Therapeutic Goods Administration in 1988 (2 mg gum) and 1997 (4 mg gum and patches), making them available over the counter (OTC) without a prescription. NRT products have been advertised directly to the public since 1998 and sold in supermarkets since 2005.

Two prescription-only quit-smoking medications, bupropion (marketed in different nations as Zyban™ or Wellbutrin™) and varenicline, also later became available. Bupropion, an anti-depressant which had been shown in clinical trials to be useful in smoking cessation, became available in the USA from 1985, and by 2021 remained the 27th most prescribed drug in the country (ClinCalc 2021) In Australia bupropion was subsidised under the Pharmaceutical Benefits Scheme from 2001.

Varenicline (sold as Champix™ and Chantix™) is a nicotinic acetylcholine-receptor partial agonist. In the presence of nicotine, varenicline blocks nicotine's ability to bind with these nicotinic acetylcholine receptors in the brain, nullifying the effects of nicotine. Its availability commenced with releases in the USA and Europe in 2006 and in Australia in 2008 (Greenhalgh, Stillman et al. 2020). A meta-analysis found that the abstinence rate at 24 weeks or more for a 12-week course of varenicline plus counselling was more than twice that of counselling alone. Pooled data from three trials found that more people were abstinent from smoking at 12 months with varenicline than with bupropion (Stead, Perera et al. 2012).

By far the greatest potential for counselling in conjunction with the provision of varenicline is the brief advice typically offered by doctors, which accompanies prescription during a consultation. A Cochrane review concluded, "Simple advice has a small effect on cessation rates. Assuming an unassisted quit rate of 2 to 3%, a brief advice intervention can increase quitting by a further 1 to 3%. Additional components appear to have only a small effect, though there is a small additional benefit of more intensive interventions compared to very brief interventions" (Stead, Buitrago et al. 2013). So a "doubling of impact" from varenicline needs to be understood as a doubling of a modest effect. In Chapter 4, I look at the extent to which doctors ever offer smokers advice on how to quit.

3 Quitting unassisted: before and after "evidence-based" methods

During the 30-plus years in which these products have been available, the pharmaceutical industry has poured huge resources into both physician-directed and general public-directed promotions. For example, in 2008 total promotional expenditure for the market leader Nicorette™ in Australia was $3.108 million, with Nicabate™ spending $4.603 million. Champix™ (varenicline) spent $4.555 million. The USA and New Zealand are the only two OECD nations which allow direct-to-the-public advertising of prescription-only medications. In Australia, pharmaceutical companies selling prescribed smoking cessation drugs have circumvented this by running advertising where the brand names are never mentioned but smokers are urged to "ask your doctor" about a drug that can help you quit.

The 2008 Champix™ launch saw over 100,000 visitors to the brand's "Outsmart Cigarettes" website during the campaign period. It encouraged 7% of all Australian smokers to make a quit attempt with Champix™, with 248,296 prescriptions being filled and $50,936,964 in sales occurring in its first year on the market. Champix™ became market leader within five months, doubling the size of the smoking cessation category (Australian Advertising Council 2009).

Figure 3.1 shows the volume of prescriptions for NRT, bupropion and varenicline in Australia from 2002 to 2020. Note that NRT can also be sold OTC, so the numbers shown are very conservative for its total use in Australia. From 2011, any smoker could obtain NRT via prescription at a subsidised price.

Between 2001 and 2020, 1.162 million scripts were issued for bupropion; between 2008 and 2020, 4.631 million for varenicline; and between 2011 and 2020, 1.792 million for NRT, all on top of unknown but certainly many millions of packs of OTC NRT. The number of smokers in Australia across this time fell from 3.6 million in 2001 to 2.9 million in 2019 despite population growth of 18.8% in that time (Australian Institute of Health and Welfare 2020h).

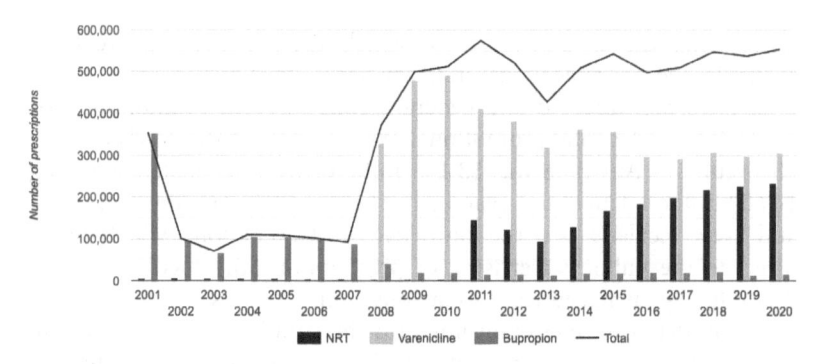

Figure 3.1 Prescriptions in Australia for smoking-cessation medications 2001–20. Source: https://www.tobaccoinaustralia.org.au/chapter-7-cessation/7-16-pharmacotherapy

How has mass use of smoking-cessation medication affected cessation at the population level?

Given this fall, an obvious question to ask is, "What has been the impact of all this prescribing and sales of these so-called effective drugs on smoking cessation across the Australian population?", always bearing in mind that there were many other policy factors designed to reduce smoking that were introduced during the same period. Particularly since 2008, in a smoking population of some 2.9 million (the 2019 figure) there has been a staggeringly high level of smoking-cessation pill swallowing, patch wearing and gum chewing among Australian smokers. With the Niagara of advertising promises of effectiveness cascading for years about these products, what has actually been the population impact? Two studies have examined this.

A 2008 examination of monthly data on Australian smoking prevalence from 1995 to 2006, which assessed the potential impact of televised anti-smoking advertising, cigarette price, sales of NRT and bupropion, and NRT advertising expenditure found that neither NRT or bupropion sales nor NRT advertising expenditure had any detectable impact on smoking prevalence across this 12-year period. Government anti-smoking campaign advertising and tobacco price did (Wakefield, Durkin et al. 2008).

The same research group updated their analysis in a second paper published in 2014 (Wakefield, Coomber et al. 2014), looking at the impact of increased tobacco taxes; strengthened smoke-free laws; increased monthly population exposure to televised tobacco-control mass-media campaigns and pharmaceutical company advertising for nicotine replacement therapy (NRT), using gross television ratings points; monthly sales of NRT, bupropion and varenicline; and introduction of graphic health warnings on cigarette packs. They used Autoregressive Integrated Moving Average (ARIMA) models to examine the influence of these interventions on smoking prevalence, and again found increased availability of these smoking cessation medications was not statistically associated with changes in smoking prevalence. They found that increased tobacco taxation, more comprehensive smoke-free laws and increased investment in mass-media campaigns played a substantial role in reducing smoking prevalence among Australian adults between 2001 and 2011.

These Australian findings echoed an earlier US analysis. A 2005 *Annual Review of Public Health* paper on the impact of NRT on smoking analysed national cigarette consumption and NRT sales from 1976 to 1998, and concluded that sales of NRT were associated with only a modest decrease in cigarette consumption immediately following the introduction of the prescription nicotine patch in 1992. However, no statistically significant effect was observed after 1996, when the patch and gum became available without prescription OTC, after which annual quit rates as well as age-specific quit ratios remained stable (Cummings and Hyland 2005).

What's the upshot from RCTs and observational studies of NRT?

In the 48 years since the first paper on NRT appeared, an immense volume of research on these three drugs has been published, with some recent renewed attention to cysteine, an antioxidant (Syrjanen, Eronen et al. 2017). Over the years, many important reviews, meta-analyses and papers have looked at questions of whether smokers using NRT or prescribed smoking cessation medications have higher quit rates than those who try to quit without using these products. Here are a selection of some of the more important of these across the years.

In 2006, Etter and Stapleton published a meta-analysis of 12 RCTs comparing NRT with placebo (Etter and Stapleton 2006). They found that while NRT performed better than placebo, "the long-term benefit of NRT is modest" and that smokers might "require repeated episodes of treatment".

In a 2011 paper, Hughes and colleagues reviewed non-RCT studies of NRT cessation outcomes reported in retrospective cohort studies of OTC NRT users versus non-users, as well as those comparing prescribed NRT with OTC NRT, including that given free to quitline callers (Hughes, Peters et al. 2011). They concluded that about half the studies "found statistically greater quitting among NRT users, and the most rigorous studies did not find greater quitting among users". They suggested that indication bias (Shiffman, Brockwell et al. 2008) (see Chapter 2) plausibly explained these findings: those using NRT were more addicted smokers who would have had lower likelihood of quitting than those attempting to quit unaided.

The Cochrane Collaboration first reviewed NRT in 2004, with its most recent update published in 2018. Only RCTs were considered. The 2018 review looked at 133 RCTs with 64,640 participants and focused on the primary comparison between any type of NRT and a placebo or non-NRT control group. People enrolled in the studies typically smoked at least 15 cigarettes a day at the start of the studies. The authors concluded:

> There is high-quality evidence that all of the licensed forms of NRT (gum, transdermal patch, nasal spray, inhalator and sublingual tablets/lozenges) can help people who make a quit attempt to increase their chances of successfully stopping smoking. NRTs increase the rate of quitting by 50% to 60%, regardless of setting, and further research is very unlikely to change our confidence in the estimate of the effect. The relative effectiveness of NRT appears to be largely independent of the intensity of additional support provided to the individual. Provision of more intense levels of support, although beneficial in facilitating the likelihood of quitting, is not essential to the success of NRT (Hartmann-Boyce, Chepkin et al. 2018).

This resounding conclusion about the superiority of any form of NRT over placebo or any control group, especially in the context of the ongoing mass sales of NRT in nations like Australia, both OTC and via prescription on government price subsidy, invites important questions about why such widespread and enduring consumption of this effective NRT appears to have not been clearly mirrored in changes in national smoking prevalence.

A 2013 US national Gallup poll reported that only 8% of ex-smokers attributed their success to NRT patches, gum or prescribed drugs (Newport 2013). In contrast, 48% attributed their success to quitting "cold turkey" and 8% to willpower, commitment or "mind over matter". Nearly 40 years earlier, a 1974 Gallup survey reported that most smokers would not attend formal cessation programs and preferred to quit on their own (Newport 2013).

In 2017 US researchers published results from two cohorts of smokers followed for a year between 2002 and 2003, and 2010 and 2011 (Leas, Pierce et al. 2018). The two population samples had many smokers who had tried to quit in the year prior to the study. These included those using smoking cessation drugs, and those not. The study found that in smokers trying to quit, there was no evidence that use of varenicline, bupropion or NRT increased the probability of smoking abstinence for 30 days or more when measured at one-year follow-up compared to those not using these drugs.

This study is of particular importance because the analysis undertaken sought to test whether indication bias (see Chapter 2) was responsible for the frequently observed outcome that unassisted quitters succeed more than assisted quitters because of confounding (i.e. those less likely to quit because of stronger addiction self-select to use medication far more than less addicted smokers). The authors in this study anticipated this issue and all smokers were assessed by what the study authors called a "propensity to quit" score (a score involving factors like smoking intensity, nicotine dependence, previous quit history, self-efficacy to quit, and whether they lived in a smoke-free home where quitting would likely be more supported).

In their analysis, those who tried to quit with drugs and those who didn't were matched on this propensity to quit score confounder, so that "like could be compared with like" in the analysis. Using these matched samples to provide a balanced comparison, there was no evidence that those using any of the three drugs increased the probability of 30 days or more smoking abstinence at one-year follow-up.

The authors concluded, "The lack of effectiveness of pharmaceutical aids in increasing long-term cessation in population samples is not an artifact caused by confounded analyses." They suggested a possible explanation of this was that counselling and support interventions often also provided in efficacy trials are rarely delivered in the general population.

Two back-to-back papers first published in the *Tobacco Control* journal in 2018 looked at (1) changes in 27 European countries in smoking prevalence and tobacco control policies between 2006 and 2014 (Feliu, Filippidis et al. 2019), and (2) changes in the use of smoking cessation assistance in the same nations between 2012 and 2017 (Filippidis, Laverty et al. 2019). In the paper looking at smoking prevalence and policies, countries with higher scores in the Tobacco Control Scale (a scale that enables ranking of nations on the extent to which they have implemented a range of tobacco control policies) (Joossens and Raw 2006) had lower smoking prevalence and higher quit ratios than those nations with low scores on the Tobacco Control Scale. The "quit ratio" is the proportion of ever smokers who have quit (so different from the prevalence of ex-smokers in a population).

One of the components that is scored in the Tobacco Control Scale is "treatment for dependent smokers" with a maximum possible score of 10/100 for that component of the scale. So while nations across Europe that were scoring high in the scale were enjoying lower smoking prevalence, what was happening to the use of assisted smoking cessation methods across time? The Filippidis et al. paper found that among current and former smokers, those who had ever attempted to quit without assistance increased from 70.3% (2012) to 74.8% (2017), while use of any pharmacotherapy fell from 14.6% to 11.1% and use of smoking cessation services (this included advice from a doctor and calling quitlines) also fell from 7.5% to 5%. E-cigarette use rose from 3.7% to 9.7%. These findings would have given little encouragement to advocates for proliferating assisted cessation across Europe.

In a 2018 paper using the US Population Assessment of Tobacco and Health (PATH) Study data (Hyland, Ambrose et al. 2017) between

3 Quitting unassisted: before and after "evidence-based" methods

Table 3.1 Smokers with persistent abstinence (>30 days) from all tobacco (numbers) by quit method used among 3,093 smokers [numbers and (percentages)]. Note: Total row numbers add up to 3370 while the total shows 3093 because the reported use of products is not mutually exclusive. Some smokers report using more than one product to help them quit.

Quit method	
E-cig user at Wave 1 ($n=200$)	11.2 (3.8%)
E-cig user sometime after Wave 1 ($n=569$)	21.1 (7.1%)
NRT ($n=533$)	32.5 (10.9%)
Varenicline ($n=156$)	15.9 (5.4%)
Bupropion ($n=92$)	9.5 (3.2%)
No aid used ($n=1820$)	227.5 (76.6%)
Total ($n=3093$)	296.9

wave 1 (2013) and wave 2 (2015), the authors reported persistent abstinence (not using any tobacco product for more than 30 days) by different quit method used at last attempt (Benmarhnia, Pierce et al. 2018). In ascending order of worst to best quitting outcomes, the quitting outcomes were (1) using e-cigarettes: 5.6% (2) NRT: 6.1% (3) varenicline: 10.2% and (4) bupropion 10.3%. But the most successful all-tobacco quit rate was for "no aid used" (i.e. cold turkey or unassisted cessation) with 12.5%.

Moreover, when we multiply these quit rates by the *numbers* of smokers using each quit method, the yield of persistent quitters who quit unaided at two years was even starker (see Table 3.1).

So in this major national cohort of US smokers, the much-maligned (see Chapter 5) and neglected unassisted cessation attempters quietly ploughed on, continuing their massive historical dominance of how most ex-smokers quit, contributing 1.5 times more quitters than all other methods *combined*, including those obtained via the much-vaunted new so-called disrupter, e-cigarettes (see Chapter 6). So not only did the supposed new heavyweight cessation champion, e-cigarettes, produce the lowest *rate* of persistent abstinence from all tobacco use after one year compared to all other quit methods, but their net contribution to population-wide tobacco abstinence was utterly *dwarfed* by all other methods (10.9% vs. 89.1%).

Australian data

In 2013–15, I was lead researcher on a three-year NHMRC grant researching unassisted smoking cessation in Australia. One of our first papers systematically reviewed all peer-reviewed research published between 2005 and 2012 about unassisted smoking cessation in Australia (Smith, Chapman et al. 2015).

We located 14 studies (11 quantitative and 3 qualitative) which reported on the number or proportion of smokers who quit unassisted. The 11 quantitative studies reported that between 54% and 78% of ex-smokers quit unassisted, and between 41% and 82% of current smokers had attempted to quit unassisted. Of the studies with representative rather than convenience samples, between 54% and 69% of ex-smokers quit unassisted and between 41% and 58% of current smokers had attempted to quit unassisted.

Two of the quantitative studies compared rates of successful cessation for smokers who used assisted and unassisted methods of quitting (Doran, Valenti et al. 2006, Kasza, Hyland et al. 2013). The Kasza et al. study found that smokers who used the NRT patch, varenicline or bupropion were more likely to maintain six-month abstinence from smoking than those who attempted to quit without medication. The odds ratios for the three medications compared to unassisted controls were 4.09, 5.84, and 3.94 respectively, which the authors noted were comparable to results from RCTs. However, this cohort study reported attrition rates of approximately 30% between surveys, with missing subjects being replenished. Attrition rates of over 20% are considered a serious threat to validity (Bankhead, Aronson et al. 2017).

Notwithstanding the different quit rates across the quit methods used, the net yield of quitting in this study was again higher for those using no medication (385) than for those using medication (326) because of the greater numbers who attempted to quit without medication.

The Australia-wide 2003–04 Bettering the Evaluation and Care of Health (BEACH) study of patients attending general practices reported a success rate (the number of former smokers divided by the total number attempting to quit for each cessation method) for smokers who quit cold turkey (defined as "immediate cessation with no method of assistance") of 40%, compared with 21% for bupropion and 20% for NRT for quit attempts since February 2001 (n=1030) (Doran, Valenti et al. 2006).

A 2011 study of recent quitters found two-thirds had used cold turkey; that it was used by a larger proportion of quitters who had been abstinent for more than six months; and that it was perceived as being more helpful than any other method (Hung, Dunlop et al. 2011).

An International Tobacco Control (ITC) Four Country study (which included an Australian arm) compared rates of successful cessation for individuals using or not using stop-smoking medications. Although the study did not differentiate between those quitting unassisted and those quitting with behavioural support, the results provide an indication of the success rate for unassisted cessation, given that the proportion of smokers who use behavioural assistance in Australia is very small (Cooper, Borland et al. 2011). The study reported that, of those who smoked 10-plus cigarettes per day and quit without medication, 14% were abstinent at six months, compared with smokers who quit with medication, of whom 16% were not smoking at six months. After controlling for differential recall bias, of those who quit without medication, 5% were abstinent at six months, compared with 14% at six months.

Trends in proportion of smokers and ex-smokers who quit unassisted

Successive Cancer Institute NSW Smoking and Health Surveys from a decade ago and a 2011 ITC study indicate that the proportion of smokers and ex-smokers quitting or attempting to quit unassisted is falling (Cancer Institute NSW 2009, Cancer Institute NSW 2011, Cooper, Borland et al. 2011). In NSW, the proportion of smokers and ex-smokers who quit or attempted to quit cold turkey on their most recent quit attempt fell from 68% to 55% between 2005 and 2012 (Cancer Institute NSW 2009, Cancer Institute NSW 2011). The ITC study reported that in Australia the proportion of smokers and ex-smokers who quit or attempted to quit without help fell from 63% in 2002–03 to 41% in 2008–09. The pharmaceutical industry's large-scale efforts to promote the use of its products appeared to be succeeding in undermining many unassisted attempts, despite the lack of evidence in populations where smoking prevalence is falling that smokers' nicotine dependency is "hardening" and is instead more likely to be softening (see Chapter 5).

Stop smoking medications in low-income nations

Pharmaceutical aids to smoking cessation became available in different nations commencing from the early 1980s. However, in many nations they remained for a long time either unavailable or priced well beyond the reach of all but the well-to-do. For example, a 2012 report on use of medications to quit in the past year found rates above 40% in the UK, USA, Canada and Australia but below 10% in Germany, Uruguay, Mexico, China, Thailand and Malaysia (Borland, Li et al. 2012).

When I visited Cambodia in 2010, a pack of 105 2-mg NRT gum was selling for US$58.10. Product information for 2-mg Nicabate™ gum advised a maximum of 20 pieces per day. Even if we were to halve that, a 30-day supply would have cost a Cambodian smoker US$166, when the average monthly income then was US$170. The corresponding cost for the same product used at the same rate for a month in the Philippines is US$140.50, where the average monthly income in 2010 was US$171. Data on the cost of NRT and varenicline in low-income nations in the Middle East and North Africa shows a similar picture (Heydari, Talischi et al. 2012). At such prices, quite obviously, NRT was utterly beyond the reach of anyone but wealthy elites in the world's poorest nations.

In a 2010 study, only 5.6% smokers in China used smoking cessation medications (Jiang, Elton-Marshall et al. 2010). Cessation treatments are unlikely to be an important factor that directly affects the quit rate or motivation to quit in China, home to the largest number of smokers in the world (Qiu, Chen et al. 2020), and in 2021 this was emphatically confirmed. In a six-city survey of men, 972 (31.5%) were unassisted cessation attempters and 535 were ex-smokers of whom 521 (97.6%) achieved abstinence without assistance. This abstinent group accounted for 18.6% of smokers (prior and current smokers) (Jiang, Yang et al. 2021).

Notwithstanding this, in Chapter 5 I'll look at an attack made on our work in a public health ethics journal where two authors tried to suggest that any detraction from the mission to encourage smokers in low-income countries to use quit-smoking medications was somehow unethical (Bitton and Eyal 2011).

Forty-two years after tobacco dependence was officially recognised for the first time in the American Psychiatric Association (APA) by its inclusion in the third edition of the *Diagnostic and statistical manual of mental disorders* (DSM-III) (Neuman, Bitton et al. 2005) and some 35 years after NRT started to be heralded as the first big hope for smoking cessation, it is time to take stock of cessation pharmacotherapy. It appears that this "treatable condition" is not responding as hoped to NRT or to the prescription smoking-cessation medications bupropion and varenicline that followed. Sadly, it remains the case that by far the most common outcome at 6 to 12 months after using such medication in real-world settings is continuing smoking.

Undoubtedly, much smoker resistance to using cessation medication is due to many smokers learning from other smokers that real-world experience of using these drugs does not produce outcomes that remotely compare with benchmarks for other drugs they use for other purposes. Few if any other drugs for any purpose with such abject track records would ever be prescribed. Despite massive publicity and (in some nations) subsidies given to NRT, bupropion and varenicline during these decades, the additional tens of millions of persons (or hundreds of millions globally) who quit smoking in this time continued to dominantly include those who quit without pharmacological or professional assistance (Fiore, Novotny et al. 1990, Pierce, Cummins et al. 2012). For the ever-optimistic evangelising assisted cessation, this is perennially explained as sub-optimal reach or message dissemination. Their solution is invariably that effort should be redoubled to facilitate greater access to assistance, improving smoker knowledge about the benefits of assistance and further individualised treatment. But after over four decades of the pharmaceutical industry's turbo-charged, no-expense-spared efforts to increase physician engagement and erode population resistance to pharmaceutical-based cessation, how many more years can the narrative of getting even more smokers to medicate retain any realistic credibility?

4
The modest impact of most popular interventions

It is now commonplace for cessation researchers to note that many smokers do not use NRT, bupropion or varenicline correctly or for sufficient duration and that professional support can improve quit rates. But how many smokers are even interested in receiving such support?

We have known for many years that smokers overwhelmingly express a preference to quit on their own. In a 1990 South Australian study, 46% of smokers were uninterested in any of the eight options for assistance with quitting. But these would have included many smokers who were not interested in quitting at all. The most preferred option (24%) was for a "program through your doctor". Only 7% were potentially interested in a stop smoking group, and 0.6% in using a quitline (Owen and Davies 1990).

In this chapter, I'll discuss some of the main interventions with mass-reach potential that smoking-cessation advocates have proposed to assist large numbers of smokers to quit, as well as what the evidence shows about the potential of each.

Quitlines

Of all smoking cessation interventions, contacting a phone quitline involves the least inconvenience and costs a smoker nothing. For decades, we have been used to calling helplines for everything from support for problems across a wide range of consumer goods and services, including appliance problems, warranties, insurance and travel. So if any form of help was to be a good candidate for attracting the most smokers, quitlines would be it.

Phone quitlines have held great promise as relatively inexpensive, highly accessible services to support smoking cessation (Stead, Perera et al. 2007). Clinicians time-pressed or lacking confidence in how best to deal with seemingly intractable smoking inpatients might feel assured by specialised referral services available in some nations. Yet, with few exceptions, the literature examining their use and outcomes shows that very few smokers (6% appears to be the best achieved) (Miller, Wakefield et al. 2003, Cummins, Bailey et al. 2007, Woods and Haskins 2007) seem prepared to even call up a quitline, despite the lines being highly publicised, including their phone number being shown on all cigarette packs in some nations. In 1993 at a time when California experienced large-scale, well-funded tobacco control campaigns, a much-publicised quitline saw only 0.05% of smokers ever call up for advice (Zhu, Rosbrook et al. 1995). In 2004–05 in the USA, an average of 1% of smokers contacted a quitline (Cummins, Bailey et al. 2007). A decade later, this had not moved, with about 1% of smokers still ever calling one up (Rudie and Bailey 2018).

But do the outcomes of quitlines match their promise even for the small proportions of smokers who ever contact them? In a nation where NRT was already free to smokers, a large English RCT (Ferguson, Docherty et al. 2012) comparing standard quitline support with (a) free NRT and (b) six follow-up calls from the service to smokers provided important information about two central questions about assisted cessation:

- What proportion of smokers wanting to quit are interested in receiving support and medication in an environment where NRT is already provided free via doctors?
- Does assisted cessation offered in real-world conditions match the outcomes achieved in clinical trials?

The data in this large study invite questions about how acceptable the offered interventions are even to smokers who express interest in quitting. Of 75,272 smokers making quitline contact and expressing interest in quitting over the recruitment period, 26,468 (35%) agreed to receive further support, but only 5,355 (7%) agreed to set a quit date. It would seem, therefore, that the vast majority of calls to quitlines may not be from those who are on the cusp of a serious quit attempt. Many may be making general enquiries on how to go about quitting but are not ready to try. In this trial, it appeared that some may also have accessed the quitline via the web or by interactive television, and so may have been less inclined to agree to a telephone-based form of ongoing support: people self-select into the mode of communication with which they most feel comfortable and online support is increasingly popular (see later on in this chapter).

Among this large group of trial participants who were motivated to quit and willing to receive further support, the authors noted that the take-up of the offered intensive telephone follow-up was similar to the use of such interventions among standard care participants. This was most likely to be because in the UK these interventions were already widely accessible. The findings here are important because they challenge the commonly expressed assumption that offering ever more intensive telephone support might increase quit rates. In fact, the study showed that there is probably an upper limit to consumer preparedness to accept more intensive support-based interventions, or to making the pathway to NRT even more accessible than it already is.

At six months, those in the study who were allocated NRT saw marginally lower self-reported cessation rates than those participating in standard telephone interaction, and quit rates were significantly worse in the group given free NRT once exhaled carbon monoxide (CO) validation of smoking cessation was taken into account: 6.6% of those in the NRT study arm were CO validated as having quit, compared with 9.4% of those in the no-NRT arm.

Unlike in clinical trials, cross-sectional and cohort studies of real-world cessation mostly show that those quitting unassisted have better success rates than those using medication and transform far more smokers into ex-smokers (Shiffman, Brockwell et al. 2008). As discussed in Chapter 2, "indication bias" may be explanatory here, with more dependent smokers who have poorer prospects for cessation being more likely to be using medication. However, this explanation does not apply in this study because smokers contacting the quitline were randomised and levels of dependency were comparable across all three arms of the trial. Yet being offered readier access to free NRT was associated with worse outcomes. This may imply that provision of NRT in this very low-effort way might have had unintended consequences: perhaps by undermining its perceived value to smokers and/or their commitment to actually using it properly. Provision of NRT is no substitute for determination to quit. Admittedly, motivation by itself is usually insufficient in most quit attempts too (Vangeli, Stapleton et al. 2011), yet quitting primarily by one's own means is the way in which the large majority of ex-smokers have finally succeeded.

North American quitlines

In the USA and Canada, quitlines are widespread. A 2018 report of the North American Quitline Consortium (NAQC) for the years 2006–17 provides a large amount of data on utilisation, costs and outcomes. Between 2006 and 2017, US$1.02 billion was provided to operate some 50 quitlines, with US$99.8 million in 2017. In 2017, 964,029 calls were made to these quitlines, with 333,919 (34.6%) being "unique" (i.e. first-time callers), and the remaining number of calls being repeat calls from these first-time callers. These numbers represented an estimated 0.87% of all US smokers, with the NAQC's target being 6% or more. In not one year between 2009 and 2017 did the reach exceed 1.19% of smokers, falling some 500% below the minimum target reach set by the consortium management.

There were 52 state quitlines invited to participate in the 2017 survey. Only 27 of these reported data on callers' self-reported quit-smoking and response rates, and of these only six reported response rates of over 50% from callers to questions about quitting. With these very major caveats, 27.6% of quitline callers who responded reported having not smoked for 30 days or more (Rudie and Bailey 2018).

The report does not provide denominator data on which the "reach" percentages were based. However, if we were to very generously assume that 27% of 0.87% of smokers living in these states quit for 30-plus days among North American smokers in the 53 states in which

4 The modest impact of most popular interventions

NAQC consortium members ran quitlines, then 0.23% of smokers in these states may have been helped to quit by these services (23 in 1000 with this figure almost certainly being much lower because of non-response bias most likely being weighted heavily toward those who did not quit).

With these low levels of reach, and even lower levels of population-attributed smoking cessation rates, it is hard to conclude that quitlines qualify as significant components of the factors which drive down smoking across populations. Those who run them of course defend them as being important ingredients in comprehensive approaches to tobacco control. They often wave cost–benefit data about, showing that the costs per smoker "treated" and helped to quit are trivial. The 2017 North American report cited above calculated this to be just US$1.81 per smoker "treated", although no figure was provided on the cost per successful quit attempt.

Stop-smoking groups and counselling

John Pinney, a former director of the Centers for Disease Control and Prevention's US Office on Smoking and Health, published estimates of the availability of quit-smoking products and services in the USA in 1995. A survey of group programs in 10 US cities found that in four of them, nothing was being offered by a major voluntary health agency because of "lack of demand". Data provided by three commercial smoking cessation vendors, SmokeEnders, Smoke Stoppers and SmokeLess showed 108,000 "cessation program unit sales" (presumably course fees paid by individuals) in 1993; "estimated sales" obtained from Marketdata (presumably a market research group) for 1993 showed a miscellany of 1,120,500 offerings provided by 14 agencies or commercial groups and two treatment modalities, hypnosis (350,000) and acupuncture (85,000). Others included the American Cancer Society (150,000 – presumably course attendance), programs offered by non-affiliated hospitals (175,000) and the Seventh-day Adventist Church (85,000) (Pinney 1995). All this occurred against a background of 47 million smokers in the USA (MMWR 1997).

A 2013 survey of contacts in 166 parties (nations) to the World Health Organization's Framework Convention on Tobacco Control (FCTC) saw 121 which responded claim that 20 had a network of treatment support covering the whole country. The authors qualified all their results in their paper by writing "for the most part, their responses could not be validated, although we made a considerable effort to identify contacts as knowledgeable as possible about tobacco cessation. Where responses were unclear we corresponded with respondents to ensure that the questions had not been misinterpreted and to clarify their responses. With some questions we acknowledge a degree of subjectivity in interpretation of their meaning" (Pine-Abata, McNeill et al. 2013). Forty of the 121 nations responded that they had nationwide treatment services.

Many nations can indeed point to examples of dedicated, specialised quit-smoking centres. But to my knowledge, only six nations, Japan, Korea, England, Ireland, Thailand and New Zealand (with dedicated services for Māori people), have in recent years implemented anything approaching what might even remotely be described as a nationwide network of such centres.

A 2014 evaluation of quit services offered in New Zealand by 32 Aukati Kai Paipa (AKP) (Māori stop smoking) providers during 2012–13 estimated that 2,035 smokers who had used these services may have quit at three months. An example of one clinic, the Ngāti Whātua Ōrākei Health Clinic in Auckland, was given where 211 smokers set target quit dates. Of these, 45% (n=95) were Māori and the abstinence rate at three months was 21%, yielding 19 quits. With obvious understatement, the report concluded, "This is clearly a small percentage of the total number of Māori smokers in Auckland, 5,637." The annual budget for these services was NZ$5.8 million.

The report concluded, "Apart from the wide variation between the District Health Boards these data demonstrate that AKP is not a means for producing mass quitting on the scale necessary for reaching the 2025 [smoking prevalence reduction] goal. Even a doubling of the numbers of quitters by AKP would not substantially impact on the numbers of smokers in New Zealand within a ten-year period." In 2013 there were 460,000 smokers including 122,000 Māori smokers

4 The modest impact of most popular interventions

and 702,000 ex-smokers in New Zealand (SHORE & Whariki Research Centre 2014).

I was told about the provision of these services in Japan in 2009 when I visited the country to give a keynote address titled "What should we do more of, and what should we do less of in tobacco control today?" at a national meeting of smoking-cessation professionals in Sapporo, Hokkaido Prefecture. Many in the audience worked in these cessation services and were not very happy hearing my message that there was very little evidence that clinics made any significant contribution to reducing smoking prevalence in any nation.

Notwithstanding the profusion of these clinics in Japan, there is scant information about their impact in English language research publications. Were there any important findings about these centres, we'd expect publications about it in English language journals. But this has not happened.

A rare evaluation of a smoking cessation clinic in a Japanese community teaching hospital reported on data from all smokers who had participated in a three-month cessation program comprising combined pharmacological treatment and cognitive behavioural therapy (Tomioka, Wada et al. 2019). During the decade 2007–17, only 813 smokers participated, with 433 (53.3%) completing. Of these, 288 (66.5%) achieved smoking cessation for four weeks – 35% of those who had enrolled. So this clinic graduated an average of just 29 quitters a year, many of whom would be expected to relapse in the months that followed, and some of whom may have quit anyway, had they never attended the clinic.

Such numbers are utterly trivial, even when multiplied many times over to account for the additional similar numbers from different clinics, when considered against the goal of maximising smoking cessation across a whole population in a country as populous as Japan.

In the opening presentation at the 13th Asia Pacific Conference on Tobacco or Health (APACT) held in Bangkok in September 2021, the opening speaker stated that Thailand has some 560 quit-smoking clinics. I've found no published assessments in English of the contribution of these clinics to reducing smoking prevalence in Thailand.

The English experience with quit-smoking centres

In April 2000, England embarked on what was almost certainly the most intensive and widespread effort the world has ever seen to set up a nationwide network of specialised smoking cessation centres. A large body of research and commentary was published about this experiment, which continues today, albeit in a much-reduced form (Action on Smoking and Health 2019).

In 2005, the journal *Addiction* published a supplement containing a collection of papers describing the establishment and early evaluation of a network of smoking treatment services and centres across England. A 1998 government white paper, *Smoking kills*, had made the case for such a network. The first paper in the supplement set out a history of the establishment and implementation of smoking-cessation services in England (McNeill, Raw et al. 2005).

Early in their paper, the authors made the remarkable statement that "Although it was not expected that smoking cessation treatment would influence smoking prevalence directly, treatment had been identified as an important and complementary approach to tobacco control." Despite this frankly underwhelming prediction of the centres' likely net impact (having no direct impact on reducing smoking prevalence), unprecedented funding was poured into their operation. Between 1999–2000 and 2002–03, £75.7 million was allocated, and £138 million budgeted between 2003 and 2006: a total of £213.7 million across seven years. Based on self-reported quitting, 518,500 smokers stopped for four weeks, although as we will see these numbers reduced dramatically when assessed at 12 months.

Another paper described the interventions offered by the treatment services. Ninety-nine percent of these recommended NRT and 95% bupropion. Group counselling was run less often in rural areas because of transportation problems. One-on-one counselling was described as the dominant mode of interaction with smokers. Coordinators of the services who were interviewed identified a variety of problems like shortages of staff with appropriate skills (51% agreed or strongly agreed this was a problem) and lack of career structure for service staff (81% agreed or strongly agreed) (Bauld, Coleman et al. 2005).

4 The modest impact of most popular interventions

In the same *Addiction* supplement, two papers described short-term and one-year quit outcomes, assessing the impact of the treatment centres. At four weeks, 53% of clients were validated by carbon monoxide testing as not smoking (Judge, Bauld et al. 2005). In two areas of England (Nottingham and North Cumbria) researchers found validated quit rates had sunk to 14.6% of those who had set a quit date by 12 months, with three-quarters having relapsed. This paper did not compare either the quit rate or quit volumes obtained with the background quit rate among smokers in a comparable population without treatment centres (Ferguson, Bauld et al. 2005).

A 2010 systematic review of 20 studies published from 1990 (before the 2000 boost in provision of services) to 2007 on UK National Health Service smoking-treatment services found 15% of participants had quit at 52 weeks (Bauld, Bell et al. 2010). And an evaluation of two Glasgow, Scotland interventions (a group counselling and one-on-one counselling with pharmacists) found carbon monoxide–validated quit rates of 22.5% at four weeks, which fell to 6.3% (group counselling) and 2.8% (pharmacists support) at 52 weeks. The authors concluded, "Despite disappointing 1-year quit rates, both services were considered to be highly cost-effective" (Bauld, Boyd et al. 2011). Twelve-month cessation rates in those who attempt to quit unassisted typically are in the vicinity of 5% (Kotz, Brown et al. 2014).

Another paper in the 2005 *Addiction* supplement assessed the cost-effectiveness of the English treatment services in 2000–01, and compared these with the benchmark cost-effectiveness of £20,000 per quality-adjusted life-year (QALY) saved set by the UK's National Institute for Clinical Excellence. Across 58 service centres assessed in the study, the median number of staff employed was 7.25 and the median annual total cost of each service centre was £214,900, of which 54% went to NRT and bupropion costs, 38% to staff costs.

Allowing for relapse, they extrapolated the costs of achieving four-week quit rates to 12-month permanent quit rates attributable to the services' intervention as being an average of £684, falling to £438 when savings in future healthcare costs were counted. These figures were thus well below the £20,000 QALY benchmark, causing the authors to conclude that the services were "a worthwhile investment for health providers compared to many other health-care interventions" (Godfrey, Parrott et al. 2005).

Given that a large majority of ex-smokers in whole populations quit smoking without any treatment from smoking cessation services, this bullish conclusion ought to have reasonably been compared to the cost-benefits of unassisted cessation. The zero costs to the government of people quitting without ever going near a professional service or using state-subsidised smoking cessation medications balanced against the benefits of this group's into-the-future healthcare cost savings would of course have produced an impressive headline, but not one that would have been welcomed by advocates of the dominant treatment paradigm in England.

Impact of English quit services on smoking prevalence

So what did all this achieve nationally? A 2005 report concluded, "Nationally, stop smoking services achieved a reduction in prevalence by 0.51% in 2003/04. If persisting up to 2010, this success would lead to a reduction in prevalence of 3.3% – i.e. from the current level of 26% to 22.4%." The report then heavily qualified this by noting that the estimates were based on self-reported quit rates recorded at just four weeks after attendance at the services but that 75% of early quitters are known to relapse by 12 months.

The authors then provided a revised contribution of the English quit services, writing, "all the estimates of reduction in prevalence ... could legitimately be divided by four – producing an overall reduction in prevalence of 0.13% per year or around 1% (from 26% to 25%) by 2010 for England" (Tocque, Barker et al. 2005).

Milne conducted a similar analysis for the English counties of Northumberland and Tyne and Wear, and concluded that "at best, current NHS smoking cessation services are unlikely to be reducing the prevalence of smoking by more than 0.1–0.3% a year". He contrasted this with what had been achieved recently in California where between 1988 and 1995, smoking prevalence fell 10% while in the rest of the USA it fell 5.5%. California focused on legislative measures for smoke-free areas, after "heavy early investment in cessation services had produced disappointing results" (Milne 2005).

4 The modest impact of most popular interventions

Irish researchers reached similar findings about the 93 quit service provider centres they were able to find in a 2009 study: "Reaching the recommended target of treating 5% of smokers does not seem feasible" (Currie, Keogan et al. 2010).

Some eight years after the 2005 evaluations, West et al. (West, May et al. 2013) reported that across 10 years (2001–02 to 2010–11), 5,453,180 smokers attended and set quit dates at English smoking cessation services operating through 151 English Primary Health Care Trusts (PHCTs). Some 92% of those who contacted PHCTs did so only once, with the remainder having more than one contact. The 5,453,180 number refers to the number of quit dates set, with some of these being set multiple times by the same individuals.

The West group applied longer-term relapse estimates to the four-week self-reported quit data, and calculated a 12-month cessation yield above that which would have been expected from just writing a prescription for a smoking cessation treatment. For the most recent year in their paper, this produced an additional 21,723 long-term ex-smokers nationally. Averaged across the 151 PHCTs, this is 144 per PHCT in a year, or fewer than three additional long-term quitters each week. At the time this paper was published, England had some 11.22 million smokers aged 16 and over, and some 33.3% made a quit attempt in 2011 (West and Brown 2012). So the maximum annual 12-month long reduction in national smoking prevalence attributable to the PHCT centres might be about 0.19% (19 in 10,000 smokers) or 0.58% of all those in England making a quit attempt.

A 2019 report from England's leading tobacco control advocacy agency, Action on Smoking and Health, lamented the 30% cut in local authority funding of specialised stop-smoking services between 2014–15 and 2017–18. It found that 89.8% of expenditure on total tobacco control was spent on specialised stop-smoking services, with the residual spent on issues like illicit trade investigation and promoting smoke-free areas. Quit rates measured at four weeks after treatment saw that the highest quit rates (414 per 100,000 smokers (0.41%) were in those local authority regions which employed specialised quit-smoking staff (Action on Smoking and Health 2019). Again, significant relapse after four weeks would be expected.

It is likely that many of these smokers attending cessation services would have stopped smoking anyway in the absence of the services, because as I have shown throughout this book it has always been the case that most people who quit smoking do so independently of any formal assistance, pharmacological or behavioural.

In England, 4.8% of people who smoked in 2010 were not smoking in 2011 (West and Brown 2012). This translates to some 538,560 ex-smokers. Those additional 21,723 who quit for 12 months after attending an English cessation PHCT centre thus represent about 4% of all those who most recently quit for 12 months.

From the variability in cessation across the PHCT centres, the authors argue that those which provided less intense support should be funded more to allow greater intensity of contact and higher quit rates to occur. If a goal of such services is to contribute meaningfully to population-wide cessation, West et al.'s data would suggest that such centres are unlikely ever to be a significant platform for reducing smoking prevalence under realistic funding increases; and exemplify the inverse impact law of smoking cessation (Chapman 2009). West has described the cessation services as the "jewel in the crown of the NHS" (Triggle 2013). If services responsible for 4% of long-term quitters are described like this, what superlatives would be appropriate descriptions for the policy and advocacy factors that motivated 96% of smokers to quit long-term without needing to access these services?

Public Health England (PHE) updated its guide to quitting smoking in 2019 and included Figure 4.1. If we were looking for a candidate graph which best illustrated the "weapons of mass distraction" metaphor for smoking cessation, this is it. If PHE had set out to answer the question, "What have been the methods used by most of England's ex-smokers when they finally quit?" the graph would have of course been completely different, with what they call "willpower" or unassisted quitting towering over all the other methods, and attendance at England's specialised smoking-cessation centres requiring a magnifying glass to help readers see their tiny contribution.

Apart from the brief embrace of quit clinics I described in the introduction which occurred in Sydney in conjunction with the 1981–83 *Quit. For Life* campaign, Australia has never been down a path proliferated with quit clinics. Indeed, there has never been any

4 The modest impact of most popular interventions

Quitting methods – what works?

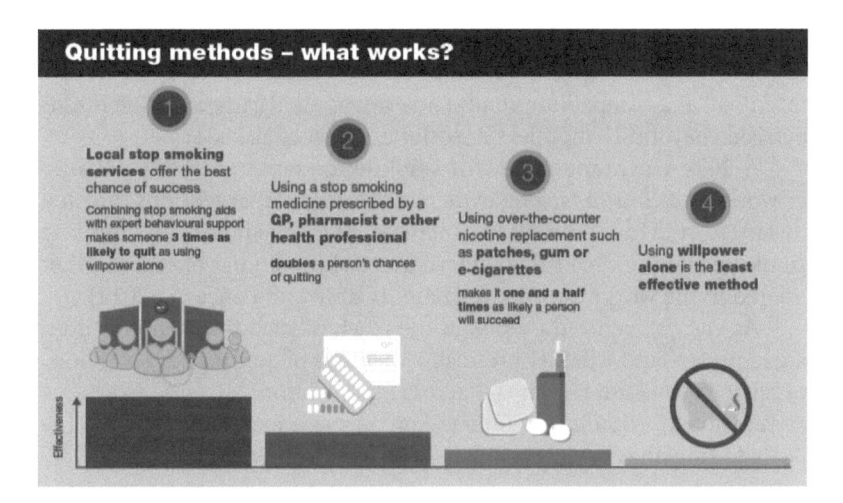

1. **Local stop smoking services** offer the best chance of success
Combining stop smoking aids with expert behavioural support makes someone **3 times as likely to quit** as using willpower alone

2. Using a stop smoking medicine prescribed by a **GP, pharmacist or other health professional** doubles a person's chances of quitting

3. Using over-the-counter nicotine replacement such as **patches, gum or e-cigarettes** makes it one and a half times as likely a person will succeed

4. Using **willpower alone** is the **least effective method**

Figure 4.1 Quitting methods: success rates. Source: (Public Health England 2019).

significant lasting clamour calling for this to happen. A census undertaken in 1992 of all Australian stop-smoking centres reported that the "throughput" (i.e. total number of smokers) attending was 8,800, representing just 0.2% of the 3.837 million Australian smokers at that time (Mattick and Baillie 1992).

Workplace smoking-cessation programs

A sibling of the dedicated smoking-cessation service is the workplace smoking-cessation program. These are typically externally run programs where smoking-cessation specialists come to workplaces either in person or virtually via online or telephone counselling, and offer assistance to smokers wanting to quit. Management offering a variety of health promotion programs and facilities (such as gyms, healthy canteen food choices, stress management) are often also keen to reduce smoking among their staff, with higher absenteeism among smokers being one motivator (Halpern, Shikiar et al. 2001).

A 2004 review of 19 papers reporting on workplace smoking cessation programs covering doctors' advice, education, cessation groups, incentives and competitions found no evidence that early cessation results persisted beyond 12 months (Smedslund, Fisher et al. 2004).

A 2014 Cochrane review of smoking-cessation programs offered in workplaces found "strong evidence that some interventions directed towards individual smokers increase the likelihood of quitting smoking", noting, "All these interventions show similar effects whether offered in the workplace or elsewhere" (Cahill and Lancaster 2014).

As always, we need to look at the reach of such interventions if we are to understand whether promising methods of quitting have any hope of having a measurable impact across a population. Here the Cochrane review noted, "Although people taking up these interventions are more likely to stop, the absolute numbers who quit are low."

GP interventions

In 1979, Michael Russell (1932–2009) from the Addiction Research Unit of the Institute of Psychiatry, University of London published a paper with colleagues in the *British Medical Journal* (Russell, Wilson et al. 1979) where they estimated a blue-sky impact on smoking cessation in England if *every* general practitioner was to urge *all* of their smoking patients to quit. Given that it is extremely doubtful that there is *any* important intervention in all of medicine which every doctor always urges all appropriate patients to use, such a benchmark was always going to be highly fanciful.

Over four weeks, the Russell group recruited all 2,138 cigarette smokers attending 28 general practitioners in five group practices in London. These were allocated to one of four groups: a control group who received nothing; another control group which was just given a questionnaire on smoking; a third group who were advised by their GP to stop smoking; and a fourth group who were given a leaflet on quitting, and told that they would be followed up by their GP. Follow-up data were obtained from 88% of patients at one month and from 73% at a year.

4 The modest impact of most popular interventions

The proportions in these four groups who stopped smoking during the first month and were still not smoking a year later were 0.3%, 1.6%, 3.3%, and 5.1%. These differences in outcomes were highly statistically significant (P<0.001).

The authors concluded that "any GP who adopts this simple routine could expect about 25 long-term successes yearly. If all GPs in the UK participated the yield would exceed half a million ex-smokers a year. This target could not be matched by increasing the present 50 or so special withdrawal clinics to 10,000".

Russell's paper, with its promise for population-wide major impact on tobacco control by the simple giving of advice and warning of follow-up to all smokers, lit a fuse of excitement among those working in tobacco control. It launched an era within tobacco control of smoking cessation research in primary healthcare settings which spread from work with GPs, to dentists, health visitors and ancillary healthcare workers. In the decades that followed, all national or international tobacco control conferences included a well-attended stream on smoking cessation in healthcare settings.

So how did things develop, with such potential being promised? Let's first look at some evidence about how many GPs even recognise which of their patients smoke.

In 1989, researchers from the University of Newcastle in Australia published a fascinating study reporting on the extent to which general practitioners identified and attempted to give brief quitting advice to smokers in their practices (Dickinson, Wiggers et al. 1989). The researchers approached 108 GPs to obtain their consent to interview patients prior to their consultation, and to tape their consultations with the doctors. Of those doctors approached, 56 consented, as did 2044 (76%) of eligible patients. The study was conducted over 18 months.

The GPs correctly identified only 56.2% of smokers, a rate just above coin-toss accuracy. Those who identified smokers gave brief counselling on smoking cessation to 78% of those who had a smoking-caused disease; 40% with smoking-exacerbated disease; and 35% of those with no smoking-caused or exacerbated diseases. Importantly, these rates were obtained while GPs were consenting to have their consultations recorded. Knowing that their clinical practices were monitored by researchers interested in public health and prevention, it is highly likely that most if not all the doctors in the study would have tried to be on their very best behaviour as diligent prevention-focused clinicians. The rates of correct identification and counselling obtained were therefore likely to be high, with the GPs' real-world, unobserved rates likely being lower than those recorded under such "be on your toes" observation conditions.

In 1996, the same research group analysed 1,075 audiotapes of patient interviews with doctors and found patient recall was systematically biased toward over-reporting of a question being asked about smoking (Ward and Sanson-Fisher 1996).

The Newcastle group returned to this issue in 2001, with only 34% of GPs who returned a questionnaire reporting that they provided cessation advice during every routine consultation with a smoker, as advised in national smoking cessation guidelines (Young and Ward 2001). In 2015, they again revisited the issue. This time, the participating GPs correctly identified 66% of their smoking patients as smokers, a big increase in the intervening years. The researchers approached 48 GP group practices with 12 (25%) agreeing to be involved. Together, these had 87 doctors of whom 51 (59%) agreed to participate. With study participant information undoubtedly explaining that this was a study about doctor–patient interactions on smoking, again, it is highly likely that those practices and doctors who declined participation were less likely to be those who knew they gave particular attention to smoking. This sample is therefore likely to be one biased toward doctors who had awareness of smoking as an important focus in primary healthcare. Yet even here, as recently as 2015, we see rates of physician engagement with smokers that remain far below Michael Russell's 1979 promise of every smoker being counselled to quit by every doctor they ever saw.

In England, a study of 29,492 smokers attending primary care in the Trent region in April 2001 found only 1,892 (6.4%) were given prescriptions for smoking cessation treatments across subsequent two years. With quintessential English understatement, the study authors concluded that this low proportion "strongly suggests that a major public health opportunity to prevent smoking related illness is being missed" (Wilson, Hippisley-Cox et al. 2005).

4 The modest impact of most popular interventions

In 2000, the US National Cancer Institute published a 230-page monograph titled *Population based smoking cessation: proceedings of a conference on what works to influence cessation in the general population* (National Cancer Institute 2000). In the first chapter, tobacco control veteran David Burns summarised the promise of physician-assisted smoking cessation:

> The gap between the effect achieved in clinical trials and the population data defines the potential that can be achieved if these modalities are delivered in a more comprehensive and organised manner and integrated with other available cessation resources. If physician advice achieves the effectiveness demonstrated in clinical trials, it could result in as many as 750,000 additional quits among 35 million smokers who visit their physicians each year. If the success rate of pharmacological interventions matched that in the clinical trials, as many as 500,000 additional quits each year could be achieved, and an even greater number could be expected if the larger numbers of smokers who are trying to quit could be persuaded to use pharmacological methods.
>
> One approach to improving the results seen with physician advice and pharmacological interventions is to increase the fraction of smokers who receive advice or use cessation assistance. However, a great deal of research and programmatic support has already been committed to increasing the frequency with which physicians advise their smoking patients to quit, and this effort has shown a substantial increase in the fraction of patients who report that their physicians have advised them to quit. Independently, pharmaceutical companies have advertised the availability of cessation treatments extensively, which has resulted in substantial demand for and use of these interventions. Both of these efforts should continue, but it is not clear that additional resources would add to the number of individuals encountering either of these two interventions, and given the limited evidence for a population based effect on long-term cessation for either of these interventions as they are currently practised, allocation of additional resource may not be appropriate ... *the promise of these interventions as*

established in clinical trials is not fulfilled in their real world applications. [my emphasis]

Anyone thinking this very blunt conclusion might have sounded the death knell for efforts to have physicians become more active in promoting smoking cessation would have been very mistaken. Those working in this area have never swerved from the pursuit of Michael Russell's blue-sky calculations where every doctor counselled every smoker.

Pooled data from the US National Health Interview Surveys between 1997 and 2003 found 84% of Americans saw a primary healthcare provider (HCP) in the past year (range across different respondent occupations 68% to 95%). Across all occupations, 53% of smokers had been advised by a HCP to stop smoking (range 42%–66%) (Lee, Fleming et al. 2007).

By 2020, the US Surgeon General's report on smoking cessation concluded that "advice from health professionals to quit smoking has increased since 2000; however, four out of every nine adult cigarette smokers who saw a health professional during the past year did not receive advice to quit" (United States Surgeon General 2020). In more than a decade, physician advice rates had only moved up slightly.

Despite these undeniably depressing findings, very clearly, any suggestion that HCPs should in any way be discouraged from advising smokers to quit would be irresponsible. Smoking is such a huge risk factor for so many health problems that the case for it being routinely noted with patients as a vital sign as important as temperature, pulse and respiratory rates, blood pressure and weight is unarguable. Yet with current rates of advice to quit from physicians being less than 60%, and over four decades having passed since Russell's famous recommendation of brief advice to quit, GP advice to quit rates remain trenchantly and scandalously low, showing little evidence of significantly rising.

Online quit interventions

The revolution in online interactive communication has seen a huge increase in the availability of programs to assist and support people

4 The modest impact of most popular interventions

wanting to improve their health in such areas as dietary change, physical activity, mental health, and substance use, including smoking cessation.

A 2017 Cochrane systematic review of 67 trials of online smoking-cessation interventions involved data from over 110,000 participants, with cessation data after six months or more being available for 35,969 smokers. The interventions ranged from simple provision of a list of smoking cessation websites to those involving internet, email and mobile phone delivered components. The review found that interactive and tailored internet programs led to higher quit rates than usual care or written self-help at six months or longer. However, the estimate of these "higher" rates in pooled results was very modest with confidence intervals crossing the null, and therefore being statistically non-significant (RR 1.10, 95% CI 0.99 to 1.22, n= 14,623), and many of the studies being classified as having moderate to low study quality and at high risk of bias. The review therefore provides very little that suggests these potentially mass-reach interventions are currently producing anything more than a good deal of *activity* rather than cessation *achievement* (Taylor, Dalili et al. 2017).

The Australian Department of Health has made available an app, My QuitBuddy, which allows smokers to see motivational and supportive data on their quitting progress. On World No Tobacco Day 2020, the Minister for Health, Greg Hunt announced that between January and May in the early months of COVID-19, the app had been downloaded more than 24,000 times, "a staggering 310 percent increase over the same time last year" (Hunt 2020). This means that in those months in 2019, it was downloaded fewer than 6,000 times. Curiously, no one I've spoken to has seen any evaluation of whether most of those downloading the app use it and whether they attribute any quitting success to it.

Contingency payments

Contingency payments in health promotion campaigns are where people receive monetary rewards or prizes for achieving particular outcomes. These can include cash, extra workplace leave, store vouchers or the return of money deposited by participants to motivate them to change. Smokers are sometimes promised incentives if they quit, typically needing to sustain this for a few months. These schemes have been run in a variety of settings, particularly in workplaces where they are sometimes bankrolled by management.

A 2021 Cochrane review of behavioural interventions found high certainty that, compared with those who received no smoking cessation support, smokers who received financial incentives had 1.5 times greater odds of successfully quitting (Hartmann-Boyce, Livingstone-Banks et al. 2021). The 2019 Cochrane review compared the financial amount of the incentives that varied between trials, ranging from zero (self-deposits) to US$1,185, although no clear direction was observed between trials offering low or high value incentives. A 2020 meta-analysis similarly found no clear relationship between the amount of financial incentives and quit rates. The incentive amount may also affect socioeconomic groups differently.

To my knowledge, these schemes have never been "upscaled" from time-limited experimental status often run by researchers to national, state or city-wide operation. This contrasts with incentives currently operating in some countries to encourage people to be vaccinated for COVID-19.

But there are important differences between a nation's concerns to have large and rapid increases in COVID-19 vaccination and national concerns to reduce smoking rates. The prevalence of active COVID-19 cases is causing massive economic damage to major sectors of entire nations. Smoking has negative economic consequences too, but these do not rain down in pandemic intensity, rather slowly percolating throughout nations year in and year out. For this reason, it seems highly unlikely that any government would invest in incentive payments to smokers for them to quit. And as I flagged earlier, many lifetime non-smokers might reasonably ask whether they too ought to be rewarded with a government financial incentive for having decided to never smoke. That prospect seems even more remote.

Quit and win lotteries

A related financial incentive smoking cessation scheme is "quit and win" (Q&W) lotteries. Here, smokers enter their name to win a

4 The modest impact of most popular interventions

sometimes substantial prize like a car or family holiday if their name is drawn at a date after the lottery entry period has closed and their non-smoking status is then confirmed by biochemical test. Those entering the lotteries are encouraged to be honest: a non-smoker entering and pretending to be a smoker could be drawn as a winner and verified as a non-smoker, although those organising the lotteries can try to minimise the chances of this happening by also requiring any winner to name a person of standing in the community (such as their doctor) to certify that they were a smoker at the time they entered.

Q&W lotteries had their heyday in the 1980s and early 1990s when their novelty energised many people working in smoking cessation to set them up in the hope that they would stimulate large numbers of smokers to enter, quit and remain ex-smokers long after the lotteries had been drawn. I was one of them. An early review of 12 lotteries in Minnesota, USA, reported that between 1% and 5% of smokers in local communities entered (Pechacek, Lando et al. 1994). In 1991, I worked with a television station in Newcastle, NSW, to run and evaluate a Q&W lottery. A local car dealer donated a small new car in return for publicity for his business. I drew and announced the winning entry, and drove with the film crew to a Hunter Valley coal-mining site where a miner was the lucky winner. I stood by in a urinal block where he supplied a urine sample for cotinine (a nicotine metabolite) testing to confirm that he was not smoking. His doctor confirmed that he had indeed been a smoker.

We published an evaluation of the lottery (Chapman, Smith et al. 1993) finding that in an estimated district population of 101,300 smokers aged 20 and over, 1,167 (1.15%) people had entered after duplicate entries were removed. We also discussed a core problem that besets most accounts of whether such interventions help smokers quit: lead time bias. This bias is sometimes called "borrowing from the future" bias and refers to the issue of whether quit lotteries genuinely increase the numbers of ex-smokers in communities in which they are run, or whether they simply provide an illusion of success by attributing a cessation effect to a researched event, when the attributed quitting volume may well have occurred in the absence of the lottery, reflecting a secular trend to quitting. Some smokers who enter these lotteries may have intended and succeeded in quitting even if the lottery had not been run. If they brought their quitting forward a few weeks or months from when it might have occurred anyway (thus borrowing from the future), the net quitting numbers across a wider time may not have been different. This is of course a question that can be asked about any intervention, and one that can only be resolved by comparing observed with expected changes over longer windows of time. Unfortunately, few research groups have sufficient resources to conduct such studies or have access to local or regional data that could help answer the question.

A year later in 1992, I had an opportunity to test whether a Q&W lottery, promoted via national television, with entry undertaken through a national chain of 4,177 pharmacies and a prize of a $30,000 car, might do any better than the earlier lottery run in Newcastle. A health magazine program, *Live it Up*, screened across Australia on Sunday evenings on the Channel 7 network. In six sequential episodes an estimated 1,466,000 people viewed all six episodes. The lottery received 7,769 entries, with about 7% being multiple entries from the same people. Forty percent of pharmacies submitted no entry forms.

So some 7,236 unique individuals from an estimated 1.446 million viewers (1 in 200) entered. I became intrigued with another question. How many entrants were trying to game the lottery by pretending to be smokers when they were not?

Several months after the Q&W lottery had been drawn, we followed up a random sample of 10% of entrants from the Sydney area ($n=300$), and had an independent experienced interviewer remind those questioned that the contest was long over (Chapman and Smith 1994). She then asked them whether they had in fact really been smokers when they entered. Nearly one-third of those questioned admitted that they had entered the lottery on false pretences, saying that they were smokers when in fact they were not. Those who said that they were smokers when they entered the lottery were asked about their smoking status at follow-up. Of 4,777 entrants who were smokers, 530 (11%) either quit during the six weeks of the program or in the three months before follow-up interview.

So here was a mass-reach intervention that saw six segments of a nationwide television program broadcast in early evening prime time on a weekend. Each program segment was designed to be maximally motivating to smokers. The substantial prize was expected to entice

4 The modest impact of most popular interventions

large-scale participation in the lottery, turbo-charging the levels of background quitting that would be expected to occur across the weeks that the program ran, had the intervention not run.

Using the most recent population data on smoking, we estimated that across the four months of the TV program and follow-up interval, some 25,328 smokers would have quit across Australia. We don't know how many of the 530 self-reported quitters who entered the lottery would have quit regardless, nor do we know how many smokers who watched and were inspired to quit but didn't enter the Q&W lottery. But making non-heroic assumptions about these numbers and remembering that many of those who reported quitting would relapse in the months and years after follow-up, it would have been very difficult to sell the story that this innovative intervention which was seen by large numbers of smokers caused anything but a tiny, one-off ripple of cessation across Australia.

How much intervention research is ever "upscaled" to become routine in mass-reach settings?

If you open the pages of public health research journals, for over 50 years, you will find a very large number of trials and evaluations of what is known as intervention research. These can include interventions in clinical settings looking at the effects of drugs, diagnostics or procedures on relevant health outcomes; interventions in community settings where groups of people in existing networks like workplaces, schools or among self-selecting community participants want to improve their health; or in whole populations as might occur with a change in laws, regulations, product standards or local government policies.

Research agencies which fund intervention research, and governments which provide those agencies with funding for competitive distribution to the best applicant research groups, invariably justify this funding as a vital step in producing evidence-based knowledge that has the best chance of improving public health. The thinking goes like this. First, what health problems are regarded as having high priority in prevention or treatment, with considerations of greater safety, effectiveness and equitable access to all relevant populations? Problems which adversely affect large numbers of people, and which cause significant burdens of death, illness and lower quality of life are often given priority status by grant bodies when they ring-fence special funding for such problems.

Second, does a research proposal describe a proposed intervention which, if successful, would be likely to attract significant interest well beyond academic research circles after it has concluded? For example, if a trial of a smoking-cessation program for hospital in-patients was found to be very successfully conducted and produced clearly higher quit rates in participants than in matched controls, would this be likely to be widely adopted in other hospitals?

Third, which researchers and groups have proven track records in both conducting and publishing high-quality research on such priority issues? Research grant agencies try to back proven research champions, and also look at the presence of early career researchers on a team who will hopefully benefit from research apprenticeship with more experienced colleagues.

Then there is a fourth consideration: one which in my experience is given far less attention by grant review committees who select and rank applications. This is the question that considers the ultimate "so what?" of research applications. It concerns the whole issue of what is the point of trialling, evaluating and publishing lots of intervention-relevant research when so little of it ever becomes adopted later? How much research ever becomes "upscaled" so that its findings change the way things are done in the world long after a demonstration research project shows it has promise? It goes well beyond asking about the reception a piece of research has had within the very cloistered world of one's national and international research peers, via metrics like high citation rates from other researchers or keynote speaking invitations to the peak global conferences or prestigious awards.

It fundamentally answers the question "Did this research change things for the better?"

I often find myself in situations where people I've just met ask me what I "do" in my work. It's easy to explain the day-to-day of teaching and research in a university. Most people understand that research is published in scholarly journals. They are very familiar with news media reports of interesting or breakthrough research, and hearing

4 The modest impact of most popular interventions

the researchers involved talk about why the research they have done is important and what it might change for the public good. But you can see the penny drop when you give illustrations of how your work actually contributed to making a difference or leveraged change in important ways.

Perhaps of all public health research, intervention research is imbued with hopes that it might produce findings of great practical importance in changing individual, clinical, institutional, educational or regulatory behaviour and practice. Despite millions of dollars being invested in intervention research each year, little is understood about how much of this research produces findings that have utility for clinicians, communities or institutional program planners. Similarly, little is understood about the characteristics of "successful" researched interventions which go on to become widely adopted in the "real world" compared to those which are never adopted.

Toward the end of my career, I led two Australian NHMRC research grants that went to the heart of these questions. The first explored the characteristics of highly "influential" Australian researchers in six fields of public health, and the second sought to understand the nature and characteristics of intervention research that has had a demonstrated impact on policy and practice, and the research translation process by which the impact of the research occurred. In short, what is it about both research and researchers whose work in public health actually makes an impact beyond the arcane world of other researchers?

With the first project, we contacted every Australian researcher who had published five or more peer-reviewed papers in the past 10 years in the fields of alcohol, illicit drugs, injury prevention, obesity, skin cancer and tobacco control. We invited them to nominate six Australian researchers in their fields who they considered to be the "most influential". We did not define "influential" but encouraged them to consider any characteristic that they believed defined influence. We then interviewed the six most nominated researchers in each field, exploring why they believed they were seen by their research peers as influential.

Finally, we interviewed a cross-section of politicians in health portfolios, their senior staff, senior health bureaucrats and heads of non-government health organisations, asking them about how they came to trust and work with researchers when it came to policy change matters. We published four papers on this work (Haynes, Derrick et al. 2011, Haynes, Gillespie et al. 2011, Haynes, Derrick et al. 2012, Chapman, Haynes et al. 2014).

In the context of our consideration about how much intervention research ever influences policy and practice, our work in this project concluded that with rare exceptions, all those nominated as most influential by their peers were those who, besides being excellent, highly productive researchers, very strongly believed that researchers had a duty and responsibility to disseminate their research as widely as possible. Almost all were well-known public advocates for change in their fields. They appeared regularly in news media, led peak committees, and actively sought to bring their work to the attention of policy makers who were in a position to support its subsequent upscaling into policy and practice.

With the second project, we focused on all NHMRC funded project grants commencing in the eight years from 2000 to 2007 that involved the conduct and evaluation of impact arising from health interventions. There were 107 of these, of which 50 research team leaders agreed to participate in our research. With those who declined to participate, we suspected that many of these were likely to have produced no evidence supporting the efficacy of their interventions and/or did not ever get subsequently implemented in relevant communities. It seemed intuitive that had an intervention proved to be successful and later taken up for use in clinical or community practice, the researchers involved would have been delighted by this and very happy to discuss it with our team. The sample of 50 comprised a mix of treatment and management (n=20), early intervention/screening (n=12) and primary prevention/ health promotion interventions (n=18), implemented in clinical and community settings. Topics reflected a wide variety of health disciplines, including medicine, psychiatry, psychology, dietetics, dentistry, physiotherapy, speech pathology, nursing and public health.

We reviewed the publications arising from these 50 projects to determine if the interventions being researched had produced results that might stimulate uptake of the interventions in relevant contexts. We then interviewed the researchers about their knowledge of any such uptake and impact and looked for evidence of any impacts of the research in a wide range of sources, just in case the original researchers were unaware that their work had inspired adoption of the interventions. We produced three papers from this work (Cohen, Schroeder et al. 2015, King, Newson et al. 2015, Newson, King et al. 2015).

We found that 56% of the projects reported at least one statistically significant intervention effect of potential interest to real-world practice and that 34% had evidence of subsequent specific policy and practice impacts (such as clinical practice changes; organisational or service changes; development of commercial products or services; policy changes) that had already occurred and were corroborated. However, mostly these were quite small examples of local or institutional intervention uptake, not state or nationwide.

What I took from this was that many researched interventions do not produce positive findings that are likely to inspire adoption in the community (hopefully, failed interventions being less likely to inspire adoption). And of course that's not a problem at all: the task of any scientific evaluation is to faithfully and transparently report all important outcomes, whether positive or negative. But our finding that for only about one in three intervention projects was there any corroborated evidence that *any part* or the complete intervention had subsequently become a routine part of prevention or treatment practice in health care settings or the community should give major pause.

This research finding was salutary. It suggests that many researched interventions which have been shown under trial conditions to "work" are, regardless of their positive outcomes, destined to never move onto any sort of real-world implementation after the research projects finish. Researchers move on to the next phase of their research careers and many do not see it as their responsibility to advocate for, or even publicise, what their research has demonstrated.

Excitement about interventions which perform well in trials or in field conditions is therefore often confined mostly to the academic research community. Any publicity that occurs at the time of publication, as occurs with all news reporting, rapidly fades. Research publications are often pay-walled and so inaccessible to the general public and journalists. Good news stories from research seldom translate into good news about the interventions concerned being upscaled for mass-reach potential impact. The lessons here need to be kept very firmly in mind when assessing the likelihood that promising interventions will simply progress through to being provided to sometimes millions in communities.

This chapter has looked at several very commonly advocated, potentially mass-reach smoking cessation interventions. Most, if not all, have fallen badly short of the promises held out for them over decades. Yet despite all this, in 2020 the US Surgeon General concluded, "More than three out of five US adults who have ever smoked cigarettes have quit. Although a majority of cigarette smokers make a quit attempt each year, less than one-third use cessation medications approved by the US Food and Drug Administration or behavioral counselling to support quit attempts." In just these two sentences, we have two important points: that stopping smoking is a widespread social phenomenon, and that most of those who succeed somehow managed to do it without using "approved" methods. In chapters 7 and 8, we'll look at how this happens.

5
"Don't try to quit cold turkey"

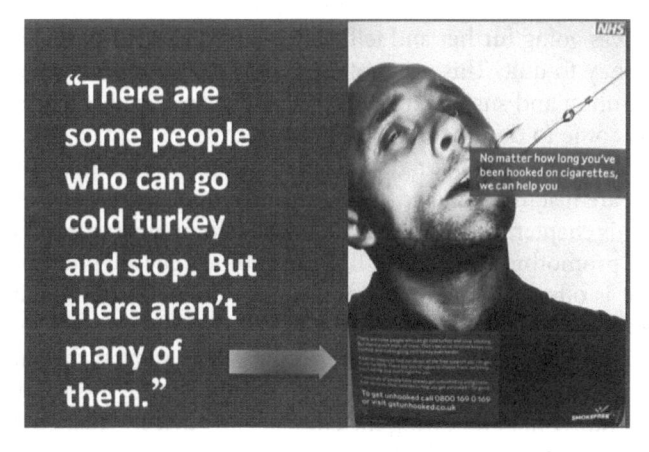

Figure 5.1 An English poster urging smokers not to try quitting cold turkey. NHS smokefree campaign 2008.

The figure above shows a poster that was used by government health services in England around 2010. I'm vague about the date because the poster has all but disappeared from public access, with only the rather distorted image shown above being locatable from Google Images. When I first saw it, I was just gobsmacked by the outrageously incorrect statement I've enlarged next to the poster in Figure 5.1. "But there aren't many of them" (who quit cold turkey) is completely and utterly wrong. It is a weapons-grade lie which, as we have seen, is easily contradicted by data from going back several decades to at least to the 1960s, showing the constant dominance of unaided quitting among former smokers.

It is also a disabling lie, because its intent was to persuade smokers that any thought they had about quitting unaided was mere folly. A smoker would be fooling themselves if they thought they could quit without help. So the intent was to undermine any sense of agency that a smoker might harbour. The message in this poster was part of a planned and sustained effort in England by health authorities to actively try to dissuade smokers from trying to quit unaided. Its message "Don't go cold turkey" (see figures 5.2 to 5.4) could not have been clearer: it told smokers that they should not attempt to stop without help. It wasn't health authorities telling smokers not to give stop-smoking medications a try; it was going further and telling them not to put any trust in their own agency to quit. This was not a one-off, isolated message, but was very common and sustained in the UK and, as we shall see, a message that has come to dominate the public narrative on how to quit. If you google "cold turkey smoking", oceans of webpages asserting the same message are instantly returned from all around the world.

In this chapter, before looking at the attacks on unassisted cessation by those promoting assistance, I'll first examine a central premise of the case that is often made for the importance of maximising the number of smokers who need to be persuaded to use assistance when quitting. I'll also summarise efforts that have been made to suggest that smokers ought to be supervised through a "tailored" progression toward quitting, rather than following the Nike slogan advice – "Just do it". And I'll also examine one of the best kept secrets in smoking cessation: a large proportion of those who quit find it surprisingly easy to do so.

I'll then critically examine the claims made by those who would like to see as many smokers as possible who are attempting to quit be supervised and medicated in their attempts, and their reactions when this is questioned.

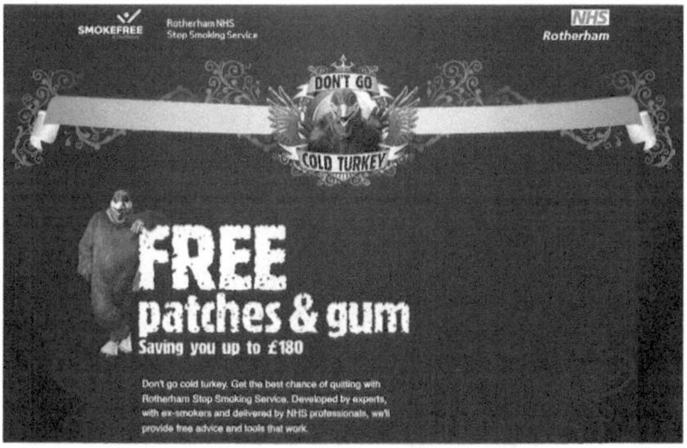

Figure 5.2 "Don't go cold turkey" promotion in England. Source: Get Healthy Rotherham.

The Don't Go Cold Turkey roadshow adopted a fun approach in order to get a serious message across.

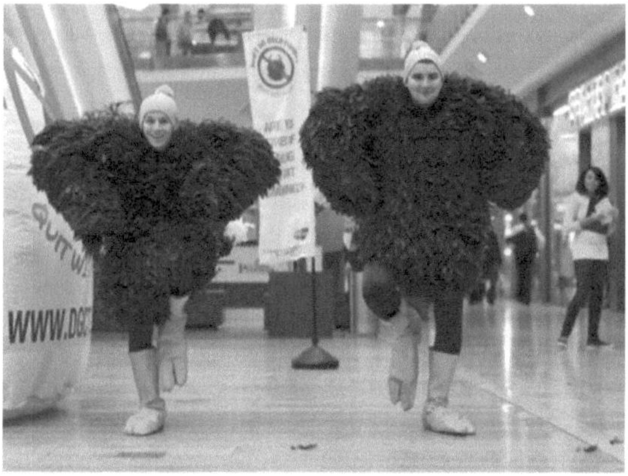

Figure 5.3 In Birmingham, UK local health workers took to shopping centres to promote their message. Source: https://www.bhamcommunity.nhs.uk/about-us/news/archive-news/cold-turkey-campaign/

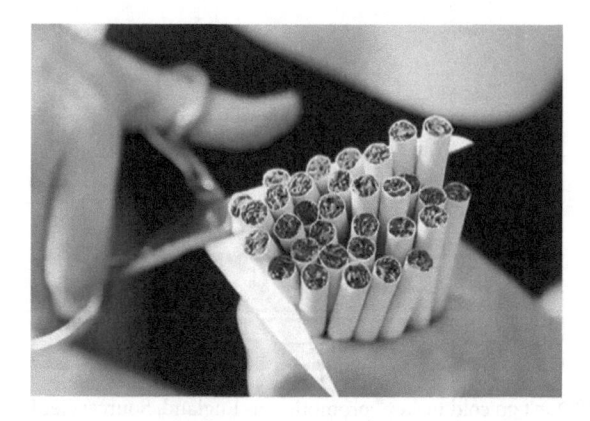

No. 2: Don't Go Cold Turkey

It's not common to successfully quit smoking by stopping immediately. Most people who quit "cold turkey" end up smoking again. Nicotine addiction can require gradual tapering to avoid withdrawal symptoms. It's hard, but the benefits of quitting are well worth it.

Figure 5.4 The "Don't go cold turkey" message persists in 2021 (Source: https://www.onhealth.com/content/1/tips_quit_smoking).

The slow death of the hardening hypothesis

As the percentage of the adult population who smoke continues its seemingly inexorable southward journey toward single-digits, it's common to see and hear comments that the smokers who remain today are nearly all "hard core". These so-called heavily dependent smokers are said to be impervious to the policies and campaigns which have caused so many millions to quit across the 60 years since modern tobacco control commenced with the publication of the 1962 Royal College of Physicians of London report and the 1964 US Surgeon General's report, both called *Smoking and Health*. The argument runs that the ripe fruit of less addicted smokers has long fallen from national smoking prevalence trees, and that today most of those still smoking are profoundly addicted to nicotine and are unresponsive to the

5 "Don't try to quit cold turkey"

traditional suite of policies and motivational appeals that in the past have been associated with continuing declines in smoking.

This argument is known as the "hardening hypothesis". It's predictably used often by pharmaceutical companies; those health workers who making a living out of promoting the idea that smokers are unwise to try to quit on their own and need their professional help; and most recently by promoters of electronic cigarettes and the growing panoply of other novel products. These promoters often highlight the spectre of smokers who they insist "can't" or won't quit but want to switch to allegedly less dangerous ways of dosing themselves with nicotine many times a day.

The "can't quit" group are said to be those who have "tried everything", sometimes many times, but have repeatedly relapsed back to smoking. A well-cited 2008 paper by Karl Fagerström and Helena Furberg looking at smoking prevalence and nicotine dependency scores on the Fagerström Test for Nicotine Dependence (FTND) in 13 countries concluded, "The significant inverse correlation between FTND score and smoking prevalence across countries and higher FTND score among current smokers supports the idea that remaining smokers may be hardening" (Fagerström and Furberg 2008). However, since that time, research on the hardening hypothesis has overwhelmingly found that it has little to no scientific support.

The most recognised way today of measuring the "hardness" of smoking is the Heaviness of Smoking Index (HSI) (Chaiton, Cohen et al. 2007). This scores smokers out of a maximum of six points, comprising a score of 1–3 for number of cigarettes smoked each day, and 1–3 on the time taken after waking to light up the first cigarette of the day.

A European study with 5,136 smokers drawn from samples of over 18,000 people found that across 18 nations, there was no statistically significant relationship between a nation's smoking prevalence and the HSI (Fernandez, Lugo et al. 2015). If the hardening hypothesis had been confirmed, nations with low smoking prevalence would have had higher HSI scores in the remaining smokers: these continuing smokers would have been smoking more cigarettes and lighting up earlier in the morning in nations with low smoking prevalence than in those with high. But they weren't.

A 2020 review by the smoking cessation maven John Hughes of published studies on hardening (Hughes 2020) found that in *none* of the 26 studies he examined was there any evidence for a reduction in conversion (or transition) from current to former smoking, in the number of quit attempts, or success on a given quit attempt, with several studies finding that these measures increased over time. These results appeared to be similar across survey dates, duration of time examined, number of data points, data source, outcome definitions and nationality. Hughes concluded, "These results convincingly indicate hardening is not occurring in the general population of smokers."

A Dutch research group went further. They calculated the prevalence of hardcore smoking in the Netherlands from 2001 to 2012. They classified smokers as "hardcore" if they satisfied each of four criteria: (1) smoked every day; (2) smoked on average greater than 14 cigarettes per day; (3) had not attempted to quit in the past year; and (4) had no intention to quit within six months. Across 12 years they found the prevalence of hardcore smoking decreased from 40.8% to 32.2% of smokers and as a proportion of the population, from 12.2% to 8.2%. Like almost all other studies, they "found no support for the hardening hypothesis", instead suggesting that "the decrease of hardcore smoking among smokers suggests a 'softening' of the smoking population" (Bommele, Nagelhout et al. 2016).

There have been several papers on hardening published using Australian data. A 2010 paper (Mathews, Hall et al. 2010) examined three series of Australian surveys of smoking (National Drug Strategy Household Survey (NDSHS), National Health Survey (NHS) and National Survey of Mental Health and Wellbeing (NSMHWB), spanning 7–10 years. The authors found that in two of the surveys (NDSHS and NHS), while smoking fell across the population, there was no change in the proportion of smokers who smoked less than daily, while in the NSMHW survey, that proportion increased from 6.9% in 1997 to 17.4% in 2007. The authors concluded that the paper presented "weak evidence that the population of Australian smokers hardened as smoking prevalence declined".

The most recent Australian paper on this issue was published in *Nature* (Buchanan, Magee et al. 2021) using data from three waves (2010, 2013 and 2016) of the Australian NDSHS. The most inclusive

5 "Don't try to quit cold turkey"

definition of hardcore smoking (i.e. being a smoker with no plans to quit) showed a significant decline between 2010 and 2016 (5.49% to 4.85%). In contrast, the prevalence of hardcore smoking using the most stringent definition (i.e., a current daily smoker of at least 15 cigarettes per day, aged 26 years or over, with no intention to quit and no quit attempt in the past 12 months) did not change significantly between 2010 and 2016. The authors concluded,"The observed trends in the prevalence of hardcore smokers (i.e. either stable or declining depending on the definition) suggest that the Australian smoking population is not hardening. These results do not support claims that remaining smokers are becoming hardcore".

A 2022 systematic review of the evidence on hardening described it as "a persistent myth undermining tobacco control" and concluded "the sum-total of the world-wide evidence indicates either 'softening' of the smoking population, or a lack of hardening" with reductions in smoking prevalence fostering even more quitting. The authors concluded "the time has come to take active steps to combat the myth of hardening and to replace it with the reality of 'softening'" (Harris et al. 2022).

Those arguing that today's smokers are increasingly heavily addicted and unable to stop, and therefore need assistance to do so, have very poor evidence supporting their case. Globally, vast numbers of smokers continue to stop or reduce their smoking every year. These include very heavy smokers and, as we will see below, many who quite suddenly stop smoking without making much if any preparation to do so.

There is also interesting evidence from Canada that people diagnosed with schizophrenia quit smoking at about the same rate as those in the wider population. Repeated surveys 11 years apart (1995 and 2006) in a community-based psychiatric rehabilitation program in Hamilton, Ontario, Canada, found that the number of quitters tripled over the past decade and the number of daily smokers decreased by almost one-third from 63% to 43% (Goldberg and Van Exan 2008).

Those who argue that it's now time we recognised that the traditional suite of population-focused policies and programs have run their course, that we are seeing diminishing returns and now need to call in the cavalry with widespread intensive, one-on-one support services and lifetime use of NRT or vaping – are blowing evidence-free and often self-serving smoke. In nations where net quitting rates may have slowed, the explanation is therefore not likely to be that remaining smokers *can't quit*, but that we may be reaching a significant rump of smokers who are best understood as *won't or don't want to quit* die-hard smokers. In Chapter 6, I'll return to this issue to consider ways in which it may be sensible to put in place policies that allow such continuing smokers to access non-combustible forms of nicotine under carefully regulated circumstances, while ensuring we do more to implement evidence-based, population-level measures that we know will reduce smoking, and do all we can to minimise the uptake of vaping by those who don't smoke (especially teenagers).

Spontaneous, unplanned quitting vs stages of change progression

Anyone working in public health since the mid-1980s who has opened a research journal in health promotion or attended a conference where health-related behaviour change is being discussed will have been unable to avoid encountering the "Stages of Change" (SOC) or "Transtheoretical" Model of behaviour change. This model posits that there are five stages at which any person with a chronic behaviour pattern like smoking, being physically inactive or having a poor diet will currently be located. The model holds that individuals move through the stages in sequence (precontemplation, preparation for change, taking action, maintenance of the change and termination) (Prochaska and DiClemente 1983).

Adherents of the model argue that understanding which stage a person is currently at allows the tailoring of interventions and support to maximise further progression through to the termination stage.

There has been no other model which has gained anything like as broad adherence among researchers of health-related behaviour, particularly when it comes to smoking cessation. In 2005 the then editor-in-chief of *Addiction*, Robert West, located 540 papers in PubMed for the search string "stages of change": 170 were about smoking, 60 on alcohol, seven on cocaine and two on heroin or opiates. However, West wrote a memorably scathing editorial calling for the model to be "put to rest" (West 2005). He summarised a large number of failings in the model, with perhaps the largest being what might be cruelly called the "No shit, Sherlock!" criticism that the theory was an unhelpful description of the obvious:

> that individuals who are thinking of changing their behaviour are more likely to try to do so than those who are not, or that individuals who are in the process of trying to change are more likely to change than those who are just thinking about it ... it is simply a statement of the obvious: people who want to plan to do something are obviously more likely to try to do it; and people who try to do something are more likely to succeed than those who do not.

West went further, describing the model as "little more than a security blanket for researchers and clinicians ... the seemingly scientific style of the assessment tool gives the impression that some form of diagnosis is being made from which a treatment plan can be devised. It gives the appearance of rigour".

"Tailoring" treatment for individuals after rigorous assessment of the stage they are at holds out the promise of greater precision in efforts to help smokers quit and so is understandably attractive to those yearning for the holy grail of much more effective approaches to cessation. But there's just a slight problem here: a 2003 systematic review comparing stop-smoking interventions designed using the SOC approach with non-tailored treatments found no benefit over those that were based on the model (Riemsma, Pattenden et al. 2003).

Perhaps the most important limitation of the SOC model is its silence on "how people can change with apparent suddenness, even in response to small triggers" (West 2005). Across the many years I edited *Tobacco Control*, we received many papers which were often simple descriptive studies about the distribution of smokers in different settings across the stages of change. The senior editorial team would roll our eyes at the plodding regularity of the PhD industry churning these out.

In 2005, we published a refreshingly original short paper from a Canadian general practitioner, Lynn Larabie from Kingston, Ontario. She had noted the dominance of using "planned" approaches to quitting in clinical guidelines encouraging HCPs to assist smokers to quit. But Larabie had gained a strong clinical impression that many quit attempts, including successful ones, were anything but planned.

She interviewed 146 of her patients who had smoked more than five cigarettes a day for at least six months and had made at least one serious quit attempt. She found that just over half (51.6%) of quit attempts were described as being unplanned or spontaneous, and that these were more common in ex-smokers than those who had relapsed (Larabie 2005). In other words, those who quit without planning to do so seemed to quit for longer than those who planned it all out.

There is mixed evidence on whether planning or "spur of the moment" quitting decisions are associated with different quitting success down the track. West and Sohal, noting that Larabie's study was the first of its kind, reported on findings from interviews with 918 English smokers who had made a serious quit attempt and 996 ex-smokers (West and Sohal 2006). They found that:

> 48.6% of smokers reported that their most recent quit attempt was put into effect immediately the decision to quit was made. Unplanned quit attempts were more likely to succeed for at least six months: among respondents who had made a quit attempt between six months and five years previously the odds of success were 2.6 times higher in unplanned attempts than in planned attempts; in quit attempts made 6–12 months previously the corresponding figure was 2.5.

These findings stimulated them to propose "A model of the process of change based on 'catastrophe theory' ... in which smokers have varying levels of motivational 'tension' to stop and then 'triggers' in the environment result in a switch in motivational state. If that switch involves immediate renunciation of cigarettes, this can signal a more complete transformation than if it involves a plan to quit at some future point." I'll return to this idea in Chapter 8 where I'll look at the importance of making quit attempts, rather than delaying them because of notions of it not being the "right time" to do so.

In 2010, a paper from the International Tobacco Control (ITC) Four Country study (Canada, US, UK and Australia) found those who reported quitting on the day they decided to do so, and those who delayed attempting to quit for a week or more had comparable six-month abstinence (Cooper, Borland et al. 2010).

A US study of 900 smokers and 800 ex-smokers recruited from a market research database were asked online about the planning involved in their most recent attempt. Just below 40% said that their most recent quit attempt involved no pre-planning (smokers: 29.5%; ex-smokers: 52.4%). Again as Larabie had found, the odds of a "spontaneous" quit attempt lasting for 6 months or longer were twice that of attempts which were pre-planned (71.7% vs. 45.6%) (Ferguson, Shiffman et al. 2009).

This paper contained a fascinating example of what can happen when researchers appear to not like the findings of their own work. All authors of this paper made declarations of support from the pharmaceutical industry and noted: "Given the evidence that use of medication can double success rates, it is surprising that *even without this assistance unplanned quitters were more likely to be successful*. [my emphasis] It seems important to find ways to combine the favorable prognosis of unplanned quit attempts with the benefit of medication, for example, by ensuring easy, rapid access to medication."

So, unplanned, unassisted smokers did better than those who were assisted with medication, but the authors still felt compelled to try to convince such smokers to use medication anyway. They also suggested the removal of barriers to NRT sale such as prescription-only or pharmacy-only status, failing to note that these barriers had already been removed in the USA where the study took place. The "surprise" expressed by the authors of this paper seems revelatory of the myopic hold that assisted smoking cessation can have on the population-wide picture of how people quit.

Understanding that smokers can and do make sudden and often successful quit attempts should invite a lot of curiosity in tobacco control circles about the possibility that there could be potent triggers which are more likely to ignite quit attempts in smokers. In Chapter 8, I'll explore what we know about such triggers that have been used in mass media campaigns to stimulate quit attempts.

How difficult is it to quit smoking?

Another major platform of the "don't try to quit cold turkey" mantra is the claim that most smokers find quitting extremely difficult. There are, of course, many smokers who do find it very hard to quit. These smokers are a much-studied group, not least because those with intense interests in selling them medications and offering professional help see them as their customer base and so they often gather intelligence about how they might best succeed in convincing them to not go it alone. Here, you'd imagine an obvious thing to do would be to study former smokers who had permanently succeeded in quitting with the goal of seeing if there were important lessons that might be used to inspire and help those trying to quit. On the rare occasions when ex-smokers have been asked about their recollections of how difficult it was to quit, we have seen distinctly myth-busting data.

Very early in my career in 1983 I read a 151-page report, *Smoking attitudes and behaviour*, by English researchers Alan Marsh and Jil Matheson and produced by the British government's Office of Population Censuses and Surveys (Marsh and Matheson 1983). The report, which is today very difficult to obtain (I found it in the US Truth Tobacco Industry Documents digital collection) was based on data obtained from 1,300 non-smokers and 2,700 smokers in Britain. They asked the respondents two questions:

1. Would you say you found giving up smoking: (*choose one*) very difficult/fairly difficult/not at all difficult
2. Was giving up (*choose one*): harder than expected/the same as expected/easier than expected

Here is what they found:

> Nineteen percent of ex-smokers say they found their effort to quit "very difficult", 27% agreed it was "fairly difficult" while a narrow majority, 53% said they found it "not at all difficult" to give up smoking. It might be said that this result supports the view that once smokers make up their minds, the effort to stop is not as great as it is supposed to be ... 15% found it "harder than they expected" to give up smoking, 38% found it much as they had

5 "Don't try to quit cold turkey"

expected while 41% found it, as best they could recall, actually easier than they expected.

Importantly, Marsh and Matheson noted that "these figures are derived from those who, however modest the length of their achievement so far, have succeeded. The majority of triers who found it 'impossible' have removed themselves from the count by resuming their habit".

Their report provides a cross-tabulated table of answers to the two questions shown above. They commented here that "the results suggest that smokers who found giving up difficult, and more difficult than they imagined it would be, are quite rare among the ex-smokers (16%). About six out of every ten of these ex-smokers say either they found the effort less difficult than they expected or that they had expected little difficulty and had experienced none". They also noted that:

> It seems that only one factor determined how hard or easy a time our ex-smokers had in giving up smoking and that is the number of cigarettes they were smoking each day when they stopped. Those smoking 10 a day or less had little difficulty with three quarters of them saying they found it "not at all difficult". Those whose former daily intake fell into the 11–20 range found more difficulty with 22% saying they found it "very difficult" and among those who gave up an even heavier habit this figure rises to 31%. Interestingly though, above 10 a day, the proportions saying "not at all difficult" remain unchanged so that among those giving up a habit of more than 30 a day, still nearly half of them (47%) say they found it "not at all difficult" to abandon a level of consumption popularly associated with an extreme and compulsive dependence. That is to say, leaving aside the lightest smokers, someone abandoning a really heavy daily consumption will be just as likely to say they found the effort "not at all difficult" as someone smoking, say, 15 or 20 a day but if they do find it at all difficult they are more likely to find it "very difficult" than will the more moderate smoker.

In the years since that report was published I have rarely seen other studies also ask questions similar to those of Marsh and Matheson. A couple of exceptions were a 2012 Tasmanian report (see Figure 5.5) reporting on the large differences between perceived and actual experienced difficulty in quitting and an unpublished paper reporting on Israeli military recruits. The majority (80%) of respondents felt that it was going to be difficult to quit smoking. However, the respondents' final quit attempt was not as difficult as first thought, with 73% reporting that it was "quite easy" or "very easy".

The Israeli study (Vered, Kedem et al. 2016) reported on all 1,574 ex-smokers in the Israeli Defence Force undergoing periodic medical examinations between September 2013 and June 2015. The great majority (83.4%) reported quitting unassisted. Cessation was reported as harder/much harder than expected by only 7.1%, easier/much easier than expected by 50%, and as expected by 42.8%. As with the research described earlier, those who reduced smoking gradually before cessation were significantly more likely to report difficulty than those who stopped abruptly.

Again, it is important to emphasise that ex-smokers have all successfully quit (for whatever length of time). We can assume that many of those who tried but relapsed would be likely to describe their experience as difficult (although some may have found it easy to quit but were tempted back into smoking after some time by lack of resolve to stay quit, rather than by finding the actual quitting experience impossibly hard).

Two things here are notable. First, that in these striking data about many ex-smokers finding the quitting experience less traumatic than expected, we rarely (if ever) hear comments or see campaigns from those in tobacco control discussing or highlighting this. We very seldom hear any efforts to de-bunk or leaven the "it's very, very hard to quit smoking" meme by pointing out that many ex-smokers were pleasantly surprised that quitting was not as tortuous as they expected. This good news story might be very motivating to some contemplating quitting but who hesitate because they have been deluged with horror stories and rarely hear alternative perspectives.

Second, given what the few rare studies which have asked ex-smokers these questions have found, it is remarkable that this issue is not routinely explored in studies of quitting. It is almost as if there is a collective "let's not go there" agreement among researchers to avoid

5 "Don't try to quit cold turkey"

Do smokers perceive quitting to be more difficult than they subsequently find it?

Section Seven – Confidence to Quit/ Stay Quit

7.1 Perceived Difficulty to Quit Smoking – Ex-Smokers

The 100 respondents who claimed that they had quit smoking in the last 12 months were asked;

Before you quit smoking, how easy did you think it would be to quit? Did you think it would be...?

Chart 19 – Perceived Difficulty to Quit Smoking
(Percentage of ex-smokers interviewed)

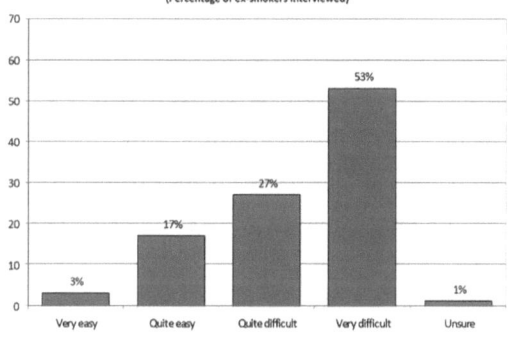

- Very easy: 3%
- Quite easy: 17%
- Quite difficult: 27%
- Very difficult: 53%
- Unsure: 1%

7.2 Actual Difficulty to Quit Smoking

The same respondents were asked;

And how easy was your last quit attempt? Was it...?

Chart 20 – Actual Difficulty to Quit Smoking
(Percentage of ex-smokers interviewed)

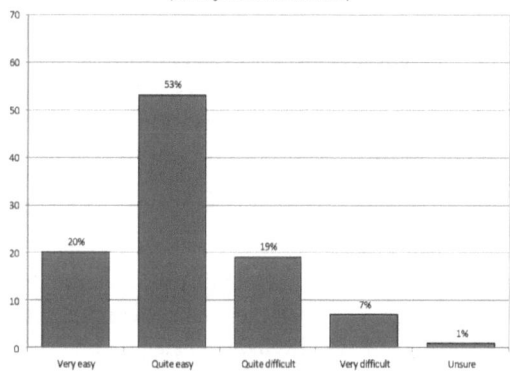

- Very easy: 20%
- Quite easy: 53%
- Quite difficult: 19%
- Very difficult: 7%
- Unsure: 1%

Figure 5.5 Perceived difficulty of quitting reported by Tasmanian ex-smokers, 2012. Source: Quit Tasmania 2012.

learning more about this. A narrative of quitting being almost always very difficult is less unsettling for those whose careers depend on assisting people to quit than one of "Hey, if you want to quit, you may be able to easily do it by yourself."

The shunning and denigration of unassisted quitting

In 2003, the American Cancer Society (ACS) published US data from 2000 showing that 91.4% of US ex-smokers had "Quit 'cold turkey' or slowly decreased amount smoked" while 6.8% had "followed recommended therapy (drug therapy and/or counselling)". For every smoker who had quit with "recommended therapy", 13.4 had successfully quit by themselves (American Cancer Society 2003). The report noted that "An estimated 44.3 million adults (24.7 million men and 19.7 million women) in the United States were former smokers in 2000. In 2000, 48.8% of US adults who ever smoked cigarettes had stopped smoking." Despite this massive ratio, the ACS report astonishingly said nothing whatsoever about this wherever-you-look, in-your-face phenomenon. Instead, across six pages it jumped into line with the established "you need help" orthodoxy and summarised the virtues of quitting with assistance.

When I spot such subversive unassisted quitting figures that seem to have quietly snuck into reports like these almost without comment or discussion, I try to imagine the conversations in the editorial writing groups who produced them. I wonder if they went something like this with the ACS report:

> *Report writer*: Are you saying that we should keep it very quiet that millions of people have and still do quit unassisted?
> *Chair of writing group*: Look, let's acknowledge the data on unassisted quitting, but not dwell on it. I suggest one line in a table or a footnote in small print up the back of the report. Can I see a show of hands? ... Good, done!

In 2019, two of the world's most cited researchers in tobacco control, Judith Prochaska and Neil Benowitz, published a 23-page review with

233 references in *Science Advances*, titled "Current advances in research in treatment and recovery: nicotine addiction" (Prochaska and Benowitz 2019). They set out to "review current advances in research on nicotine addiction treatment and recovery, with a focus on conventional combustible cigarette use and evidence-based methods to treat smoking in adults". It contained copiously referenced summaries of what is known about the efficacy and effectiveness of various pharmacotherapies, e-cigarettes, brief and intensive counselling, quitlines, mobile phone and internet technologies, and financial incentives. But nowhere in the entire article did it mention that the method that has produced by far the most ex-smokers well before and continuously since the 1960s has been unassisted cessation.

A similar review published in *The Lancet* in 2008 also gave unassisted cessation only cursory attention – a mere nine words in a nine-page review ("Although most smokers will give up on their own ...") (Hatsukami, Stead et al. 2008). It is common to see unassisted cessation framed as a challenge to be eroded by persuading more to use pharmacotherapies. For example: "Unfortunately, most smokers ... fail to use evidence-based treatments to support their quit attempts" (Curry, Sporer et al. 2007). Prominent English physician John Britton wrote in *The Lancet*, "If there is a major failing in the UK approach, it is not that it has medicalised smoking, but that it has not done so enough" (Britton 2009).

Both the 2019 Prochaska and Benowitz and the 2008 *Lancet* reviews were written as information for those involved in tobacco *treatment*, but importantly also concerned *recovery* from nicotine dependency. With the majority of smokers "recovering" unaided from being smokers, the assumption that this unavoidable, large-scale and enduring phenomenon should have zero or negligible reference in reviews and guidelines on how to quit is seriously, remarkably and quite appallingly bizarre. Yet unassisted quitting is almost always ignored in cessation clinical guidelines written for health professionals on how they might best help their patients to quit. While the US National Center for Health Statistics routinely included a question on "cold turkey" cessation in its surveys between 1983 and 2000, it mysteriously disappeared in 2005 (National Center for Health Statistics 2008), despite unassisted cessation remaining the method used by most successful quitters (Shiffman, Brockwell et al. 2008).

If a smoker asked their doctor the perfectly sensible and understandable question, "How have most ex-smokers quit?", failure to emphasise that most have always stopped unaided would be like explaining that most cyclists, roller skaters and surfboard riders have professional tuition rather than being self-taught in these skills, that most people who exercise do it under supervision of a trainer or in a class, that most entirely competent domestic cooks attended cooking classes and that most guitarists in thousands of the world's bands were fully trained in music schools rather than being self-taught or having a few early lessons (Pierce and Chiareza no date).

I know of no campaigns and only rare health promotion messages that highlight the fact most ex-smokers quit unaided even though hundreds of millions have done and continue to do just that.

Drivers of the medicalisation of smoking cessation

In 2010, I published a paper with Ross MacKenzie in *PLOS Medicine* titled *The global research neglect of unassisted smoking cessation: causes and consequences* (Chapman and MacKenzie 2010). We set out to test a broad hypothesis I had described in a short *Lancet* paper in 2009: *The inverse impact law of smoking cessation* (Chapman 2009). This posited that "the volume of research and effort devoted to professionally and pharmacologically mediated cessation is in inverse proportion to that examining how most ex-smokers actually quit. Research on cessation is dominated by ever more finely tuned accounts of how smokers can be encouraged to do anything but go it alone when trying to quit – exactly opposite of how a very large majority of ex-smokers succeeded." We tested the hypotheses that support for research into unassisted cessation and non-pharmaceutical interventions is less common and that research on pharmaceutically mediated cessation is frequently conducted by researchers supported by pharmaceutical companies.

We searched Medline for "smoking cessation", limiting results to English language original articles, meta-analyses, and reviews published in 2007 and 2008. We found 511 papers which were studies of cessation interventions. Of these, 467 (91.4%) reported the effects of assisted cessation and 44 (8.6%) described the impact of unassisted cessation. Of the studies describing assisted interventions, 52.9% involved pharmacotherapy and 47.1% non-drug interventions. Of the papers describing cessation trends, correlates, and predictors in populations, only 11% contained any data on unassisted cessation.

Of the 84 papers for which competing interest information was available, 48% of pharmacotherapy intervention studies and 10.3% of non-pharmacotherapy intervention studies had at least one author declaring support from a company manufacturing cessation products and/or research funding from such a company – but no unassisted cessation study did.

We argued that there are three main synergistic drivers of the research concentration on assisted cessation and its corollary, the neglect of research on the natural history of unassisted smoking cessation. These are: the dominance of interventionism in health science research; the increasing medicalisation and commodification of cessation; and the persistent, erroneous appeal of the "hardening" hypothesis, discussed earlier in this chapter.

The dominance of interventionism

Most tobacco control research is undertaken by individuals trained in positivist scientific traditions. As I described in Chapter 2, hierarchies of the quality of evidence give experimental evidence more importance than observational evidence (Rychetnik, Frommer et al. 2002); meta-analyses of RCTs are given the most weight. As I'll develop more in Chapter 8, cessation studies that focus on discrete, easily quantifiable proximal variables, such as specific cessation interventions, provide "harder" causal evidence than those that focus on distal, complex and interactive influences which coalesce across a smoker's lifetime to end in cessation. Specific cessation interventions are also more easily studied than the dynamics and determinants of cessation in whole populations (Chapman 1993). Experimental research focused on proximal relationships between specific interventions and cessation poses fewer confounding problems and sits more easily within the professional norms of scientific grant assessment environments, which are populated largely by scientists working within the positivist tradition.

The dominance of the experimental research paradigm is amplified by pharmaceutical industry support for drug trials. More than half the papers we found on assisted cessation were pharmaceutical studies and, unsurprisingly, these were much more likely than papers on non-pharmacological interventions to have industry-supported authors. Companies have an obvious interest in research about the use and efficacy of their products and less interest in supporting research into forms of cessation that compete with pharmacotherapy for the cessation market.

The availability of pharmaceutical industry research funding – often provided without the lengthy processes of open tender or independent peer review – can be highly attractive to researchers understandably intent on keeping their soft money funded teams employed. Furthermore, it is often observed that "research follows the money", with scientists being drawn to well-funded research areas (Russo 2005). Researchers steeped in clinical backgrounds where medication is nearly always indicated as the way that health problems are resolved may self-select to seek funding. The large pool of research funding for pharmacotherapeutic cessation may cause researchers to gravitate toward such studies while those interested in the natural history of smoking cessation have to secure funding through highly competitive public grant schemes.

This greater availability of funding for certain sorts of research produces a distorted research emphasis on pharmacotherapy that, when combined with the industry's formidable public relations and marketing abilities and direct-to-consumer advertising, concentrates both scientific and public discourse on cessation around assisted pharmacotherapy. *Fortune Business Insights* put the global NRT market value of NRT at US$2.81 billion for 2020, saying that the demand for NRT during the 2020 COVID pandemic grew 12.2% and was projected to increase to US$3.92 billion in 2028. Eighty percent of the global market was in North America and Europe, with 80% of market share held by two companies, GlaxoSmithKline and Johnson & Johnson Inc (Fortune Business Insights 2021). Chantix™/Champix™ (varenicline) earned Pfizer US$918 million in revenue worldwide in 2020 (Pfizer Inc 2020).

With this sort of money swirling around, it comes as no surprise that messages about cessation frequently focus on drugs. An early study found the pharmaceutical industry placed more messages about quitting in front of smokers than any other source: in the USA, there were 10.37 pharmaceutical cessation advertisements per month but only 3.25 government and NGO cessation messages (Wakefield, Szczypka et al. 2005).

The medicalisation and commodification of cessation

Iconoclast Ivan Illich was one of the first to discuss the tendency toward the medicalisation of everyday life in a paper in the *Journal of Medical Ethics* in 1975 (Illich 1975). On 3 October 2021 a PubMed search for "medicalization or medicalisation" returned 581 papers in the peer-reviewed health and medical literature, with the first mention published in 1974. Many concerns previously perceived as normal human differences or problems have now been defined as tractable illnesses that can benefit from diagnosis and often lifetime drug taking (Conrad 1992, Deyo and Patrick 2005, Moynihan and Cassells 2005). These include shyness and sadness (Horwitz and Wakefield 2007, Lane 2007), tallness in girls (Rayner, Pyett et al. 2010), baldness in men (Jankowski and Frith 2021) and many, many more normal human differences and phases of life. Le Fanu has described galloping medicalisation as an iatrogenic catastrophe (Le Fanu 2018).

In 1975, Renaud wrote of the fundamental tendency of capitalism to "transform health needs into commodities … When the state intervenes to cope with some health-related problems, it is bound to act so as to further commodify health needs" (Renaud 1975). The pharmaceutical industry creed is that wherever possible, problems coming before physicians need to be pathologised as biomedical problems that need to be treated with medication. Tobacco use, like other substance use, has become increasingly pathologised as a treatable condition as knowledge about the neurobiology, genetics and pharmacology of addiction develops. The burgeoning commodification of smoking cessation by manufacturers of both effective and ineffective drugs seems to have induced a kind of professional amnesia in tobacco control circles about the many millions who quit in the decades before the dominance of the contemporary smoking cessation discourse by pharmacotherapy.

The NRT industry in particular has been well served by a plethora of studies which recommend an ever-expanding menu of ways and times to consume NRT. These include:

- NRT for light smokers (Rahmani, Veldhuizen et al. 2021).
- NRT for both "pre-quit" and "post-quit" (Lindson and Aveyard 2011, Przulj, Wehbe et al. 2019).
- Multiple, combination, dual-form NRT (Tulloch, Pipe et al. 2016).
- NRT long after stopping to prevent relapse (Agboola, McNeill et al. 2010).

One Pfizer-sponsored study examined the effect on quit attempts of varenicline when used by smokers with no immediate intention of quitting, suggesting that thinking may be circling the challenge of promoting pharmacotherapy even to those unmotivated to quit (Hughes, Rennard et al. 2011).

It appears that there is no smoker, regardless of how much or little they smoke, and regardless of whether they are not at the point of trying to quit, actively trying to do so or have long stopped smoking, for whom medication and especially NRT is not recommended. It is in the interests of that industry to persuade as many smokers as possible to use pharmaceutical aids for as long as possible.

All smokers should use NRT: a promotional case study

From December 2009 until February 2017, the transnational pharmaceutical giant GlaxoSmithKline (GSK) published a website called *Path2Quit*, an online, interactive website designed to assist smokers to understand which pathway to quitting was optimal for their personal smoking profile. The website is available today on the Wayback Machine (GlaxoSmithKline 2009). The home screen showed three statements:

- Quitting is really hard.
- Different smokers need different solutions.
- Discover which path is right for you and start your journey on the right track.

5 "Don't try to quit cold turkey"

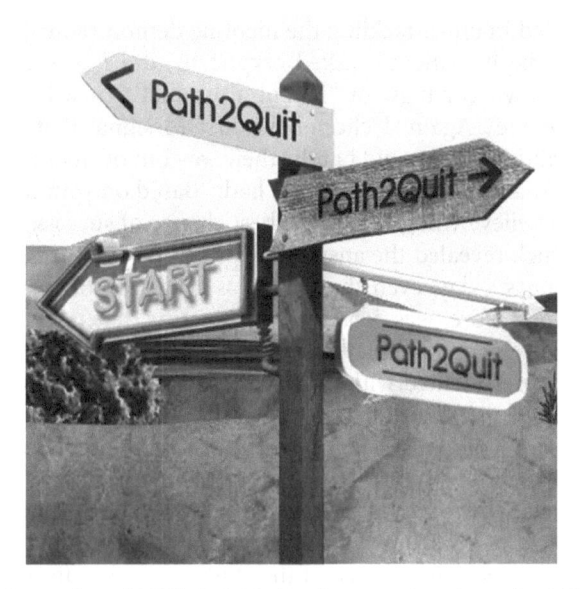

Figure 5.6 Screenshot of GSK's Path2Quit web promotion, Australia, 2009–17.

GSK manufactures the Nicabate™ NRT brand. I decided to put the site to the test of what it would advise a light smoker, who'd never tried to quit smoking, who was not very addicted to nicotine and was confident of their ability to quit.

A signpost (Figure 5.6) showed three different potential pathways which by clicking "start", smokers would discover the best route for them. The next screen asked, "Have you ever tried to quit smoking?" with four options (never, once, 2–4 times and 5-plus). I clicked "never". The next screen asked, "How many cigarettes do you smoke a day?" The options were less than 10, 10–14, 15–19 and 20-plus. I clicked "less than 10". The third screen fished for nicotine dependence, asking, "How long after waiting do you reach for your first cigarette?" ("less than 30 minutes or 30 minutes or more") I clicked the less urgent time.

The next three screens probed confidence and preferred pace in quitting, asking whether a smoker was ready to quit now and give up all cigarettes immediately, was anxious about quitting altogether suddenly, or preferred to "take one step at a time" (I opted for the first to suggest

129

that I believed in crash-tackling the nicotine demon rather than trying to slowly tame it.) Another asked cryptically, did I "want to actively manage my own cravings" or "I want a product that will manage my cravings for me". Again, I clicked the first to signal that here was a smoker confident they could handle their way out of smoking.

The next and penultimate screen had: "Based on your answers, the product we believe will give you the best chance of success is ... ") and one more click revealed the answer. Surprise! I should use a Nicabate™ patch 24 hours a day, even though I was a light smoker who'd never tried quitting before, was probably not nicotine dependent and had a sleeves-rolled-up, confident attitude to quitting.

I then experimented with different responses to the questions and – you guessed it – it didn't matter which option I clicked, every combination of responses recommended that I use Nicabate™. All Path2Quit directions amazingly lead to the same destination: using NRT. Predictably, the website never mentioned quitting unassisted.

At the time that this website was published, the Cochrane systematic review stated, "Most of the studies [on the efficacy of NRT] were performed on people smoking more than 15 cigarettes a day" and demonstrated "no benefit for using patches beyond 8 weeks".

Attacks on my work on unassisted cessation: perspectives from the woods and the trees

Between 2010 and 2013, my work with other authors on unassisted cessation (Chapman 2009, Chapman and MacKenzie 2010, Chapman and Wakefield 2013) was subjected to five extended attacks, mostly by doyens of the English smoking-cessation research community who had all been long-standing researchers and public advocates for assisted cessation. Most, but not all, had declared histories of support from pharmaceutical companies with skin in the smoking-cessation game.

The first cab off the rank was a gratuitous swipe by English smoking-cessation researcher John Stapleton in a commentary on Banham & Gilbody's *The scandal of smoking and mental illness* where he wrote, "There are some who argue that the sort of effective help to stop smoking described in this issue of *Addiction* and in other reviews should be denied people with mental illness, and all smokers. They argue that viewing tobacco dependence as a disorder and helping smokers individually in the way caring societies normally help those with health-related disorders is unnecessary and counter-productive" (Stapleton 2010). Our *PLOS* paper (Chapman and MacKenzie 2010) was cited in support of this claim.

We set fire to this straw-man argument (Chapman and MacKenzie 2012), noting that our paper made no reference at all to smokers with mental illness, contained no discussion about smoking as a disorder and emphatically said nothing about denying treatment to anyone. One of the final statements in our paper was that "NRT, other prescribed pharmaceuticals, and professional counselling or support also help many smokers, but are certainly not necessary for quitting" (see more on this in Chapter 8).

M'lud, the accused is charged with spreading four "fallacies"

The next salvo was fired in an editorial in *Addiction* (*Should smokers be offered assistance with stopping?*), signed by nine authors, led by the journal's editor-in-chief, Robert West (West, McNeill et al. 2010). The editorial was translated into French, Spanish and Mandarin and displayed prominently for months on the homepage of the pharmaceutical-industry-sponsored website, www.treatobacco.net. It seemed that the English assisted-cessation officers' mess had decided that our upstart arguments needed to be jumped on from a great height. The editorial set out four "fallacies" they believed we were promoting. Triumphantly, they declared that after the application of their blowtorch, these fallacies were now "out of the way". We were not invited to respond to the editorial, despite this being customary and common in most serious journals, including *Addiction*.

They claimed that the first fallacy illustrated that we "misunderstood arithmetic" because anyone numerate could surely see that if 5% of 1000 smokers quit without assistance, the resultant 50 ex-smokers clearly were an inferior outcome to a 20% success rate in 100 (i.e. 20) assisted smokers quitting. They wrote, "So in this example, more than twice as many smokers will have stopped without assistance as with it, despite the fact that doing it this way was four times less effective."

The authors' supercilious reasoning here of course depended entirely on their criterion for success: higher quitting success *rates*, not higher quitting *numbers*. As I discussed in Chapter 4, no evaluation of the English smoking-cessation special services has ever shown that their contribution to reducing smoking prevalence has been anything more than minor and a pale shadow of the numbers who have quit decade after decade without ever going near a smoking-cessation professional or using medication. So, if the goal here is all about pointing to impressive quit *rates* in cessation settings, which, in aggregate, barely caused a blip in national smoking prevalence, then we wave the white flag. But of course in the goal of increasing national smoking cessation, the proof of the pudding is not success *rates*, but total success *numbers*. So we kept our white flag furled.

Our second egregious fallacy was to argue that denigration of unassisted cessation as inferior and something to be actively advised against might actually cause many hearing those messages to do just what was being advised: *to not try to quit on their own*. That is plainly the intent of any message saying, "Do not go cold turkey". Here the authors argued that in a nation where assisted cessation was strongly promoted and cold turkey disparaged, there was no evidence of smokers reducing their quit attempts. Perhaps not. But hundreds of millions of ex-smokers globally know a thing or two about successful unassisted quitting. Yet they are perpetually disenfranchised by professionals, and hear and read constantly that the way they actually quit is not recommended and not "evidence based". But the evidence is all around us in plain sight. There are many experienced quitters out there who possess wisdom, but it is mostly ignored.

Self-change scholars Harald Klingemann and Mark and Linda Sobell are explicit about the importance of taking self-changers far more seriously. They note that public awareness of self-change dominating cessation of problem behaviours is often limited and argue that "disseminating knowledge about the prevalence of self-change could be a type of intervention itself" (Klingemann, Sobell et al. 2010). What if such news actually empowered people to try to change?

5 "Don't try to quit cold turkey"

Many critics start from the premise that unassisted cessation attempts are far less successful than those assisted by professionals and/or medication, and by reason of that, it would be wrong-headed if people are led to try to stop using less effective methods when they would have chosen more effective ones.

To this I would say that the bottom line on "more effective" is far less sanguine than a good deal of the messages that are sent to smokers, which are mostly based on clinical trial outcomes with all the problems I discussed in Chapter 2. The group-think here is "Let's all keep quiet about this and jump hard on those who give this subversive message any major oxygen." Hustlers for assisted cessation write about unassisted cessation as if it is hopeless, a shocking recipe for failure. How perplexing then that for decades it has continued to deliver so many more successes each year than combined yields from the anointed "evidence-based" methods backed by assisted-cessation advocates.

Those who argue this believe they should never compromise and recommend anything but the very best. I'm reminded of the adage that the perfect should not be the enemy of the good. On several occasions I'd been taunted by critics suggesting that my logic would require that I would not recommend antibiotics for the treatment of pneumonia, as if there were obvious parallels between being ill with pneumonia and being a smoker who wanted to stop. But there are important differences between the two which make the comparison very misleading. When you have pneumonia it needs to be urgently treated. Before the advent of antibiotics, pneumonia killed very large numbers of infected people often quite quickly, particularly the aged. The same cannot be said about untreated smoking: the great majority of smokers who keep smoking will not die today, this week, this month or even this year from a disease caused by smoking. The health risks of smoking accumulate over decades, and while many thousands of smokers die every day around the world from smoking-caused and exacerbated diseases, no one argues that it was the recent cigarettes they smoked which killed them or that, as often occurs with untreated pneumonia, death occurs quickly. And that's before we even get to questions I've looked at throughout this book about whether the real-world effectiveness of stop smoking medications are in any way comparable to the value of taking antibiotics for pneumonia.

In 2010, three papers addressing the stubborn problem of unacceptably low rates of US smokers using assisted cessation were published back-to-back in a special supplement of the *American Journal of Preventive Medicine* (Abrams, Graham et al. 2010, Levy, Graham et al. 2010, Levy, Mabry et al. 2010). These detailed papers explored every conceivable way that the intransigence of American smokers in resisting the promises of medications and professional supervision might be eroded. One paper modelled the huge population-wide health benefits that would follow if this came to pass. It all had a very familiar ring to it.

But it's plainly the case, with the promotion of assisted cessation having now been on full throttle since the late 1980s with pharmaceutical industry general practitioner promotions, pharmacy in-store promotions and displays, massive direct-to-consumer advertising saying don't try to do it alone, and endless efforts to reduce barriers to health care professionals engaging more in identifying and assisting smokers that the assisted-cessation camp has fired off its full arsenal of strategies, many, many times. Does anyone seriously imagine that there are big rabbits still left in hats that will see a far bigger proportion of smokers want to avail themselves of cessation services and medications than has happened so far? There is no evidence from anywhere for this hope.

The West group's third alleged fallacy we were spreading was that RCT evidence is not mirrored in real-world outcomes (for all the reasons set out in Chapter 2) and that longitudinal cohort studies provide greater guidance on how well different cessation methods actually perform when used in conditions that post-RCTs, they will always be used in. The West-led nine authors' counter arguments here argued that recall bias plagues such studies and that confounders like nicotine dependence levels are often uncontrolled in cohort studies. Recall bias is certainly an issue when it comes to recall of quit attempts (as I discussed in Chapter 2) but it is not a major problem when recall of final, successful quit attempts is the key outcome of interest. Smokers remember how they finally quit, but often don't recall failed quit attempts that may be little more than gestures rather than serious tries.

In Chapter 2, I also discussed the peculiar sleight-of-hand argument often used by assisted-cessation stalwarts concerning "indication bias".

5 "Don't try to quit cold turkey"

Here, when trying to explain why smoking-cessation medications and NRT often do less well than unassisted quitting in real-world studies, it's argued that no one should be surprised that heavy smokers fare badly when trying to quit. The sleight of hand here is, of course, that it's the more dependent smokers who are typically highlighted as the very smokers who most need assistance to quit. So they are especially urged to use medications. But when data show they often do worse than unassisted quitters, the post hoc explanation then dragooned into explanation is that we should not have expected them to succeed because of the very same reason they were recommended to be used.

The West nine authors' gotcha moment then came by citing *one* evaluation (Ferguson, Bauld et al. 2005) which showed assisted quitters did better than typical unassisted quitters. Chapter 3 of this book discussed a good deal more evidence inconvenient to that one citation.

Our fourth fallacy was apparently to argue that mass-media campaigns are a better investment than setting up national networks of smoking-cessation centres. The latter attract very small percentages of all smokers while well-funded, mass-reach campaigns find and influence huge numbers of the whole population and, as I will discuss in Chapter 8, motivate many smokers to make quit attempts.

The editorialists insisted that comparing the respective contributions of stop smoking services and media campaigns was a "false dichotomy" because they worked synergistically, and along with policy initiatives like tax rises and smoke-free public areas, together were driving down smoking across the population. But this stock response hides the evidence I described in Chapter 4 which shows that the attributed contribution made by English quit-smoking services to national falls in smoking prevalence was very small. Expenditure on media campaigns on smoking in England between June 2008 and February 2016 averaged £5.58 million per year (Kuipers, Beard et al. 2018), while that allocated to cessation services between 1999 and 2006 averaged £30.53 million per year (McNeill, Raw et al. 2005). English local health authorities in 2014–15 and 2017–18 allocated 89.8% of expenditure on total tobacco control to specialised stop-smoking services (£121.2m in 2014–15 and £85.2 (Action on Smoking and Health 2019). Clearly, important questions need to be asked about the opportunity costs of allocating such disproportionate expenditure to methods of increasing cessation when the track record of cessation services is and is realistically destined to remain small.

"Unsupported by the facts"

On 13 October 2011 a third damp squib salvo was fired by Jacques Le Houezec, a French consultant to pharmaceutical companies manufacturing smoking-cessation treatments, who posted to the now-defunct global tobacco control listserv, Globalink. Signed by ten senior researchers in tobacco control, eight of whom were English, and seven of whom signed the 2010 *Addiction* editorial, the post read:

> It is regrettable that Professor Chapman persists with the fallacies dealt with in the editorial by West and colleagues (West, McNeill et al. 2010). The editorial is open access and points out that the optimum approach to cessation is to encourage smokers each time they try to stop to use the most effective method available to them. Unaided cessation has been found in clinical trials, clinical observational studies and population level studies to be less effective than using either pharmacotherapy under supervision or behavioural support or ideally a combination of the two. To argue that an approach to quitting is the best one because it is the most common is illogical and unsupported by the facts.

John Britton, Professor of Epidemiology and Director, UK Centre for Tobacco Control Studies, University of Nottingham

Linda Bauld, Professor of Socio-Management, University of Stirling

Dorothy Hatsukami, Forster Family Professor in Cancer Prevention, University of Minnesota

Martin Jarvis, Emeritus Professor of Health Psychology, University College London

Jacques Le Houezec, Special Lecturer, University of Nottingham, Manager www.treatobacco.net

Ann McNeill, Professor of Health Policy, University of Nottingham

Hayden McRobbie, Reader in Public Health Interventions, Queen Mary University of London

Martin Raw, Special Lecturer, University of Nottingham

5 "Don't try to quit cold turkey"

John Stapleton, Senior Research Associate, University College London
Robert West, Professor of Health Psychology, University College London

I replied to the listserv the next day:

This debate is ultimately a debate between those who are fixated on success *rates* and those who are more interested in success *numbers*; a debate between those with orientations that are inescapably clinical and those whose ultimate criteria for "the best" is population focused; between those who look at the net cessation yield of various cessation modalities in a population, and see what is obvious (unassisted remains not only more preferred but produces far more successes), and those who get more excited by success rates of some of those modalities but seem blind to their continuing failure to collectively deliver more successes.

Advocates for assisted cessation have had something like 30 years to show that they can persuade smokers to take drugs, call quitlines, attend clinics and abandon silly notions that they might succeed in quitting without all this. Despite the billions of dollars that must have been spent globally in this time on advertising to physicians, direct-to-consumers, in continuing medical education, attracting government subsidies and funding consultants (like most of the signatories), it remains the case that most who quit today do not quit with these forms of assistance. None of these signatories deny this. They instead denigrate it as "illogical" that smokers should ever be told this or that it is undeniably, potentially empowering good news.

They use lame analogies with other forms of pharmacotherapy for other illnesses, trying to paint a spurious equivalence between the treatment of diseases which seldom improve without drugs, and smoking, where we know that most ex-smokers have always stopped without drugs or other assistance.

If the final test of "optimum" cessation policy is the decline of smoking in whole populations and the "how" stories told by most of those who stopped, then we can look at the evidence. In Australia, we today [2010] have 15.1% of 14+ adults smoking daily – and significantly less than this in two states. Both prevalence and cigarettes per day have never been lower and are showing no signs of slowing. We have a handful of UK-style clinics here which collectively contribute an insignificantly small number of ex-smokers to the number who quit each year. What's the score in the UK, the world's assisted cessation capital? Isn't the tail trying to wag the dog?

My final question about smoking prevalence in England in 2010 was rhetorical. In 2010, Australian smoking prevalence (including even very occasional use, and including all forms of combustible tobacco) was 18% (Australian Institute of Health and Welfare 2020c). In England it was 20% for cigarettes and roll-your-own cigarettes only (National Statistics 2012). The most common "lame analogy" I was referring to was about the best way to treat pneumonia, discussed earlier.

A fourth attack

A fourth smackdown appeared in 2013 in a short paper in *Nicotine & Tobacco Research* journal (Raupach, West et al. 2013), again including Robert West among the authors. They wrote:

> One argument used by these authors is that unaided quit attempts are effective because many former smokers report to have quit without help. This argument is based on a logical fallacy, which ought to be obvious, but clearly is not.

They then provided data from the Smoking in England study showing that smokers who had used assisted approaches to quitting had the highest rates of successful quitting at their last quit attempt, while those who had tried to quit unassisted had the lowest rates. From this, they argued – yet again – we had got things completely around the wrong way and were blind to our most egregious, irresponsible error. It was obvious all that mattered in answering any question about "success" in quitting was to use a head-to-head comparison of assisted methods

5 "Don't try to quit cold turkey"

and unassisted methods and see who fared best in terms of *rates* of success. So if we took 100 smokers using assistance and 100 not using assistance, we could see which approach yielded the highest success rate at the most recent quit attempt. What more was needed to answer the question? It was *that* simple and we couldn't get our limited heads around that, apparently.

We replied, suggesting that there was a myopic "not seeing the woods for the trees" problem with their critique (Chapman and MacKenzie 2013). We wrote:

> Those with a clinical focus are often understandably preoccupied with the question of which smoking cessation approaches are most efficacious. If assisted approaches triumph in such comparisons, the task then becomes how to increase use of such assistance in significant proportions of the smoking population. For nearly 30 years there has been a constant refrain from proponents of assisted cessation that they just need to work better to improve desultory participation in clinics, premature abandonment of medication, low single-digit percentages of smokers ever calling quitlines and stagnant levels of sub-optimal interventions by primary care workers. This Sisyphean task is seemingly endless, but meanwhile the hardening hypothesis appears to be largely discredited and rogue nations like Australia which fail to heed the English wisdom continue to be perplexed about the virulence of the criticism directed at our recalcitrance while smoking prevalence continues to fall faster than theirs.
>
> By contrast, those with a "woods" orientation start with a different question which combines effectiveness with reach or participation to answer the question, "What approaches to tobacco control reduce smoking most in a population?"

Population-focused analysts can see great merit in approaches which might not have the highest head-to-head efficacy, but which have far higher consumer acceptance and so greater net population impact. They are less concerned with *failure rates* than with *net success numbers*.

Raupauch, West and Brown epitomised the myopic "trees" orientation when they boasted that England has "probably the highest assisted quitting rate anywhere in the world" before turning to the comparative failure rate of those who try to quit unassisted. But the profane rhinoceros in the room which apparently must never be acknowledged let alone commended by assisted-cessation proponents (who are very often supported by the pharmaceutical industry), is that despite all this "failure", unassisted cessation unarguably is and always has been the approach used by the large majority of people who have quit smoking successfully. It is undeniably the "most" successful strategy if your frame of reference is actual population impact. Our heresy has been to point this out and to suggest that it is in fact an instructive, good news message, not one that should be deemphasized or attract denigrating campaign slogans like "Don't go cold turkey". Globally, hundreds of millions of unassisted ex-smokers' experiences testify to this, something which did not prevent a 2008 English NHS poster containing the flagrant misinformation that "There are some people who can go cold turkey and stop. But there aren't many of them" (see Figure 5.1).

Quitting "attempts" are often half-hearted. So much so, that unassisted attempts are frequently not even recalled (Kasza, Hyland et al. 2013). But a preoccupation with failures in such attempts seems to blind some to the net effect of all this failure: that despite it, unassisted cessation delivers nearly twice as many ex-smokers as all other approaches combined (Shiffman, Brockwell et al. 2008).

Finally, in a candidate for a "pots calling kettles black" award, Raupauch, West and Brown claimed that we selectively cited observational studies that "do not show benefit for treatment". But they then selectively cited studies that support their position. Again, their words mischaracterised what such studies show: treatment does benefit many, but in "real-life", this can be actually less than the unassisted success rate because of indication bias, where more severely dependent smokers with a higher probability of relapse receive a treatment and less dependent smokers do not.

5 "Don't try to quit cold turkey"

It is "unethical" to not promote treatment for smoking in low-income nations

A fifth attack landed in 2011 in the journal *Public Health Ethics* (Bitton and Eyal 2011). Two authors mounted a lengthy critique (titled "Too poor to treat? The complex ethics of cost-effective tobacco policy in the developing world") that Ross MacKenzie and I, in our 2010 *PLOS Med* paper, were condemning smokers in low-income nations to lack of access to NRT and quit-smoking medicines.

We published a reply (Chapman and MacKenzie 2012) to their paper. In it, we rehearsed many of the arguments in this book but focused on the twin issues of the dismal real-world performance of smoking-cessation medications and the stratospheric cost of these products in nations where incomes are very low.

Warner and Mackay have argued that "We can have our cake and eat it too", stating that further resources and emphasis should be given to treating tobacco dependence *as well as* to public-health, population-focused approaches to promoting cessation (Warner and Mackay 2008). Wealthy nations arguably can afford both approaches, although as I wrote earlier, there are few if any drugs which attract the epithet "successful" when 90% or higher of those who take them still have the problem a year after treatment.

However, today's largest smoker populations are nations with massive populations on low incomes for whom quit-smoking aids are prohibitively expensive. This was emphasised in a 2011 survey of tobacco treatment across 121 nations (Pine-Abata, McNeill et al. 2013), interestingly co-authored by Asaf Bitton, the first author on the "Too poor to treat?" paper questioning the ethics of smoking treatments being often unavailable in low-income nations.

In the 2011 survey, just 19 of the 121 respondents providing information on the provision of different elements of smoking-cessation support in their nations were from low-income nations. Twelve of the 19 said their nations "had no specialized treatment at all" for smokers; one had a quitline; and none had nationwide tobacco dependence treatment services. The authors concluded, "A third of countries had no specialized treatment services at all. Availability of medications was limited, and they were frequently perceived to be unaffordable … Overall, tobacco cessation support and treatment appear to be a low priority for most

Parties, especially lower-income countries ... Unfortunately, most countries' health care systems do not cover the cost of tobacco cessation medications and in some countries even NRT, one of the less expensive medications, is far more expensive than cigarettes."

Ten years on from this assessment, I've seen no updated data suggesting that much has changed. A packet of 210 pieces of 4 mg Nicorette™ gum was selling from an Indonesian online pharmacy in November 2021 for 959,000 rupiah (A$90.13). Nicorette's manufacturers suggest 20-a-day smokers wanting to quit should use 1–2 gums per hour, up to a maximum of 20 day. Assuming a smoker used 10 gums a day, then a month's supply would cost A$128.76. With average monthly earnings for Indonesians in December 2020 being A$228, the average Indonesian would need to outlay 56% of their earnings on nicotine gum if they used it as recommended (CEIC 2022).

So in Indonesia, the world's fourth most populous nation, NRT is way out of the reach of all but the wealthy. NRT and prescribed medications would thus seem to be largely irrelevant to population-wide cessation goals in many low- and middle-income nations. Such nations emphatically cannot afford "both" and are often still struggling to fund basic primary health care, and public-health and sanitation infrastructures. Population-oriented, mass-reach tobacco control policy and programs are the exceptions in such nations. In my view, it would be a disaster for tobacco control progress if such nations were to be influenced to proliferate the labour-intensive UK-style models of assisted cessation I discussed in Chapter 4 before they implemented comprehensive and sustained population-focused cessation policies and programs. In most nations, tobacco control is in its nascent phase. Siphoning resources and scarce personnel into smoking-cessation strategies that reach relatively few and help even fewer would be grossly inequitable. And *that* is a serious ethical problem.

In summary, if most ex-smokers quit unaided and many as we have seen early in this chapter don't find it too difficult to do so, this is a very important, empowering message that should be shouted from the rooftops to smokers instead of "You need help! Don't try doing it alone!" It is a message that should be used to balance the overwhelming dominance of the pharmaceutical and vaping industry driven messaging about cessation: that most smokers will find it hard to quit and that most

5 "Don't try to quit cold turkey"

need assistance in the form of drugs or professional oversight to do it. What we get instead is widespread denigration of going cold turkey, a message plainly encouraged by Big Pharma which sees cold turkey as "the enemy", as it was put to me once by a GSK executive. It is seriously depressing to see this situation persist year after year.

Why does Big Tobacco never attack assisted smoking cessation?

Finally, across my entire career I cannot recall a single instance of any tobacco company or "independent" astroturf group or sock puppet doing the industry's bidding, which has ever launched an all-out attack on or even mildly criticised any smoking cessation treatment service, quitline or any of the other cessation approaches described in Chapter 4.

Even more telling is the seemingly bizarre involvement of the tobacco industry in actually running quit-smoking programs. McDaniel et al. summarised their motivations well in a 2017 paper (McDaniel, Lown et al. 2017) showing that these quit programs and other mundane corporate social responsibility gestures served wider purposes of:

> enhancing the industry's image and credibility (Apollonio and Malone 2010); marginalizing public health advocates (Landman, Ling et al. 2002); creating allies among policymakers and regulators (Landman, Ling et al. 2002); forestalling effective tobacco control legislation and preventing enforcement of existing tobacco control laws (Landman, Ling et al. 2002, Apollonio and Malone 2010); providing a litigation defense (Mandel, Bialous et al. 2006); and directing funds away from programs that work (e.g. those that directly confront the tobacco industry) and toward programs in which the industry could be a partner (Mandel, Bialous et al. 2006).

Article 5.3 of the WHO's Framework Convention on Tobacco Control concerns tobacco industry interference in tobacco control (Assunta and Dorotheo 2016). The history of industry interference has included trenchant attacks often lasting decades on policies, laws and regulations which threaten to seriously stimulate large-scale quitting, reducing the number of cigarettes smoked by continuing smokers, preventing uptake or denormalising smoking by expanding smoke-free public spaces. Some of the most sustained opposition has been levelled against tobacco tax rises, advertising and promotion bans, pack warnings (particularly graphic health warnings), plain packaging, smoke-free laws, point-of-sale display bans, ingredient disclosures and duty-free limits.

Hard-hitting mass-reach campaigns with substantial budgets have also been attacked. An early example of this was an attempt to stop a pioneering campaign operating on the North Coast of New South Wales. "All printed advertisements were suspended for 15 weeks from October 1979 (four months after the start of the antismoking campaign) after complaints to the Media Council of Australia by the three major tobacco manufacturers. One television commercial was also suspended pending a change in wording." All of the complaints concerned issues of advertisements disparaging smoking (Egger, Fitzgerald et al. 1983).

Against all of this, the tobacco industry has never opposed or even criticised anything to do with assisting smokers to quit whether this be efforts by governments, health agencies or pharmaceutical companies. Its indifferent behaviour to these activities has been similar to its typical silence on school health education curricula about smoking, mandatory signs in shops about it being illegal to sell to children, and laws on minimum age of tobacco purchase. Indeed, it has often trumpeted its own corporate social responsibility efforts to dissuade children from smoking through initiatives it privately described as "a phony way to express sincerity [to governments about tobacco control] as we all know" (Assunta and Chapman 2004, Knight and Chapman 2004).

The tobacco industry's reaction to policies that in any serious way threaten its bottom line (sales) has long been shorthanded in global tobacco control as the "scream test". If the industry screams loudly in the media, in its lobbying of governments and in its efforts through the courts to stop, reverse or neuter tobacco control policies, this is an unfailing litmus test of its understanding of which policies are potent ways of reducing smoking. The corollary of this is that when it stays silent on any development, it understands these things are inconsequential. Its silence on quit-smoking treatments and services is deafening.

6
Vaping to quit: the latest mass distraction

Electronic cigarettes (e-cigarettes or ECs) and heat-not-burn nicotine vaping products (NVPs, which include ECs) have become immensely popular in some parts of the world since their first appearance in China in 2004. In the UK and USA, they are now the most common aid being used in cessation attempts (West, Kale et al. 2021). Market analysts Grand View Research estimated the global vape market size at US$15.04 billion in 2020 and expected this to expand at a compound annual growth rate of 28.1% from 2021 to 2028 (Grand View Research 2021). The boundless hype megaphoned by NVP marketers and enthusiasts about these products is that they are as near as possible to being perfectly benign health-wise; that they are peerless in their effectiveness as a means of quitting smoking; that they are a massively disruptive product in the way that digital cameras were to film cameras and electric vehicles are fast becoming to fossil-fuel-powered cars; and that they are capable of saving a billion lives this century, in people who are forecast to die from smoking (A billion is the number of smokers who've been estimated will die from smoking-caused diseases by the end of this century) (Peto and Lopez 2001).

That final modest claim assumes that all the world's smokers would permanently switch to NVPs and never return to smoking, with combustible tobacco use disappearing without a trace, and that these products will also prove to be as benign as fairy dust into the long-term.

As I will discuss in this chapter, widespread sightings of porcine aviation seem about as likely.

Big Tobacco butts in

All transnational tobacco companies have lost no time investing heavily in the development and marketing of NVPs (Tobacco Tactics 2020a). Some of these companies have made statements that they hope to one day stop selling combustible tobacco products. But tellingly, unlike the car manufacturing industry where ten companies have now announced dates for them to stop manufacturing fossil-fuelled cars (Nicholson 2021), no tobacco company has set a target date for the end of cigarettes. And just as tellingly, they continue to do all they can to maximise cigarette sales and as they've done for 70 years, thwart any evidence-based government policies which seriously threaten to put a brake on the uptake of smoking or accelerated quitting.

Far from turning off its efforts to produce and market cigarettes, Philip Morris International (PMI) continues to expand its cigarette business wherever it can. In March 2018, PMI opened a new factory in Tanzania with capacity to produce 400 million cigarettes a year "to cater for the local and international market" (Tanzania Invest 2018). In October 2021, Turkish conglomerate Sabanci Holding took steps to turn over its shares in Philip Morris Sabanci Cigarette and Tobacco Inc (PHILSA) and Philip Morris Sabanci Marketing and Sales Corp (PMSA) to its parent company, PMI, thus consolidating PMI's interests in tobacco (Daily Sabah 2021).

In Indonesia, the world's fourth most populous nation with huge rates of male smoking and feeble tobacco control, PMI owns the Sampoerna cigarette company but local sales of its IQOS NVP are very small. PMI's president for South and Southeast Asia, Stacey Kennedy, explained on PMI's website:

> If we packed up and left Indonesia tomorrow it doesn't change anything for smokers. They just pick up a different cigarette. Cigarettes don't go away until we give adult smokers an alternative ... How we go from a small scale to a large scale is the journey

that we're trying to tackle now. We're absolutely on the path to transition from conventional cigarettes to smoke-free products in Indonesia, just like we are everywhere else in the world. It takes time. Every country's path is unique, because there's different levels of awareness and support, country by country (Kennedy 2019).

Kennedy was adamant that it's "simply not true" that PMI only focuses on its heated tobacco products in wealthy nations:

We want to bring smoke-free alternatives to all adult smokers in Indonesia over time. That's a pretty big ambition and it starts with being able to understand what adult smokers need and want ... I can absolutely tell you that I spend the vast majority of my time focused on Indonesia and other countries in Southeast Asia and how we can convince adult smokers who won't otherwise quit to switch to our reduced-risk products.

But Kennedy's words are hard to reconcile with what PMI does in concert with other cigarette manufacturers in Indonesia when it comes to local tobacco control policies. In Indonesia, Gaprindo, the white (non-kretek) cigarette manufacturers association, represents the interests of transnationals like PMI, British American Tobacco (BAT) and Japan Tobacco International (JTI). Gaprindo routinely lobbies to oppose tobacco control policies like tax increases, as does the tobacco industry globally. In November 2018, it fought advertising bans and opposed tax increases (Cahya 2018). The head of Gaprindo said that the cigarette industry has in the past few years experienced a sales volume decline of 1–2%. In 2015, Gaprindo said, "Increasing excise tax on cigarettes twice a year will just harm the [tobacco] industry growth" (Amin 2015).

PMI has even gone as far as saying that they want their customers to stop using *all* forms of nicotine: "To be clear, PMI's core message is: For adults who use nicotine in any form it is best to quit completely" (Kary and Gretler 2020). Here, we are meant to believe that the company wants its cigarette customers to stop smoking and switch to its heat-not-burn IQOS brand (which contains tobacco). But it says it wants even these customers ("it is best") to also quit IQOS. This sounds as credible as a motor vehicle company urging owners of its petrol-powered vehicles not just to switch to its fully electric models, but to also then abandon those and not own cars at all. Only a tobacco company could have the weapons-grade gall to make such a statement publicly.

In a 2019 presentation to investors, BAT emphasised that dual and poly-using next generation product (NGP) users were of vital importance to its mission. Sixty-five percent of EC users and 55% of heated tobacco product (HTP) users are dual users. These products allowed nicotine "moments being regained" in places where "smoking is not allowed or socially unacceptable, such as in a shared office, at home with family, or in public social spaces" (Tobacco Tactics 2021). In 2018, BAT's boss, Nicandro Durante, said that dual use had become "the key consumer dynamic", growing from 13% to 23% in less than one year. Another BAT presentation identified most popular "new occasions" for EC users were "when I can't smoke cigarettes" (86%), "in the car" (62%) and "inside pubs and restaurants" (47%) (Durante 2018).

So BAT, like all tobacco companies, knows very well that its bread is being buttered far more by the pursuit of dual and poly NVP and NGP use than by just concentrating on cigarettes. And like all of them, it's very happy to do whatever it can to maximise sales of all its addictive products.

In late 2021, the US Federal Trade Commission published its annual report on total cigarette sales (including promotional giveaways) and marketing expenditure in the USA, drawing on data supplied by the four largest tobacco companies operating there (United States Federal Trade Commission 2021). US tobacco sales were up for the first time in 20 years with 203.7 billion cigarettes sold or given away. The US tobacco industry has been experiencing an unstoppable haemorrhaging of sales for over 20 years. The small 2020 rise needs to be seen in context of the 48.9% continual fall that had been happening since 2001.

The industry does all it can to stem this bleeding. Its advertising and promotional expenditures rose 2.8% in 2020 to reach US$7.84 billion, with the biggest spend being discounts paid to cigarette wholesalers and retailers (a whopping 88.5% of all promotional expenditure) to keep the price of cigarettes as low as possible for smokers to encourage sales. Remember this next time you hear anyone in the tobacco industry unctuously intoning that they want to get out of selling combustible tobacco while vaping proliferates.

6 Vaping to quit: the latest mass distraction

Those who promote vaping typically focus their pitch around five arguments for why they believe NVPs are a revolutionary disruptive technology which promises to reduce the galactic harm caused by smoking:

1. NVPs are all but 100% safe ("E-cigarettes are about as safe as you can get ... E-cigarettes are probably about as safe as drinking coffee. All they contain is water vapour, nicotine and propylene glycol [which is used to help vaporise the liquid nicotine]" (Hickman 2013).
2. It's not too early to declare that NVPs will not have long-term serious health consequences.
3. Nearly all teenagers who vaped before they started smoking would have smoked anyway.
4. Flavours are a vital factor explaining the popularity of vaping and therefore governments should let a million flavours bloom with minimal regulation.
5. NVPs are peerless as an effective way of helping smokers quit permanently.

Pulling all these together, who could possibly be in any doubt that in NVPs we have the ingredients for a major milestone in the entire history of public health. Or so the hype goes. Indeed, one vaping champion, the hyperbolic David Nutt, has gone as far as declaring breathlessly that e-cigarettes are "the most significant advance [in medicine] since antibiotics" (National Institute for Health Innovation 2013); are "the greatest health advance since vaccinations" (BBC News 2014); and that those rejecting the opportunity of harm reduction from vaping are engaging in "perhaps the worst example of scientific denial since the Catholic Church banned the works of Copernicus in 1616" (Caruana 2020). While I've yet to see a single authoritative source endorse or even repeat any of these comparisons, Nutt was apparently being serious.

The focus of this book is smoking cessation, the fifth of the pitches for vaping I listed above. So the bulk of this chapter will examine the evidence for this claim, highlighting the conclusions of reviews of recent evidence for smoking cessation which have been published since 2017; the evidence for cessation from randomised controlled trials; and papers coming out of the large US Population Assessment of Tobacco and Health (PATH) prospective cohort study which commenced in 2013 and provides the most important data on transitions in nicotine use across the years since (Hyland, Ambrose et al. 2017).

I'll look at challenges in assessing the role played by vaping in reducing smoking at the population level, when many other variables known to put downward pressure on smoking are also in play at the same time. I'll also consider the question of whether vaping might actually hold more people in smoking, than providing a large-scale off-ramp out of it. If this were the case, the interests of the tobacco industry in eagerly promoting NVPs would be obvious. I'll also look at evidence that vaping reduces smoking frequency (how many cigarettes are smoked each day) in those who keep smoking while vaping (dual users) and whether reduced use actually reduces harm in those who cut down rather than quit all smoking.

But before turning to these questions, let's briefly look at the four other core claims about NVPs.

"95% less dangerous than smoking"

A claim relentlessly asserted by vaping advocates is that NVPs are far less dangerous than smoking, most commonly phrased as "95% less dangerous" than smoking. This figure emerged from a meeting held in London in 2014 of twelve selected participants, several of whom had track records as tobacco harm-reduction advocates. Some had tobacco industry connections (Gornall 2015). David Nutt chaired the group. The published paper in which this resoundingly large, unforgettable number first appeared provided no data or calculations on how it was arrived at, beyond describing a process where the participants ranked different nicotine products against cigarettes, using 16 criteria on harm (Nutt, Phillips et al. 2014).

Specifically excluded from the list of harms were drug-specific and drug-related mental impairment so that the potential of various nicotine delivery devices to initiate and perpetuate nicotine addiction was not included in the assessment, despite tobacco use disorder or dependence being included in the International Classification of Diseases (ICD) of the World Health Organization, and the *Diagnostic and statistical manual of mental disorders* (DSM), compiled by the American Psychiatric Association.

However, deep in the paper's discussion section, the authors stated, perhaps at the insistence of reviewers' and editors' comments, "A limitation of this study is the lack of hard evidence for the harms of most products on most of the criteria" used to rank the harmfulness of different nicotine delivery products.

Let's pause here and roll that sentence around in our minds again. In my over 40 years of academic life in public health, including editing a research journal (*Tobacco Control*) for 17 of these which currently has the highest impact factor in its field, and having reviewed hundreds of research papers, I don't recall ever reading such a deeply self-eviscerating "Actually, we have almost no hard evidence" caveat about the very foundations of an exercise in supposed scientific risk assessment. This caveat is frankly a public suicide note for the credibility of the paper's central take-home message. But it is not an admission which has given NVP "true believers" even the slightest pause to keep megaphoning it as much as possible over the past seven years.

With others, I have critiqued the provenance of the "95% less dangerous" statement in the *American Journal of Public Health* (Eissenberg, Bhatnagar et al. 2020) and in greater detail in my blog (Chapman 2019). I showed how it has been uncritically repeated and even pushed beyond 95% by some, with all referencing leading back to the original Nutt group report with its sweeping "there's no hard evidence" caveat. A factoid is an item of unreliable information that is reported and repeated so often that it becomes accepted as fact. The 95% claim is a vampire-like factoid which just won't die and derives its status from its mass repetition as an article of faith in what I've often heard described as vaping theology.

Too soon to know the true health risks of vaping

When confronted with their 95% emperor's lack of evidential clothing, vaping advocates frequently retort, "Well, if it's not 95% safer, what's your figure then?" Those who believe this question can actually be answered today could only be ignorant of the nature of risk assessment of chronic diseases and the history of our evolving understanding of the risks of smoking. Or perhaps they believe that scientific risk assessment is properly approached by guesswork.

Cigarette use exploded at the beginning of the 20th century after mechanisation in factories replaced handmade cigarettes. This made smoking very affordable to even those on the lowest incomes. But tobacco-caused diseases didn't start showing up in large numbers until 30–40 years later. US surgeon Alton Ochsner, recalling attendance at his first lung cancer autopsy in 1919, was told he and his fellow interns "might never see another such case as long as we lived". He saw no further cases until 17 years later in 1936 – and then saw another nine cases in six months (Ochsner 1971). Since the 1960s, lung cancer has been by far the world's leading cause of cancer death with 18% of all cancer deaths in 2020, ahead of the next most frequent killer, liver cancer, with 8.3% (Sung, Ferlay et al. 2021).

The chronic diseases caused by smoking take many years before manifesting clinically. They are not like infectious, communicable diseases such as COVID-19, influenza or HIV where there is typically a very short period between exposure to the infectious agent and the onset of symptoms and sometimes death. Instead there are long latency periods that can stretch for several decades when smokers may not have any signs or symptoms of emerging disease (Smith, Imawana et al. 2021).

The incidence of lung cancer rose rapidly in the decades 1930–80 but it was not until 1950 that seriously compelling case-control evidence was published in the USA (Wynder and Graham 1950) and England (Doll and Hill 1950). These reports were foundational in the emerging consensus that long-term smoking caused lung cancer. Knowledge about smoking's causal role in many other diseases followed and continues to consolidate, with the smoking attributable death rate increasing in recent years from half of long-term smokers (Doll, Peto et al. 2005) to two in three (Banks, Joshy et al. 2015).

If any scientist had declared in 1920 that cigarette smoking was all but harmless, as vaping advocates insist today about NVPs, history would have judged their call as heroically and dangerously incorrect. But this is the cavalier call that many vaping advocates routinely make, after just 10 years or so of widespread use in some nations. For example, English vaping advocate Clive Bates put it simply in a 2017 interview produced for the government agency Public Health England (PHE): "Almost none of the [news media] stories holds any water or should give anyone any cause for concern" (Public Health England 2017). And Professor Robert Beaglehole went a step further in a video interview with a vaping advocacy group, at one point referring to "the supposed harm of nicotine and vaping" while theatrically gesturing air quotes around "supposed harm". He then said, "A lot of that information is incorrect. *All of it is incorrect.* And based on very poor science and vested interests" [my emphasis] (Chapman 2021).

All of it is incorrect? *All* of it? So any published evidence that has concluded that there are any concerns about vaping being harmful or not very effective in helping smokers quit it is all wrong, apparently.

With vaping having been around in large numbers for only about ten years, it is predictable and unsurprising that we have as yet seen little clinical disease caused by e-cigarette vaping. As acknowledged in 2021 by 15 presidents of the global Society for Research on Nicotine and Tobacco, "High-quality clinical and epidemiological data on vaping's health effects are relatively sparse. There are no data on long-term health effects, reflecting the relative novelty of vaping and the rapid evolution of vaping products. Determining even short-term health effects in adults is difficult because most adult vapers are former or current smokers" (Balfour, Benowitz et al. 2021). However, recent reviews of cardio-respiratory impacts of vaping may be pointing to sick canaries in this coalmine (e.g. Tsai, Byun et al. 2020, Wehrli, Caporale et al. 2020, Keith and Bhatnagar 2021).

Professor John Britton from the University of Nottingham acknowledged this in the same 2017 PHE compilation interview as Clive Bates' statement, saying, " Inhaling vapour many times a day for decades is unlikely to come without some sort of adverse effect. And time will tell what that will be" (Public Health England 2017).

A colleague of mine, Sydney respiratory physician Professor Matthew Peters, summarised recent research this way:

Ween et al. recently reported findings of a carefully conducted study on the effects of e-liquid exposure in human bronchial epithelial cells (Ween, Hamon et al. 2020). There were three key findings. E-cigarette (EC) liquids, with a variety of constituents, induce damage that manifests as necrosis and apoptosis; macrophage efferocytosis, an adaptive mechanism that clears apoptotic cells, is compromised; and purchasers of EC liquids can have no confidence in the constituents that they are exposing their lungs to – with three versions of apple flavour having very different chemical mixes. The observations of Ween et al. have even greater pertinence after the report of histopathology from 17 cases within the current outbreak (Butt, Smith et al. 2019). Open biopsy findings suggest that the dominant pathology is a form of airway-based chemical pneumonitis and not exogenous lipoid pneumonia as previously believed by some (Peters 2020).

These findings complement an NIH-funded comprehensive 2017 review by Chun et al. on the effects of EC on the lung, which examined a combination of in vivo and in vitro studies (Chun, Moazed et al. 2017). Since that publication, we have also seen the seminal work of Ghosh et al. who observed airway inflammation in a man in vivo, describing the proteomic characteristic of bronchial tissue in smokers, EC users and controls (Ghosh, Coakley et al. 2018). In summary, considering significant positive and negative changes, there were 292 changes seen with smoking, of which 78 were also seen with EC use. Importantly, there were 113 separate proteomic changes that occurred only with EC use. This would not be unexpected by an open mind because the nature of the lung exposure is very different.

A 2020 *New England Journal of Medicine* report of serious pulmonary disease in two US states in 53 vapers, with a median age of just 19, found that 17% of these patients reported vaping only nicotine products (Layden, Ghinai et al. 2020). British NVP advocates were quick to point out that none of these cases were being reported in the UK where vaping is also prevalent. Soon afterwards the *British Medical Journal* (*BMJ*) published a case report of a young woman with respiratory failure from lipoid pneumonia, suspected of being caused by her vaping (Viswam, Trotter et al. 2018). In October 2021, the *Medical Journal of Australia* published a case report of a 15-year-old girl hospitalised with diagnostic criteria consistent with Electronic Cigarette or Vaping Product Use-Associated Lung Injury (EVALI) (Chan, Kiss et al. 2021). She had vaped two to three times a week for seven months, had smoked cannabis through a water pipe and also smoked cigarettes, like a majority of vapers do. But she had never vaped cannabis and her vaping device contained no traces of cannabis nor vitamin E acetate, agents known to be present in many, but not all, cases of EVALI (Winnicka and Shenoy 2020).

In February 2022, ABC TV in Australia reported on an autopsy conducted on a 71-year-old man who had switched to daily vaping 10 years earlier and had died after collapsing and being put into a coma with acute lung failure. The autopsy described "acute lung injury superimposed on chronic lung disease and a probable cause of EVALI – meeting three of the four criteria". The man's intensive care doctor described "huge cystic lesions at the apex of the lung" and noted that with emphysema, the typical presentation of lung injury was throughout the lung (Atkin 2022).

When many have pointed out this fundamental "too soon to know" problem, vaping defenders snort derisively that toxicological science has progressed exponentially in the years since the connection of smoking with cancer was first authoritatively established. The implication here is that we can now tell very early with a high degree of certainty if a drug or chemical combinations such as those found in NVPs are likely to cause disease down the track.

That certainty would be informed by all that advanced crystal-balling toxicology capable of early detection of long-term risk so brilliantly that between 1953 and 2014, 462 drugs initially assessed as being likely to be safe and let into the market have been withdrawn with some causing very serious health problems or death (Onakpoya, Heneghan et al. 2016). Remember the global thalidomide birth defects tragedy? (Sjostrom and Nilsson 1972).

All but the most impoverished and chaotic nations have drug assessment, scheduling, adverse event reporting, and the possibility of recall and bans because pre-registration drug trials can never provide data on the consequences of long-term use. That of course is not a sensible reason to ban all new drugs, but it is the primary reason why new drugs are almost invariably scheduled as prescription-only so that monitoring of any adverse reactions can be better undertaken. Many prominent vaping advocates have been stridently opposed to NVPs being scheduled as prescription items. They appear to embrace a peculiar kind of regulatory exceptionalism, strongly supporting drug regulation in general but not when it comes to vaping.

In 2017 vaping activists on social media were jubilant about a 3.5 year follow-up study of just nine subjects (with another seven having dropped out) which – hey presto – showed no "long term" ill-effects (Polosa, Cibella et al. 2017). "Case closed: study shows no lung damage from vaping" gloated one report on a pro-vaping channel (Stafford 2017). Such a baby-steps follow-up between exposure and pathology compares with the 9 to 11-fold greater 30–40 years that passed before the huge upswing in smoking in the first decade of the 20th century began to show lung cancer in case-control studies in the early 1950s.

A good example of the common "nothing to worry about" promotion of vaping can be seen in the online promotion in Figure 6.1 promising "risk free" vaping, with one mouse click past the first page we find a remarkably self-contradictory sentence that vapers can "entirely avoid the harm" while "lessen[ing] the possibility of inducing danger on your lungs". Reckless calls to just allow unregulated NVPs to flood corner stores and be promoted with advertising like that is the sort of risk assessment we are supposed to embrace by flatulent arguments that the risks of vaping are already known.

If NVPs are really so safe and so effective, their manufacturers would surely have nothing to fear by applying for registration through regulatory bodies like the Australian Therapeutic Goods Administration (TGA). Why is it then, that no such applications have been received? What might these manufacturers know or fear that the TGA's assessment process might conclude?

6 Vaping to quit: the latest mass distraction

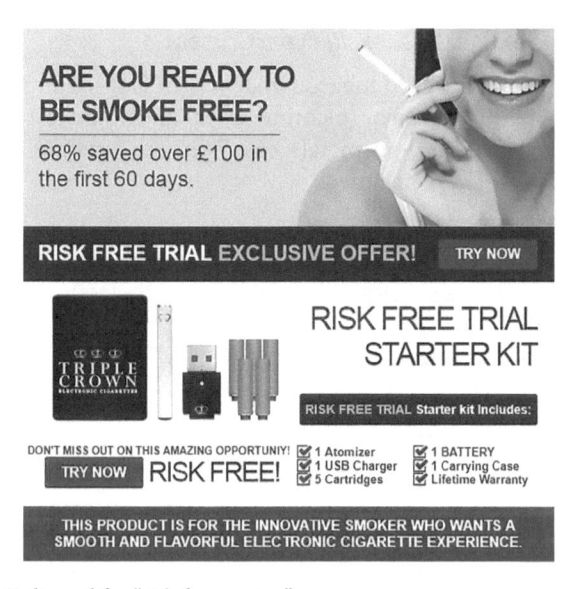

Figure 6.1 Online ad for "risk free vaping".

PATH data on toxicant exposure: never-tobacco users vs. smokers vs. exclusive vapers vs. dual users

Information of immense importance to the debate about the net contribution of vaping to toxicant exposure was published in 2018 using data obtained from the US longitudinal PATH study (Goniewicz, Smith et al. 2018). The authors compared concentrations of tobacco-related toxicant biomarkers among e-cigarette users with those observed in cigarette smokers, dual users of e-cigarettes and cigarettes, and those who had never used tobacco in any form. They compared mean concentrations of 50 individual biomarkers from five major classes of tobacco product constituents: nicotine, tobacco-specific nitrosamines (TSNAs), metals, polycyclic aromatic hydrocarbons (PAHs) and volatile organic compounds (VOCs). Following is a summary of their main findings.

Never-tobacco users vs. exclusive EC users

Those who had never used tobacco in any form had significantly lower concentrations of all major nicotine metabolites and total nicotine equivalents, all TSNAs, four metals, one PAH and four VOCs than did exclusive vapers. These included:

- NNAL (the tobacco-specific carcinogen 4-(methylnitrosamino)-1-(3-pyridyl)-1-butanol): 81% less
- Metal exposure: lead (19% less), cadmium (23% less)
- Pyrene: 20% less
- Acrylonitrile: 67% less

Exclusive EC users vs. exclusive smokers

Exclusive EC users had significantly lower concentrations of all major nicotine metabolites, two minor tobacco alkaloids, all TSNAs, one metal (cadmium), all PAHs and 17 VOCs (markers for toluene, benzene and carbon disulfide) than did exclusive smokers. These included:

- Total nicotine equivalents: 93% less
- NNAL: 98% less
- Cadmium: 30% less
- Naphthalene: 62% less
- Pyrene: 47% less
- Acrolein: 60% less
- Acrylonitrile: 97% less

Dual users vs. exclusive cigarette smokers

Claims are often made that dual users replace some of the cigarettes they once smoked with ECs and are thereby predicted to be reducing their total toxicant load. But contrary to that claim, dual users in this study were found to have significantly *higher* concentrations of most biomarkers, including most major nicotine metabolites, 3 TSNAs, two metals, five PAHs and 13 VOCs than exclusive smokers. These included:

- Total nicotine equivalents: 36% more
- NNAL: 23% more

- Pyrene: 15% more
- Acrolein: 10% more
- Acrylonitrile: 15% more
- Lead and cadmium levels were equivalent

So in summary, if you have never used tobacco in any form, unsurprisingly you are likely to have far lower biomarkers for tobacco use than those who use ECs. If you exclusively use ECs, you'll have far lower tobacco toxicant levels than if you smoke. And if you both smoke and vape (dual use), you'll have higher levels than those who only smoke. So if dual use is the Mount Everest of toxicant exposure, then smoking is the K2 exposure, vaping is the Matterhorn and never smoking or vaping is the toxicant exposure at sea level.

Adding to this, another paper using PATH data (Christensen, Chang et al. 2021) found that dual users have a greater concentration of an oxidative stress marker, F2-isoprostane, than smokers. Exclusive EC users have biomarker concentrations at similar levels to those of former smokers, and lower than those of exclusive cigarette smokers.

Johns Hopkins University researchers applied liquid chromatography–high-resolution mass spectrometry (LC–HRMS) and chemical fingerprinting techniques to characterise e-liquids and aerosols from a selection of popular EC products (Mi-Salt™, Vuse™, Juul™ and Blu™) (Tehrani, Newmeyer et al. 2021). They found nearly 2,000 chemicals in these products, the vast majority of which were unidentified. Six potentially hazardous additives and contaminants, including the industrial chemical tributylphosphine oxide were identified. The authors noted, "Existing research that compared e-cigarettes with normal cigarettes found that cigarette contaminants are much lower in e-cigarettes. The problem is that e-cigarette aerosols contain other completely uncharacterized chemicals that might have health risks that we don't yet know about" (Johns Hopkins University 2021).

Many vaping advocates appear to believe they are on a messianic mission to save a billion lives. All tobacco companies now marketing NVPs are delighted to buy into that framing of what vaping is all about, while just down the corridor in their tobacco divisions they continue trying to maximise demand for the cigarettes that will cause the same billion deaths they claim vaping could prevent.

Armed with that moral imperative, like all evangelists they believe that no impediment should be placed in the way of their lifesaving work. But medicine of course has a very long history of claims being made by purveyors of a multitude of miracle cures who also believe their crusades are far too important to be regulated by the dead hand of bureaucracy in government agencies (Barker Bausell 2007). Most people readily understand why consumer protection laws often include specific provisions about outlawing health and medical claims for which there is little or no evidence. Quack claims for treatments for cancer, HIV/AIDS, COVID-19, asthma and many other life-threatening diseases have long been exposed and prosecuted by governments or their drug regulatory agencies.

But NVP advocates constantly make claims for both the safety and the efficacy of vaped products, despite them never having been declared as such by any regulatory agency. In October 2021, the US Food and Drug Administration (USFDA) announced that for the first time it had authorised the marketing of a limited number of NVPs. In doing so, however, the USFDA was explicit that about what this authorisation did *not* mean:

> While today's action permits the tobacco products to be sold in the US, it does not mean these products are safe or "FDA approved". All tobacco products are harmful and addictive and those who do not use tobacco products should not start (US Food and Drug Administration 2021b).

In 2021 Australia's TGA published a similar fundamental caveat on its new prescription-only access to NVPs (see Chapter 8):

> There are currently no nicotine vaping products approved by the Therapeutic Goods Administration (TGA) and registered in the Australian Register of Therapeutic Goods (ARTG). Medicines that are not in the ARTG are known as "unapproved" medicines. There are established pathways for consumers to legally access unapproved nicotine vaping products, with a valid prescription, but these medicines have not been assessed by the TGA for safety, quality and efficacy (Therapeutic Goods Administration 2021b).

Safety and efficacy are the two core considerations on which drug regulation is based. But many vaping advocates believe their case should somehow place them above all this. There is much evidence of trying to walk on both sides of the street here. NVPs are better than NRT for cessation, they say, thus making a therapeutic claim. "Oh no, we are not making any therapeutic claim because NVPs are a 'consumer product', not a pharmaceutical product," comes their reply. "Those using NVPs are not sick, so why should they be regulated by therapeutic agencies?" they continue. But those who take other smoking-cessation products like bupropion or varenicline aren't "sick" either. Yet no one has called for these products to be sold over the counter at convenience stores.

However, the question of the safety of products claiming to help people stop smoking is tangential to the focus of this book: smoking cessation in real-world use. Readers wanting far more detailed information on developments are referred to authoritative reports like that of the 2018 doorstopper-sized report on ECs from the US National Academies of Sciences, Engineering and Medicine (National Academies of Sciences, Engineering and Medicine 2018). Among its conclusions on product safety were:

- There is *substantial evidence* that EC aerosols can induce acute endothelial cell dysfunction, although the long-term consequences and outcomes on these parameters with long-term exposure to EC aerosol are uncertain.
- There is *substantial evidence* that components of EC aerosols can promote formation of reactive oxygen species/oxidative stress. Although this supports the biological plausibility of tissue injury and disease from long-term exposure to EC aerosols, generation of reactive oxygen species and oxidative stress induction is generally lower from e-cigarettes than from combustible tobacco cigarette smoke.
- There is *substantial evidence* that some chemicals present in EC aerosols (e.g., formaldehyde, acrolein) are capable of causing DNA damage and mutagenesis. This supports the biological plausibility that long-term exposure to EC aerosols could increase risk of cancer and adverse reproductive outcomes.

Insignificant uptake by teens and no gateway to smoking?

A third platform of vaping theology sees vaping advocates dismiss all concerns about any reports of dramatic uptake of vaping by teenagers and those even younger by a three-step argument: first (as just discussed), vaping is all but benign, so there's almost nothing to worry about when children vape. Second, nearly all children who take up smoking after first vaping would have taken up smoking anyway if NVPs had never appeared on the scene (so-called common liability theory) (Vanyukov, Tarter et al. 2012). And third, vaping "protects" children from starting to smoke, so we should perhaps even encourage it. This is an argument so bereft of evidence that it is usually only explicitly voiced by those from the twilight zone of vaping advocacy.

Australian vaping advocate Alex Wodak put much of this together in 2021 in a comment to the press when he likened teenage vaping to past harmless yoyo and hula-hoop fads: "In 2023 they'll be on to hula hoops or yoyos, they'll drop vaping. There are fads and fashions. Regular frequent vaping by young kids is not a problem and where young people vape, they have almost always been smokers first" (Hansen 2021). Wodak and other vaping advocates have often described concern about teenage vaping as a confected "moral panic". They argue that it's better that teenagers vape than smoke, that their vaping is preventing them from smoking, and so isn't teenage vaping therefore nothing but positive?

This attempted framing is happening against a background where teenage smoking rates in nations like Australia have fallen to the lowest levels ever recorded, thanks to decades of success in tobacco control policies reducing uptake (Greenhalgh, Winstanley et al. 2019). As the tobacco industry watches a diminishing proportion of each birth cohort's potential future smokers fail to take up smoking, the vital importance of addicting as many of these nicotine-naïve children to nicotine through vaping for the commercial viability of the tobacco industry is all too obvious and urgent (Chapman 2015).

New Zealand and Canada are cases in point. In New Zealand, following an unsuccessful 2018 challenge by the Ministry of Health over Philip Morris International's plans to sell the NVP HEETS product (Reuters Staff 2018), the government was forced to allow the marketing

6 Vaping to quit: the latest mass distraction

Regular smoking and vaping prevalence, Year 10 (14-15 years), New Zealand 2012-2019

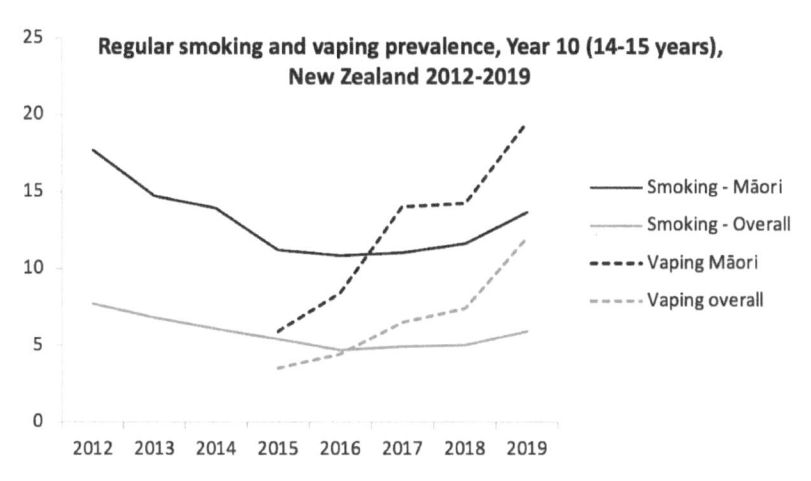

Figure 6.2 Regular smoking and vaping prevalence (per cent Y axis) Year 10 (14–15 years), New Zealand 2012–19 (Source: Action on Smoking and Health NZ 2021).

of NVPs, including no age restrictions for purchase, no advertising constraints and no accountability for retailers.

Figure 6.2 shows what has been occurring with 14–15-year-olds' regular smoking and vaping prevalence in New Zealand. Between 2012 and 2015, prior to the widespread availabilty of vaping, overall smoking fell by 21% from 6.8% to 5.5% and by 37% from 17.7% to 11.2% in Māori teenagers. But after the advent of vaping, the decline changed to a growth of 9% between 2015 and 2019, with Māori smoking rising 21%. While this was happening, regular vaping was rising dramatically: between 2015 and 2019, the prevalence of regular vaping rose 173% (5.4% to 12%) and by a roaring 261% in Māori teens (5.4% to 19.5%).

Canada similarly opened the EC floodgates in 2018. Statistics Canada released survey results from the national Canadian Tobacco and Nicotine Survey (CTNS) in July 2021. Although Canadian youth and young adults (aged 15 to 24) make up only 15% of the surveyed population, they accounted for 40% of those who vape. An estimated 425,000 teenagers vaped in Canada. About 1.46 million Canadians vaped in the previous month. Of these, one-third (485,100) were former smokers. The remainder were those who'd never smoked

(438,500, 30%) or current smokers (532,400 dual users, 38%) (Statistics Canada 2021).

Immediately, both the New Zealand and Canadian governments started furiously backpedalling. From August 2021 new regulations in New Zealand "banned retailers such as dairies (small owner-operated convenience stores), service stations and supermarkets from selling vaping products in flavours other than tobacco, mint and menthol. Only specialist vape retailers will be able to sell other flavours. From 28 November, vaping and smoking in motor vehicles carrying children will be banned" (Verrall 2021). All advertising was prohibited, as was distribution of free NVPs and discounting (Ministry of Health New Zealand 2021b).

From the summer of 2019, only a year on from opening the floodgates and allowing a broad range of EC advertising, the Canadian government severely restricted promotions (Government of Canada 2021). In June 2021, Health Canada commenced public discussion of its intent to restrict vaping flavours options to tobacco and mint or menthol (Cision 2021) and reduced the maximum nicotine concentration in vaping liquids to 20 mg/ml in line with the European Union limit.

When asked about the rise in teenage vaping, extreme vaping advocates shrug with supreme indifference. More moderate advocates, intoning with socially responsible concern, typically call for policies that will target reducing youth uptake. Here, we encounter all manner of hopelessly naïve and discredited suggestions, such as retailer education, tougher and more explicit signage in shops advising that vaping is not for under 18s, marketing regulation that makes adult-directed advertising somehow magically invisible to youth, greater "education" and vigilance in ensuring that all online marketing is accompanied by site entry buttons requiring all potential visitors to declare that they are over 18 years old. That will stop them! All of these proposals had of course been trotted out for decades by the tobacco industry with its fingers firmly and cynically crossed behind their backs, knowing how ineffective each of these suggestions was (Knight and Chapman 2004).

As I'll discuss in Chapter 8, requiring prescription authority to access NVPs combined with bans on all sales without prescription, all backed by seriously deterrent fines seem likely to be the only feasible ways of greatly reducing youth access.

While youth vaping rates are booming, there had been until recently (see Figure 6.2) no convincing evidence yet published of any substantial increase in uptake in adolescent smoking or stalling of its decline in any nation (although the very recent New Zealand data cited above are cause for concern). This has given succour to vaping advocates who like to point out that this lack of evidence is incompatible with the core prediction of gateway theory: if youth smoking rates are falling while vaping rates are rising, vaping cannot be acting in any significant way as a gateway. This argument is slippery with sophistry.

In a critique I wrote with Wasim Maziak and David Bareham of repudiations of the gateway hypothesis involving vaping and smoking, we pointed out:

> declining trends of smoking among youth were apparent well before the introduction of e-cigarettes. Moreover, associations in population trends are known to be prone to the ecological fallacy; i.e. what is true at the population level may not be true at the individual level, especially when other population-level attributes are not considered (e.g. effective tobacco control policies). Specifically, the ecological argument relies on an assumption *that the population net impact of any putative gateway effect of e-cigarette use would be larger than the combined net impact of all other policies, programs and factors which are responsible for reducing adolescent smoking prevalence* (e.g. tobacco tax and retail price, measures of the denormalisation of smoking, exposure of children to adult-targeted quit campaigns, retail display bans, health warnings and plain packaging). *This is an extremely high bar that gateway critics demand that anyone suggesting gateway effects needs to jump over.* The combined impact of such factors in preventing uptake could, thereby, easily mask considerable smoking uptake that might not have occurred in the absence of e-cigarettes [my emphasis] (Chapman, Bareham et al. 2019).

Systematic reviews and meta-analyses on youth uptake

For this reason, cohort studies which follow the same individual adolescents across a number of years are of critical importance for they provide relevant data at the individual level as well as at the cohort group level. There have been several recent systematic reviews and meta-analyses on the question of whether young people who vape have a higher probability of later taking up smoking compared to those who never vape (Khouja, Suddell et al. 2020, O'Brien, Long et al. 2020, Yoong, Hall et al. 2021).

Khouja et al. included 17 studies in their meta-analysis and found strong evidence for an association between e-cigarette use among non-smokers and later smoking (OR: 4.59, 95% CI: 3.60 to 5.85) when the results were meta-analysed in a random-effects model.

The Irish Health Research Board, in an analysis of nine cohort studies conducted with follow-up periods between four and 24 months, also found that adolescents who ever used ECs were four times more likely to start smoking cigarettes. The strength of association was statistically significant across all primary research studies. They commented that "the findings build a case towards a causal relationship as the findings are consistent across all studies included in the meta-analysis" (O'Brien, Long et al. 2020).

Common liability theory holds that those who use drugs share common latent traits which account for or explain much of their drug use. This theory is probably the favourite objection used by vaping advocates who often crudely paraphrase it by saying that "kids who try stuff, will try stuff" or "kids who will smoke, will smoke". This glib response has been repeatedly held aloft in arguments like an omnipotent crucifix before the evil gateway hypothesis vampire. It holds that children who are attracted to experiment with, say, vaping, may be more likely to have a propensity to be willing to try smoking and perhaps other "forbidden fruit" as well. These responses are voiced as self-evident truisms, with their circularity being seductive at first blush. However, any cessation researcher offering the equally trite "smokers who will quit, will quit" as a serious contribution to understanding the complexity of transitioning *out* of smoking, would be rightly pilloried for their primitive understanding of the complexities involved in reaching permanent smoking cessation.

There is a vast literature on the efficacy of smoking-cessation interventions where relevant mediating variables (for example: level of addiction, self-efficacy, levels of personal and professional support, planned versus unplanned and gradual versus rapid quit attempts) are measured, and then adjusted for in estimates of the contribution of the cessation drug or intervention. Yet common liability supporters argue that the hypothesis can explain all the main claims of the gateway hypothesis: all we need to say about anyone who smokes regularly is that they had a "propensity" to do so. If this hard determinism was all that was needed to be invoked in understanding smoking uptake, how then do we explain the dramatic falls in uptake that have been seen in nations which have robust tobacco control programs? What eroded that "propensity" to smoke so dramatically? Liability to nicotine dependence may well be a predisposing factor. But what of the known tractable reinforcing and enabling factors that tobacco control has so successfully identified and addressed over decades?

Most importantly and very awkwardly for this hypothesis, several longitudinal studies have reported that the strongest association between EC use and smoking initiation is among youth with the lowest risk of smoking (Primack, Soneji et al. 2015, Barrington-Trimis, Urman et al. 2016, Wills, Knight et al. 2017). Moreover, evidence using US National Youth Tobacco survey data shows that a third of youth who start with ECs have risk profiles that make them unlikely to start smoking (Dutra and Glantz 2017).

A 2021 paper in *Addiction* (Staff, Kelly et al. 2021) looked at adolescent EC use and tobacco smoking in the UK's huge Millennium Cohort Study. It concluded:

> Among youth who had not smoked tobacco by age 14 ($n = 9,046$), logistic regressions estimated that teenagers who used e-cigarettes by age 14 compared with non-e-cigarette users, had more than five times higher odds of initiating tobacco smoking by age 17 and nearly triple the odds of being a frequent tobacco smoker at age 17, net of risk factors and demographics.

Very importantly, the paper also knocked the stuffing out of the glib "kids who try stuff, will try stuff" common-liability theory adherents' dismissal of the concern that vaping acts as training wheels for later smoking uptake. In their analysis, the authors controlled for a rich constellation of "propensity" to smoke factors that have been suggested by common liability theory adherents to predict smoking uptake in youth. These included parental educational attainment and employment status; parental reports of each child's behaviour during the prior six months using the Strengths and Difficulties Questionnaire, with indicators of externalising behaviours (i.e. conduct problems, hyperactivity, inattention), and internalising behaviours (i.e. emotional symptoms, peer problems); parental smoking; whether a child spent time "most days" after school and at weekends hanging out with friends without adults or older youth present. Young people, via confidential self-reports, indicated whether they had ever drunk alcohol (more than a few sips), ever engaged in delinquency (e.g. theft, vandalism) and whether their friends smoked cigarettes. The authors concluded:

> we found little support that measured confounders drove the relationships between e-cigarettes and tobacco use, as the age 14 e-cigarette and tobacco cigarette estimates barely changed with the inclusion of confounders or in matched samples. Furthermore, early e-cigarette users did not share the same risk factors as early tobacco smokers, as only half the risk factors distinguished e-cigarette users from non-users, whereas age 14 tobacco smokers were overrepresented on almost all the antecedent risk factors. If there was a common liability, we would expect similar over-representation for users of both forms of nicotine.

Flavours and vaping

NVPs have many aspects of appeal that differentiate them from cigarettes, NRT and other smoking-cessation pharmaceuticals. These include claims about them being much less harmful, being generally less expensive than cigarettes, being less astringently malodorous than cigarettes and providing continuity of the hand-to-mouth cigarette ritual. But perhaps the most prominent of the appeals is the cornucopia of beguiling flavours available to vapers which drives huge consumer demand, including among adolescents. I recently asked my 11-year-old granddaughter about what she thought attracted some of her Year 6 classmates to vaping. Instantly she replied, "You can get lemonade flavour!"

NVP flavours are very relevant to the focus of this book because if evidence demonstrated that vaping was an effective way to obtain a significant population level increase in quitting, and flavours were an important factor in attracting smokers to switch to vaping, then this would be an important argument in their favour.

However, we would still need to consider any potential downsides to the proliferation of vaping (such as non-smoking teenagers commencing vaping) in any risk–benefit analysis of their likely net effect. And here e-cigarette flavours wave a large red flag. A huge clue to one of these downsides lies in looking at the non-use of flavours in medicines that are inhaled daily all over the world.

Why aren't asthma inhalers flavoured?

Australia, with a population of some 25 million, has about 2.7 million people living with asthma (Australian Institute of Health and Welfare 2020a), and some 464,000 with chronic obstructive pulmonary disease. Most of both groups use salbutamol inhalers ("puffers") for relief, sometimes at lifesaving moments. But significantly, none of the asthma drugs that are inhaled come in flavours which might make them more palatable. Respiratory medicine colleagues tell me that many users, particularly children do not enjoy their distinctive medicinal taste. We'd therefore imagine that the manufacturers of inhaled medicines would jump at any opportunity to add flavours to puffers if this would encourage more people to use them when needed. It is unimaginable that pharmaceutical companies manufacturing them would not have long been aware of this unpleasant taste downside to their products and tried to find any way possible to have drug regulatory agencies allow them to add flavours as we see happen with infant cough mixtures, for example.

But none has done so.

One of the big reasons for this is undoubtedly because asthma products have to go through therapeutic goods regulation. The two considerations there are efficacy and safety. Efficacy refers to how well a drug performs in doing what it is supposed to do – so here, helping smokers quit. As we will see later in this chapter, when it comes to the question of how well vaping performs in helping smokers quit, the answer is 'very poorly'. The pharmaceutical industry knows it would struggle to demonstrate that inhaling flavours is acceptably safe in the ways they would be used by vapers.

In 2014, there were already 7,764 unique vaping flavour names being sold online (Tierney, Karpinski et al. 2016). In 2016–17 this had more than doubled to 15,586 (Hsu, Sun et al. 2018). In 2017 Professor Robert West was confident this was unlikely to be a problem: "Now some concerns have been raised about the risk that might be attending to the flavourings in e-cigarette vapour but again, these are flavourings that have been tested and the concentrations are sufficiently low that we wouldn't expect them to pose a significant health risk" (Public Health England 2017).

So is it indeed the case that these flavouring chemicals have all been "tested" and cleared by government food and drug regulatory bodies as safe to inhale? Well, no.

The peak flavour manufacturers association in the USA, the Flavor and Extracts Manufacturers Association (FEMA) stated in 2021:

1. There is no apparent direct regulatory authority in the United States to use flavors in e-cigarettes. In this context, it is important to note that the "generally recognized as safe" (GRAS) provision in Section 201(s) of the Federal Food, Drug, and Cosmetic Act (FFDCA) applies only to food as defined in Section 201(f) of the Act.
2. None of the primary safety assessment programs for flavors, including the GRAS program sponsored by the Flavor and Extract Manufacturers Association of the United States (FEMA), evaluate flavor ingredients for use in products other than human food. FEMA GRAS status for the uses of a flavor ingredient in food does not provide regulatory authority to use the flavor ingredient in e-cigarettes in the US.
3. E-cigarette manufacturers should not represent or suggest that the flavor ingredients used in their products are safe because they have FEMA GRAS status for use in food because such statements are false and misleading (Flavor and Extracts Manufacturing Association (FEMA) 2021).

6 Vaping to quit: the latest mass distraction

In summary, some flavouring chemicals likely to be used in EC liquid may have been assessed as safe to ingest, but not to inhale.

The FEMA statement above is worth thinking about. Here is an association representing an industry which exists to promote and safeguard the interests of manufacturers of chemical flavours. Vaping would represent a massive additional source of demand for flavouring chemicals for the chemical companies in that industry. Yet here we have FEMA going out of its way to explicitly warn that no one should ever suggest that inhaling vapourised chemical flavours is safe as this would be false and misleading.

Flavours are a major factor in attracting people to vape. For example, 83% of New Zealand vapers named flavouring as a main reason they took up vaping (Gendall and Hoek 2021). We also know that flavours are a big factor that attract children and adolescents to vaping (Ranney 2019). Liquid nicotine manufacturers have paid close attention to these appeals. Here are a few examples of flavours that would be a big hit when announced at any five-year-old's birthday party: Cherry Crush, Vivid Vanilla, Banana Split, Cotton Candy, Rocket Pop, Gummy Bears (Campaign for Tobacco-Free Kids 2014).

Vaping advocates argue that regulators should keep their hands off flavours because they are a major factor attracting smokers to try to keep vaping, which these advocates of course believe should be very much encouraged. As the then head of the Foundation for a Smoke-Free World, an agency entirely funded by the tobacco company Philip Morris International, tweeted on 21 February 2021, "E-cigarette flavor bans will drive more people back to smoking – InsideSources. Responsible regulators should take note. In their zeal to address youth vaping they may well undermine the health of millions of smokers seeking to switch. @US_FDA" (Yach 2019).

So apparently, those concerned to stem the dramatic rises in regular vaping by teens in several nations which have followed the opening the e-cigarette access floodgates should get their priorities right. They should always put the interests of adult vapers ahead of preventive efforts to reduce the uptake of vaping by children.

The US Food and Drug Administration (USFDA) in late August 2021 took a decidedly different view of the risk–benefit balance when it came to flavoured vapes. Announcing that it had issued marketing denial orders over 55,000 flavoured vaping products submitted by three manufacturers, it said the applications "lacked sufficient evidence that they have a benefit to adult smokers sufficient to overcome the public health threat posed by the well-documented, alarming levels of youth use of such products" (US Food and Drug Administration 2021a). By September 2021, 295 Marketing Denial Orders had been issued by the USFDA for flavoured NVPs which impacted an estimated 1,089,000 flavours (Tobacco Business 2021).

Jordt et al. using gas chromatography, mass spectrometry and nuclear magnetic resonance spectroscopy and observed that:

> flavour aldehydes such as vanillin (vanilla flavor) and benzaldehyde (berry/fruit flavor) rapidly undergo chemical reactions with the E-liquid solvents PG and VG after mixing. The chemical adducts formed, named aldehyde PG/VG acetals, are carried over into the aerosol and are stable at physiological conditions.
>
> Toxicological tests reveal that these compounds activate the sensory irritant receptors TRPV1 and TRPA1, involved in triggering cough, secretions and cardiovascular reflexes to irritant inhalation. The aldehyde acetals activate these receptors more robustly and potently than the parent aldehydes. Comparison of the cytotoxic effects of parent aldehydes and acetals in cultured bronchial epithelial cells demonstrate that acetals induce cell death at lower concentrations. Analysis of mitochondrial respiration and glycolysis reveal that flavor aldehyde acetals suppress mitochondrial oxygen consumption and ATP production.
>
> These findings suggest that electronic cigarettes release unstable chemical mixtures containing a large variety of chemical products with unexpected toxicological properties (Jordt, Caceres et al. 2020).

In summary, the authors found that "flavourings combine with solvents in e-cigarettes to produce new toxic chemicals that irritate the airways, triggering reactions that can lead to breathing and heart and blood vessel problems". The lead author commented, "This is the first demonstration that these new chemicals formed in e-liquids can damage and kill lung cells and probably do this by damaging their

6 Vaping to quit: the latest mass distraction

metabolism. Although, in some cases, more than 40% of flavour chemicals are converted into new chemicals in e-cigarettes, almost nothing was known about their toxicity until now" (European Lung Foundation 2020).

Despite such evidence, a 2021 review of 58 research reports on e-cigarette flavours and young people found "no included reports of adverse effects of flavours" in studies where the "quality of the evidence was very low". The authors nonetheless found that the evidence "suggested that flavours are important for initiation and continuation of vaping. Qualitative evidence shows interest and enjoyment in flavours" (Notley, Gentry et al. 2021), which explains a great deal about why vaping interest groups defend flavours to the death.

In November 2020, Clive Bates gave evidence to the Australian Senate's inquiry into vaping (Australian Senate 2020a):

> Senator Urquhart: A lot of these flavourings are approved for ingestion in foods but not for inhalation into your lungs.
> Mr Bates: You're right. Many of them haven't been evaluated for inhalation. They are generally recognised as safe as food additives and they're added to these products to make them appealing. So you're right. They don't have —
> Senator Urquhart: I don't want to cut you off. I don't want to do that at all, but I am pressing for time. I just want to try and get the justification for how it can be safe to inhale stuff that is not meant to be inhaled into your lungs ...
> Mr Bates: ... With vaping, they're not moving to a situation where they're inhaling chemicals we know to be dangerous – where there are known dangers, the manufacturers tend not to put them in – but they're moving to inhaling chemicals that at least at one level have been recognised as safe for ingestion. But you're perfectly correct; most of the flavours have not been evaluated as safe for inhalation.

This is why the vaping industry and its facilitators have fought proposals for therapeutic regulation and instead want their products to bypass safety standards that they would try in vain to demonstrate.

Instead, they effectively argue that the public health and human rights imperatives to allow unimpeded access to vaping are so stratospherically important that e-cigarettes should be accorded exceptional status, allowing them to be exempted from any regulations that might prevent maximum uptake. This of course is an argument that has often been made by purveyors of quack cures for a wide range of deadly diseases, including cancer, HIV and COVID-19 (Dyer 2018, Australian Associated Press 2021). No sensible person believes that breathless claims and testimonies for these shonky and often dangerous treatments should raise them above regulatory scrutiny, but many evangelical vaping advocates believe NVPs are too important to be seriously regulated.

Without the choice of thousands of untested flavours, they argue that many vapers would abandon vaping, regardless of their conviction that these products are saving their lives. Yet people living with asthma who know that salbutamol is critical for control of asthma attacks don't abandon their unflavoured puffers because they don't taste the best.

How many puffs a day do vapers take?

Finally, there is also an important difference between inhaling flavoured nicotine and using an asthma puffer or attending a theatre performance once in a while when theatrical fog using propylene glycol (also found in EC vapour) might waft into the audience for a minute or two. People who use asthma puffers are advised that it is safe to use them 4–6 times a day maximum. Let's contrast this with the number of times that the average vaper fills their lungs with propylene glycol, nicotine and flavouring chemicals, all vaporised from the liquid that is heated by the metal coil heated by the e-cigarette battery.

A 2020 study monitoring vaping found those who were exclusive vapers pulled this cocktail deep into their lungs from point-blank range on average 173 times a day – 63,188 times a year. Those who were dual users (i.e. who vaped but still smoked) basted their lungs 72 times a day with their e-cigarettes in addition to the smoke from their smoking (Yingst, Foulds et al. 2020). Another study found the average daily number of puffs taken was 200, with a range up to 611 (Martin, Clapp et al. 2016). A third study, where researchers observed vapers using their normal vaping equipment *ad libitum* (as often as they pleased) for 90 minutes, reported the median number of puffs taken over 90 mins was 71 (i.e. 0.78 puffs per minute or 47.3 per hour) (St Helen, Ross et al. 2016). If a person vaped for 12 hours a day at that rate, this would translate to 568 puffs across a 12-hour day or 207,462 times in a year.

We can contrast this with the number of puffs today's average 12-cigarettes-a-day smoker inhales. One study observing puff frequency in those smoking in social settings recorded an average of 8.7 puffs per cigarette with an average 38.6-second gap between puffs (Chapman, Haddad et al. 1997). At 12 cigarettes a day, this would translate to 104 puffs per day or 38,106 per year. So vapers' puffing compared to smoking occurs at an almost frantic rate, making a mockery of the bizarre denialism often seen in vaping chat rooms insisting that vaped nicotine is not addictive.

Evidence on the effectiveness of e-cigarettes in smoking cessation

On 6 July 2017 submissions closed on an Australian House of Representatives committee considering the regulation of e-cigarettes. The 332 submissions included many individuals' personal stories explaining that e-cigarettes had succeeded in helping them quit when other methods had failed (House of Representatives Standing Committee on Health, Aged Care and Sport 2017). Many wrote passionately about having tried and failed with other ways of stopping smoking. Some made statements about their health rapidly improving. They wanted to spread their good news and encourage others to try to do what they had done. Many of these stories would have been very real: most of us have heard of someone who has quit through vaping.

It is certainly true that around the world there are many such cases. But just as we would never conclude that drink-driving was not risky after counting the number of people who drove after drinking and suffered or caused no harm, we should never conclude that any given method is an effective way to quit smoking by listening only to those who say they have benefitted from it.

Parliamentary inquiries into quackery such as homeopathy and naturopathy would doubtless see passionate submissions from former smokers about how these methods had helped them quit. But the public policy question is whether such strategies actually make smoking cessation more likely when studied under suitably controlled research conditions.

As I discussed in Chapter 2, we do not assess evidence on smoking cessation by only considering examples of success. There were no submissions to the House of Representatives committee from the smokers who had switched to vaping but failed or did not even attempt to quit, as there were no such submissions to yet another inquiry held by the Australian Senate in 2020 (Australian Senate 2020b). Yet in 2019, there were close to half a million such people in Australia who had started vaping but no longer did, almost double the number of current daily vapers (see Table 6.1).

The 2019 national data in Table 6.1 are sourced from the Australian Institute of Health and Welfare's national household survey where the AIHW describes "current" vaping (in a footnote to Table 2.23) as including people who reported "using electronic cigarettes daily, weekly, monthly or less than monthly". So that means "current vaping" in the last year includes people who might have had a puff or two at a party out of curiosity, 15-year-olds passing an e-cigarette around after school once or twice at the local skate ramp and those who bought vaping gear, tried it a few times and then put it in the drawer with other seemed-like-a-good-idea-at-the-time, five-day wonders.

Had I been swept up in such an AIHW sample a few years ago, the "current vaping" cohort also would have included me because I once had a pull on an e-cigarette to see what it was like. So are many of these 527,000 people any more meaningfully "current" vapers than I am a current Aston Martin driver (because I've driven one once), a current Chateau Laffite drinker (I shared one with friends once) or a current guest at Australian prime ministers' houses (because I attended a fundraiser at one once)?

Vaping advocates pitch their most emotional appeals for policy change around profiles of heavy smokers who they say have often tried to quit and failed. This profile could only reasonably be applied to daily vapers, not those who smoke every day and vape very occasionally, nor those who are not nicotine dependent and neither smoke nor vape every day. So this means we are talking about some 222,000 Australians 14 years and over who are daily vapers in a population of some 25 million

Table 6.1 Vaping status of Australian e-cigarette users (Source: Australian Institute of Health and Welfare 2020c).

Vaping status	% of those who have ever vaped	Estimated number
Daily	9.4	222,000
At least weekly (but not daily)	5.1	127,447
At least monthly (but not weekly)	3.4	80,298
At least monthly	17.9	422,744
Less than monthly	4.4	103,915
"Current" vaping		526,659
I used to use them, but no longer use	18.1	427,468
I only tried them once or twice	59.6	1,407,573

people. A substantial proportion of this group will be dual users who continue to vape *and* smoke and, importantly, have no plans to quit.

This is because it is very wrong to imply that all who are vaping today are former and current smokers who started vaping to quit smoking. The 2019 AIHW survey (at Table 2.32) reported that 51.2% of current e-cigarette users vaped to try and help them quit smoking. A recent paper from the ITC Four Country Survey (Australia, USA, UK, Canada) found that "among smokers who also vaped, 46% planned to quit smoking within six months, 30% planned to quit in the future, but beyond six months, with the remaining 24% reporting that they did not know or did not plan on quitting, suggesting low motivation to quit smoking among many of the concurrent [both smoking and vaping] users" (Gravely, Cummings et al. 2021). "Planning to quit" is also a very soft, rubbery measure, liable to be pregnant with social desirability response biases and often not full of much conviction.

So it is very clear that many dual users (who both vape and smoke) are not at all desperate or even interested in quitting smoking. We need to strongly oppose regulatory policy which puts the flavour-experimenting interests of vapers who don't intend to quit ahead of policies that keep beguilingly flavoured vapes well out of the reach of children.

Recent reviews of the evidence on cessation

I'll now summarise what we know from the best evidence available about how well NVP users go with quitting smoking. The following 17 reviews of the evidence and position statements by professional health associations published since 2017 have concluded that the evidence for e-cigarettes being effective for smoking cessation is inconclusive, insufficient, weak or inadequate:

- (2021) Wang et al: Meta-analysis of 55 observational studies: "As consumer products, in observational studies, e-cigarettes were not associated with increased smoking cessation in the adult population" (Wang, Bhadriraju et al. 2021).
- (2021) Zhang et al: "Evidence from 9 cohort studies showed that e-cigarette use was not associated with cessation" (Zhang, Bu et al. 2021).
- (2021) WHO: "To date, evidence on the use of ENDS [Electronic Nicotine Delivery Systems] as a cessation aid is inconclusive" (World Health Organization 2021).
- (2021) US Preventive Health Services Task Force: "The USPHSTF concludes that the current evidence is insufficient to assess the balance of benefits and harms of e-cigarettes for tobacco cessation in adults." (Krist, Davidson et al. 2021).
- (2021) WHO Study Group on Tobacco Product Regulation (TobReg): "There is insufficient evidence that HTPs (heated tobacco products) aid a switch from smoking. Therefore, claims should not be made to that effect. Even if future evidence supported HTPs as effective switching aids (i.e. substituting one tobacco product for another), they should never be considered as treatment for smoking cessation, which includes quitting nicotine use" (WHO Study Group on Tobacco Product Regulation 2021).
- (2021) European Commission's Scientific Committee on Health, Environment and Emerging Risks (SCHEER): "There is weak evidence for the support of electronic cigarettes' effectiveness in helping smokers to quit while the evidence on smoking reduction is assessed as weak to moderate" (Scientific Committee on Health 2021).

- (2020) United States Surgeon General's report on smoking cessation: "there is presently inadequate evidence to conclude that e-cigarettes, in general, increase smoking cessation" (United States Surgeon General 2020).
- (2020) Ireland's Health Research Board: "there is no evidence of a difference in effect on incidences of smoking cessation. There is a low-level of certainty in these results due to low successful event rates and high rates lost to follow-up in all studies" (Quigley, Kennelly et al. 2020).
- (2020) Australian National University (preliminary report): "there is insufficient evidence that nicotine-delivering e-cigarettes are efficacious for smoking cessation, compared to no intervention, placebo existing nicotine-replacement therapy or other best-practice interventions" (Banks, Beckwith et al. 2020).
- (2020) Thoracic Society of Australia and New Zealand: "Smokers who enquire about using e-cigarettes as a cessation aid should be provided with appropriate information about approved medication in conjunction with behavioural support (as these have the strongest evidence of efficacy to date). E-cigarettes are not the first-line treatment for smoking cessation" (McDonald, Jones et al. 2020).
- (2021) Grabovac and others (Effectiveness of Electronic Cigarettes in Smoking Cessation: a Systematic Review and Meta-Analysis): "nicotine-ECs may be more effective in smoking cessation when compared to placebo ECs or NRT. When compared to counselling alone, nicotine ECs are more effective short-term but its effectiveness appears to diminish with later follow-ups. Given the small number of studies, heterogeneous design and the overall moderate to low quality of evidence, it is not possible to offer clear recommendations" (Grabovac, Oberndorfer et al. 2021).
- (2020) Public Health England: "The data presented here suggests [sic] that vaping has not undermined the declines in adult smoking." Note that they presented no evidence that vaping, endorsed and widely promoted by PHE, had accelerated the decline in smoking in the UK. This is to my knowledge the first time that PHE has taken such a lukewarm position on the impact of vaping on smoking rates (McNeill, Brose et al. 2020).

- (2019) European Respiratory Society: "There is not enough scientific evidence to support e-cigarettes as an aid to smoking cessation" (Bals, Boyd et al. 2019).
- (2018) US National Academies of Science, Engineering and Medicine – a "review of reviews". "Conclusion 17-1. Overall, there is limited evidence that e-cigarettes may be effective aids to promote smoking cessation" (National Academies of Science, Engineering and Medicine 2018).
- (2018) European Public Health Association: "e-cigarettes may help some smokers quit but, for most, e-cigarettes depress quitting" (European Public Health Association 2018).
- (2018) CSIRO Australia: "While many smokers and former smokers state a preference for e-cigarettes as a smoking cessation method, the effectiveness of this method compared with other smoking cessation methods is not known" (Byrne, Brindal et al. 2018).
- (2017) El Dib et al.: A systematic review and meta-analysis of three RCTs and nine cohort studies concluded: "There is very limited evidence regarding the impact of [e-cigarettes] on tobacco smoking cessation, reduction or adverse effects: data from RCTs are of low certainty and observational studies of very low certainty. The limitations of the cohort studies led us to a rating of very low-certainty evidence from which no credible inferences can be drawn" (El Dib, Suzumura et al. 2017).

It remains true that, as summarised in the 2020 US Surgeon General's report on smoking cessation, and cited as recently as October 2020 in an authoritative article by the heads of the US Centers for Disease Control, the Food and Drug Administration and the National Cancer Institute in the *New England Journal of Medicine*, "there is presently inadequate evidence to conclude that e-cigarettes, in general, increase smoking cessation" (Redfield, Hahn et al. 2020).

Randomised controlled trials (RCTs)

A 2021 Cochrane update of the evidence from three concluded randomised controlled trials on e-cigarettes in smoking cessation concluded that there was "moderate-certainty evidence, limited by imprecision, that quit rates were higher in people randomized to nicotine

EC than in those randomized to nicotine replacement therapy (NRT) (risk ratio (RR) 1.69, 95% confidence interval (CI) 1.25 to 2.27; 3 studies, 1498 participants)" (Hartmann-Boyce, McRobbie et al. 2021).

In terms that the general public might better understand, the review stated, "For every 100 people using nicotine e-cigarettes to stop smoking, 10 might successfully stop, compared with only six of 100 people using nicotine-replacement therapy or nicotine-free e-cigarettes, or four of 100 people having no support or behavioural support only." Or to put it another way, if we take 100 smokers participating in an RCT, 90 would still be smoking six months later if they used e-cigarettes, compared with 94 who used NRT, and 96 who just tried to quit alone or got some "behavioural support".

Australian vaping advocates tried valiantly to spin this as e-cigarettes having been "proclaimed by the gold standard of RCT evaluation as being 70% more effective than NRT", presumably taking the RR of 1.69 as being the most flattering angle that they could find.

But there can be few if any other drugs, used for *any* purpose, which have even come close to the dismal success rate of e-cigarettes or NRT in achieving their main outcome. If we went along to a doctor for a health problem and were told, "Here, take this. It has a 90% failure rate. But let's both agree to call this successful," we would understandably take the view that "success" when used in this context was not the way that it is used in any other treatment context, or indeed *any* context.

Importantly, as we saw in Chapter 2, results obtained from RCTs do not reflect those obtained in real-world use where "success" is often even much worse. RCTs exclude many people from high smoking prevalence population sub-groups (e.g. those with mental health problems, drug and alcohol problems); participants in RCTs are subject to a wide range of cohort retention strategies to prevent them dropping out of the trial – as happens commonly in real-world use; and participants are paid and given free quit-smoking medication (including e-cigarettes).

When considered together, all the above problems make the match with RCTs on smoking cessation a far cry from the way smokers use NRT and e-cigarettes in the real world. But this has not stopped wide-eyed commentaries about "effectiveness", as if these artificially constructed trials bore any resemblance to the spread, patterns and conditions of use in communities.

Let's look in more detail at one of the most recent RCTs.

In February 2019, Hajek and others published results in the *New England Journal of Medicine* of an RCT of nicotine replacement therapy (NRT n=446) versus use of a second-generation refillable e-cigarette device (n=438). Subjects were all self-selecting attendees at UK National Health Service stop-smoking services (Hajek, Phillips-Waller et al. 2019). Randomisation into the different arms of the RCT began after they had set a quit date. Astonishingly, dual users (the most common way that e-cigarettes are used) were excluded. So this was a study of smokers who were anything but a random sample of smokers from the UK smoking population.

The paper attracted considerable attention as it was a randomised study with an active control arm and used modern e-cigarette devices. Compared to previous RCTs which used earlier generation e-cigarettes, it had a substantially greater effect size with a relative risk of 1.75–1.84 (depending on adjustments and exclusion of certain subjects) for the primary outcome variable of continuous abstinence at 52 weeks. In media coverage, this effect was often rounded up to a doubling of smoking cessation compared to NRT.

Largely unreported in news coverage of this study was that ongoing use of e-cigarettes by 80% of subjects in the EC arm did not prevent relapse – the relative risk of relapse by 52 weeks in those who quit with EC rather than NRT was 1.27.

Significantly, all trial participants also received "weekly behavioural support for at least 4 weeks", with the authors noting in their conclusion that "E-cigarettes were more effective for smoking cessation than nicotine-replacement therapy, *when both products were accompanied by behavioral support*" [my emphasis]. This support "involved weekly one-on-one sessions with local clinicians, who also monitored expired carbon monoxide levels for at least four weeks after the quit date". Eighty-one percent of participants received four or five support sessions. So this was far from being a "brief advice" intervention situation.

However, in real-world use of either NRT or e-cigarettes for smoking cessation, only a tiny proportion of smokers ever receive such support. Important questions therefore arise about the relative contributions of NRT and NVPs, compared with that of the support which all trialists received. A study of a national English prospective cohort of 1,560 smokers found "the adjusted odds of remaining abstinent up to the time of the six-month follow-up survey were 2.58 times higher in users of prescription medication in combination with specialist behavioral support". Notably though, the use of NRT bought over the counter was associated with a lower odds of abstinence (odds ratio, 0.68), compared with smokers not using NRT (Kotz, Brown et al. 2014). In other words, using NRT without behavioural support might be actually *preventing* some from quitting. It's possible that the same might be true for e-cigarettes. But because all participants received behavioural support, we will never know.

Late in 2021, results of an Australian RCT were published (Morphett, Fraser et al. 2021). In a pragmatic trial that sought to assess quitting outcomes in as naturalistic conditions as possible (reflecting many of the concerns I raised in Chapter 2), smoking participants were randomised into three groups. One group was offered free first generation (cigalike), unflavoured ECs and/or NRT. At seven months' follow-up a desultory 1.3% (8 of 619) assigned to that group self-reported that they were no longer smoking. Vaping advocates will shrug off this result, pointing out the irrelevancy in 2021 of a trial of first-generation, unflavoured cigalikes, which very few vapers use today. But an interesting question remains: why did a trial which was conducted in 2014–15, with 12 months' follow-up, take until December 2021 to be published? It is difficult to imagine any circumstance where a trial showing positive results would have remained unpublished for such a time.

Cessation and dual use (vaping and smoking)

Before looking further at the evidence from longitudinal cohort studies of the effectiveness of NVPs in smoking cessation, it's important to note that there is evidence of under-reporting of continuing smoking among vapers. Using biomarker data on the tobacco-specific nitrosamine NNK from those who provided it in the PATH study, Goniewicz and Smith estimated that one in six of those self-reporting as exclusive vapers were still smoking (Goniewicz, Smith et al. 2018). This major caveat should be kept in mind when reading summaries of the research on quitting to follow.

Unlike NRT, where persistent use is uncommon after six months (2.3% of NRT gum users, 0.9% for patch, with 0.4% persistent use of any NRT after 24 months) (Shiffman, Hughes et al. 2003), those who take up vaping can stay with it for years.

And importantly, a majority of those who vape also smoke (dual use). A stock tenet of vaping advocacy theology is that anyone who is a dual user should always be understood to be perpetually in the process of transitioning to completely quitting smoking. It doesn't matter how long they have been vaping: if they are still smoking, they are still working hard on quitting smoking and should never be seen as a person who is smoking and vaping and not planning to stop either. Repeat often: dual users should always be counted as success stories in progress. If you follow a dual user down the track from when a cohort study first counts them as a dual user, at some future follow-up when they are interviewed, they are highly likely to have kicked smoking and now be an exclusive vaper, so the theology goes.

US PATH cohort study findings

Unfortunately for that argument, we have excellent longitudinal cohort data from the USA that shines bright warts-and-all-revealing light on its veracity. The US Population Assessment of Tobacco and Health (PATH) project (funded by the USFDA and the National Institutes of Health) has been collecting national cohort data on 46,000 Americans since 2013 (Hyland, Ambrose et al. 2017). These are the best data we have on real-world use of NVPs, and with PATH's longitudinal design involving interviews with the same individuals every year, analyses from the data are peerless as a guide to the effectiveness of NVPs, unconstrained by the many limitations of RCTs that I discussed in Chapter 2.

I noted earlier that many who vape and keep smoking have little serious interest in quitting. With this being the case, analyses of quit rates among *all* who vape are bound to be heavily diluted by the inclusion of such vapers in the denominators of the studied population.

Many dual users continue to smoke and vape at follow-ups because they were never interested in quitting. This has seen researchers report results for frequent vapers apart from those of all vapers, reasoning that infrequent vapers were probably far more likely to be smokers not trying to transition. A PATH report by Glasser and colleagues analysed three waves of PATH data from 2013 to 2016. Like other PATH studies, the odds of quitting when all vapers were included, were found to be insignificantly different to those smokers who didn't vape. But "consistent and frequent e-cigarette use over time is associated with cigarette smoking cessation among adults" (Glasser, Vojjala et al. 2021). So it follows that frequent use of e-cigarettes being associated with higher quit rates should be seen as encouraging news, yes? Undoubtedly, except when we take a close look at the desultory numbers involved.

There were 5,894 participants using e-cigarettes at the beginning of the study. But only 78 (1%), were "consistent and frequent" users of e-cigarettes. For that 1% of users, quitting with e-cigarettes was more successful, but this was hardly a finding signalling that we are looking at results portending a major population-wide tsunami of quitting via vaping in the USA. If we take all who vape together, there's no net story about way more quitting than when we compare smokers who don't vape.

And another question we might ask here is about how many vapers who were trying to quit smoking also stopped using e-cigarettes by the 2016 follow-up? The Glasser paper does not provide that data. But Pierce and colleagues, analysing the same PATH data sets across the same years did look at this question (Pierce, Benmarhnia et al. 2020). Are you ready?

"None in the daily e-cigarette use group ($n=56$) and 45% of the no e-cigarette group ($n=162$) were abstinent from all tobacco (including e-cigarettes) for 12+ months at Wave 3." Not one e-cigarette user who was using e-cigarettes to quit was able to quit both cigarette and e-cigarettes after three years. The heat generated from the excited rubbing of hands together in Big Tobacco boardrooms on learning this must have been formidable.

Another PATH paper by Coleman and others reported on a 12-month follow-up (Wave 1 to Wave 2) of 2,932 vapers (Coleman, Rostron et al. 2019). Table 6.2 using data from the paper shows that

Table 6.2 Summary of e-cigarette transitions from Wave 1 to Wave 2 by cigarette smoking status (n=2932) derived from (Coleman, Rostron et al. 2019).

Positive outcome at Wave 2 n=524 (17.9%)	Negative outcome at Wave 2 n=1116 (38%)	Remained the same n=1291 (44%)
143 dual users who quit EC and smoking	886 dual users who relapsed to smoking exclusively	902 dual users continuing as dual users
104 dual users who became exclusive EC users	109 exclusive EC users who progressed to smoking	389 EC users continuing as exclusive EC users
277 exclusive EC users who quit EC	121 exclusive EC users who progressed to dual use	

for every person vaping at the Wave 1 assessment who benefitted across 12 months by quitting smoking and/or e-cigarettes, there were 2.1 who either relapsed or took up smoking having not been a smoker at baseline. The single most populous subgroup in the cohort were those who were dual users at wave 1 and remained dual users at Wave 2.

Ongoing dual use is not a beneficial, harm-reduction outcome from using e-cigarettes (I will look at the evidence for reducing smoking as compared with not smoking later in this chapter). So if we add these "stayed the same" dual users to those with negative outcomes in the left-hand column of the table, then for every positive outcome (left column), there were 3.85 negative outcomes in this cohort. Most disturbingly, in this adult cohort, nearly one in four of those who had never been established smokers took up smoking after first using e-cigarettes.

Another PATH paper (Dai and Leventhal 2019) found that in *long-term* quitters, relapse to smoking was 1.8%, 10.4%, 9.6% and 15% among never, prior, current occasional and current regular baseline e-cigarette users respectively. So regardless of how long people had vaped, relapse to smoking was between five and eight times higher than in those smokers who had quit but had never vaped. Big Tobacco could only be delighted by the 10% lapsing of long-term ex-smokers and 15% of vapers back to smoking. These were people they probably considered they had lost forever.

Still another PATH longitudinal paper (McMillen, Klein et al. 2019) reported that former smokers who had quit a long time ago but who vaped were far more likely than those who had never vaped to relapse back to smoking and that vapers were far more likely than those who had never vaped to have transitioned from being never smokers to smokers:

> Distant former combustible cigarette smokers who reported e-cigarette past 30-day use (9.3%) and ever use (6.7%) were significantly more likely than those who had never used e-cigarettes (1.3%) to have relapsed to current combustible cigarette smoking at follow-up ($P < .001$). Never smokers who reported e-cigarette past 30-day use (25.6%) and ever use (13.9%) were significantly more likely than those who had never used e-cigarettes (2.1%) to have initiated combustible cigarette smoking ($P < .001$). Adults who reported past 30-day e-cigarette use (7.0%) and ever e-cigarette use (1.7%) were more likely than those who had never used e-cigarettes (0.3%) to have transitioned from never smokers to current combustible cigarette smokers ($P < .001$). E-cigarette use predicted combustible cigarette smoking in multivariable analyses controlling for covariates.

Across 12 months follow-up, PATH data from 1,082 dual users of tobacco cigarettes and e-cigarettes, found 88.5% of dual users continued smoking, although the odds of being smoke-free at follow-up were higher among dual users who vaped every day (Miller, Smith et al. 2020).

As I've emphasised, not all vapers are trying to quit, so it is important to focus on long-term abstinence among those who tried to quit with and without use of e-cigarettes as a cessation aid. Another PATH paper looked at 2,535 adult smokers in 2014-2015 (baseline assessment), who, in 2015–16 reported a past-year attempt to quit and the cessation aids used, and then reported smoking status in 2016–17 where continuous abstinence from smoking for 12 months or more was the key outcome (Chen, Pierce et al. 2020). They found that among smokers using e-cigarettes to quit, 12.9% succeeded in long-term abstinence. But this was no different to the results seen in those trying to quit who did not use e-cigarettes. And some two-thirds of e-cigarette users who quit smoking kept vaping.

Again using PATH data from Waves 1-3 (2013-16), Osibogun et al (2020) examined transitions of adult dual users. Among 1,870 adult dual users at Wave 1, after two years, 55.2% had relapsed to smoking, 25.7% remained dual users (so 80.9% were still smoking) 7% were exclusively vaping and 12.1% reported no past-month smoking or vaping. They found that greater nicotine dependence was associated with decreased relative risk of no past-month tobacco use (Osibogun et al 2020).

In late 2021, Kasza et al. reported from PATH data from waves 2-5 (October 2014 to November 2019) that daily vapers who expressed no interest in quitting at Wave 1 were more likely to quit cigarette smoking than those who did not vape, while non-daily vapers were less likely to quit (although this effect was not statistically significant). The major limitation of this paper was the very small number of quitters – just three among the non-daily vaping group and 17 among those who vaped daily. Across the years of the study there were 2,489 data records from 1,600 individuals, so by only focusing on those smokers who indicated no intent to quit at the beginning of the wave series studied, and considering attrition from the cohort, this left a very small group with the outcomes described. A footnote to a table warned "Estimate should be interpreted with caution because it has low statistical precision" (Kasza et al. 2021).

A 2020 paper from the ITC Four Country Survey (Australia, USA, UK, Canada) found that after 18 months:

> smokers with established concurrent use [smoking and vaping] were not more likely to discontinue smoking compared to those not vaping … *it is clear that the rates of transitioning away from smoking remain unacceptably low*, and perhaps current vaping tools at best bring the likelihood of quitting up to comparable levels of less dependent smokers. The findings of our international study are consistent with the findings of the US PATH transition studies, and other observational studies, in that *most smokers remain in a persistent state of cigarette use across time, particularly the daily smokers* [my emphases] (Gravely, Meng et al. 2020).

Big Tobacco, now with major investments in NVPs, would have had all its fingers crossed in the hope that dual use would be as common as it is. And if they are wise investors, they would be also very confident that the net effect of vaping proliferation throughout the population will be to keep far more people in smoking than are tipped out of it, and that it will provide high adoption of nicotine-addiction training wheels to many children and adolescents who have never used any form of nicotine and probably never would have done.

Is vaping the primary cause of falls in smoking prevalence in nations where vaping is prevalent?

There are many factors which can combine to cause changes in smoking prevalence over time. Vaping advocates argue that nations with widespread vaping are seeing their falls in smoking prevalence accelerate mostly *because of* vaping.

Figure 6.3 is constructed from Smoking in England data (West, Kale et al. 2021) and suggests that the role of e-cigarettes in accelerating the downward trend in smoking in England could only be modest. The dramatic upsurge in smokers using e-cigarettes in quit attempts commenced in late 2012. Use has more or less plateaued since mid-2013 and does not appear to have had any marked association with the downward slope of the historically declining smoking prevalence rate.

However, if we look at the data on smoking prevalence and changes in tobacco affordability in the UK, we can see a rather different picture (Figure 6.4) (National Health Service Digital 2020). Smoking prevalence was falling well before vaping commenced and there is a close relationship between the decline in the affordability of tobacco and the fall in smoking prevalence. Cigarettes were 27% less affordable in the UK than they were in 2009. Vaping grew rapidly from around 2011 in the UK and did not alter the relationship between smoking prevalence and tobacco affordability.

Researchers from the Smoking in England project published a step-by-step estimation of the number of English smokers whose smoking cessation in 2014 could be attributed to e-cigarettes (West, Shahab et al. 2016). They took into account factors like an estimated 70% relapse back to smoking and the fact that e-cigarettes displace

Smoking rates vs Use of EC in quit attempts

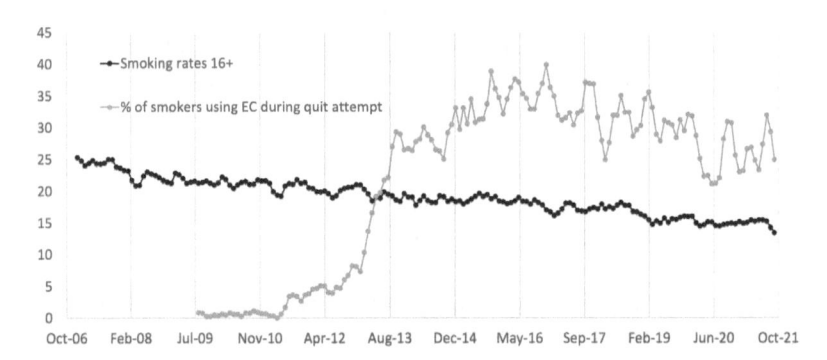

```
45
40    ──Smoking rates 16+
35
      ──% of smokers using EC during quit attempt
30
25
20
15
10
 5
 0
  Oct-06  Feb-08  Jul-09  Nov-10  Apr-12  Aug-13  Dec-14  May-16  Sep-17  Feb-19  Jun-20  Oct-21
```

Figure 6.3 English smoking prevalence and quit attempts using e-cigarettes (Source: Data extracted from Smoking in England website.) Note: From April 2020, data were collected by phone and from people 18 years and over. Before then, data were collected by household visits from people 16 years and over.

success rates that would have occurred via other methods (which fewer people use with the rise of e-cigarettes).

The group estimated that 16,000 smokers quit permanently in a population of 8.46 million adult smokers. That's about 0.19% shaved off England's smoking population in one year by e-cigarettes – just one in 529 smokers in a year quitting permanently.

For perspective, in Australia where the prevalence of regular vaping in the same data period examined by the above report was very marginal (only 1.5% of Australia's daily smokers and 0.8% of ex-smokers used e-cigarettes daily), smoking prevalence in those aged 14+ had declined over the 10 years between 2007 and 2016 (from 19.4% to 14.9%), an average of 0.45% a year. This decline reflected both smokers quitting and dying, and reductions in uptake.

Smoking prevalence has indeed fallen rapidly in England in recent years while e-cigarette use has increased. But it is simplistic to assume this is the only explanation needed. The trajectories for smoking prevalence and quit attempts differ from that for prevalence of use of e-cigarettes.

6 Vaping to quit: the latest mass distraction

Adult Smoking vs Tobacco Affordability – UK 2000-2019

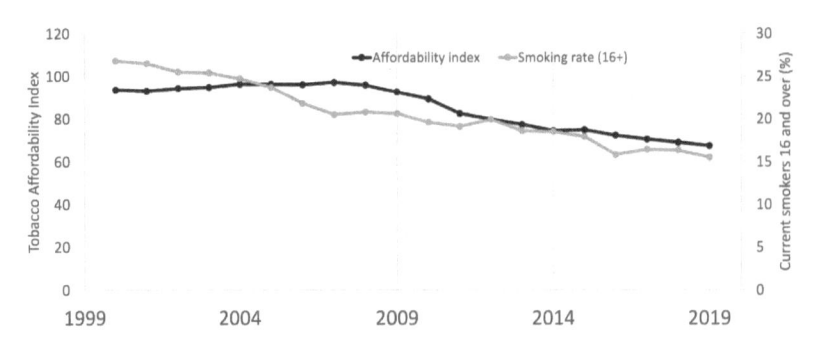

Figure 6.4 Changes in smoking prevalence in persons aged 15 and over and tobacco price index relative to retail price index (all items) 2000–19, UK. Source: Statistics on Smoking, England 2020; Smoking prevalence in the UK and the impact of data collection changes: 2020.

In fact, the reduction has occurred concurrently with a comprehensive program to reduce smoking. During that time there had been a spectacular decline in tobacco affordability, with cigarettes being 27% less affordable in 2016 than in 2006 (NHS Digital 2017) (see Figure 6.4).

Schooled by English experts

The Australian Senate Select Committee on Tobacco Harm Reduction's report was published in 2020 (Australian Senate 2020b). I was lead author on a submission to the Senate inquiry along with Mike Daube from Curtin University and Matthew Peters, a professor of respiratory medicine (Chapman, Daube et al. 2020). Four English tobacco control experts, Ann McNeill (McNeill 2020) and Jamie Brown, Lion Shahab and Robert West (Brown, Shahab et al. 2020) read our evidence and wrote to the committee, seeking to advise them of our errors in understanding the impact of vaping on declining smoking prevalence in England. We were invited to reply. The exchanges are very relevant to this section of the chapter.

Response to letters from Professors Brown, Shahab and West, and Professor McNeill

Professors Brown, Shahab and West's brief letter entitled *Impact of e-cigarettes on smoking in England* (Brown, Shahab et al. 2020) provides different conclusions from the data on the impact of e-cigarettes on smoking prevalence in England. They claim these conclusions as "the correct analyses". We would, however, note that:

In their 2016 *BMJ* paper (cited in their letter) they wrote:

> With quit attempts at 32.5% of eight million smokers (2.6 million) in 2015, and prevalence of e-cigarette use in quit attempts at 36% in that year, *this equates to 54,288 additional short to medium term quitters in 2015 compared with no use of e-cigarettes in quit attempts. We would expect up to two thirds of these individuals to relapse at some point in the future, so we would estimate that e-cigarettes may have contributed about 18,000 additional long term ex-smokers in 2015.* This figure is similar to that estimated indirectly using the estimated effect size of e-cigarettes and the numbers using them. Although these numbers are relatively small, they are broadly similar to previous estimates, and are clinically significant because of the huge health gains from stopping smoking. A 40 year old smoker who quits permanently can expect to gain nine life years compared with a continuing smoker. *This number of additional quitters is unlikely to produce a detectable effect on smoking prevalence in the short term, but might be picked up over a period of several years* [our emphases in italics] (Beard, West et al. 2016).

In their paper in *Addiction*, first published in 2019, they wrote:

> 845,152 smokers used e-cigarettes in quit attempts; this equates to 50,700 ... additional past-year smokers who report that they are no longer smoking as a consequence of e-cigarette use in a quit attempt in 2017. This is broadly similar to the estimate which we reported for 2015 (Beard, West et al. 2020).

We note that in their *Addiction* paper, the authors did not discount that figure by two-thirds relapsing in the future, as they did in their *BMJ* paper. If we apply that discount to the 845,152 smokers who used e-cigarettes in a quit attempt (50,700 who were not smoking in 2017 x 0.33) we get 16,731 (2%) ... who, by the authors' 2015 assumptions, would have quit in the long-term. (Expressed differently, 98% of smokers using e-cigarettes in quit attempts in England in a year are estimated to not quit in the long-term). This is a proportion very close to the quit rate (4%) for quit attempters allocated to no quitting support arms in the recent Cochrane trials update (Hartmann-Boyce, McRobbie et al. 2021).

So 16,731 of 7 million English smokers were additional long-term quitters in one year because of e-cigarettes: 1 in 418 of all English smokers. We heartily concur with Professors Brown, Shahab and West in their *BMJ* paper that "This number of additional quitters is unlikely to produce a detectable effect on smoking prevalence in the short term". The number span 16,000–18,000 is not well expressed as "tens of thousands a year" as they wrote in the preface to their submission, so we remain curious about why they believe our interpretation of their data is incorrect.

Brown et al.'s *BMJ* paper states that there were 8 million smokers in England in 2015 and their *Addiction* paper says this number had fallen to 7 million in 2017 (a fall of approximately 12.5% or 6.25% per annum). If we assume there were three full years encompassed in the 2015–17 period, there were three years of approximately 17,000 estimated additional long-term quitters between 2015 and 2017, then some 51,000 (5.1%) of the extra 1 million who were not smoking in 2017 might be attributable to e-cigarette use. The other 949,000 fewer smokers would be attributable to deaths of smokers, cessation by smokers other than via e-cigarettes, and increasing numbers of never smokers thanks to prevention policies and programs.

Recent US longitudinal data from the PATH cohort study across five years 2013–17 (Brouwer, Jeon et al. 2020) found:

> Cigarette use was persistent, with 89.7% (95% CI 89.1% to 90.3%) of exclusive cigarette users and 86.1% (95% CI 84.4% to 87.9%)

> of dual users remaining cigarette users (either exclusive or dual) after any one year

and

> Among all W1 (Wave 1 or baseline) daily smokers, there were no differences in discontinued smoking between daily smokers who vaped (concurrent users) and exclusive daily smokers.

A preliminary report of a Swiss study of over 5,000 young men (Gmel, Wicki et al. 2020) found no cessation effects and that non-current smokers (never- and ex-) and smokers at baseline were more likely to be smokers four years later if they subsequently had started vaping. The authors concluded that:

> Some smokers may have benefitted from using ECs, but they were few. At the general population level, ECs are not predominantly used in a way which might optimise reducing or ceasing smoking. Therefore, the public health effect on the general population of using ECs may be questionable, as may policy measures to facilitate EC use.

The 2020 *Addiction* paper showed that the proportion of smokers in England making quit attempts fell from almost 40% in 2013 to about 34% in 2017 (Beard, West et al. 2020). The definitions of quit attempts differ somewhat between the surveys used in different countries and quit rates will fall after periods when large numbers of smokers have already successfully quit (for instance, immediately following large tax increases). Nevertheless, in contrast to the 29% of smokers in England who made a quit attempt in 2019 (West, Kale et al. 2021) – the proportion of current smokers who report having attempted to quit in the previous 12 months in Australia – a country with much lower rates of use of e-cigarettes – was about 50% in 2007 and 2013 and was still 51% in 2019 (Australian Institute of Health and Welfare 2020d).

If the proportion of smokers trying to quit in England was approximately 50% rather than approximately 30%, an additional 1.4 million smokers would be making quit attempts each year, with an additional 56,000 likely to succeed even assuming no additional cessation support. The challenge for tobacco control in both nations is to simultaneously increase *both* the numerator of quit successes *and* the denominator of quit attempts.

All major companies in the global tobacco industry are now promoting putative harm-reduced products, while continuing to aggressively promote cigarettes. It is clearly in the industry's interests to sell as much of both types of product as possible. If e-cigarettes put quitting in a prolonged holding pattern for many smokers and relapse to smoking is widespread, vaping may be holding many in smoking who might otherwise have quit.

Further data

Since we wrote that response, further salient information has come to hand from the UK Office for National Statistics data on the percentage of current smokers who have never vaped (Office for National Statistics 2020b). If widespread vaping was driving large-scale smoking cessation, it would follow that the proportion of current smokers who have never vaped would rise with time. Vapers who progressed to being ex-smokers would leave the pool of continuing smokers and persistent smoking would become concentrated in those who had stubbornly never vaped. Tables 6.3 and 6.4 show the data on the proportion of current UK smokers who have never vaped for the years 2015–19 – a period of heavy e-cigarette promotion.

However, these data and the trend within them could also be explained, or contributed to, by vaping leading to smoking. So it is important that we look at them the other way. If vaping were effective at a population level, the proportion of ex-smokers who had never been vapers should be declining. The ex-smoker pool should be enriched by current or past vapers who have recently quit and older ex-smokers who quit before the advent of vaping die off. Again, data on the proportion of ex-smokers who have never vaped is inconvenient to a narrative about vaping driving smoking cessation.

With England seeing major declines in the use of varenicline (−69.2% from peak in 2010) bupropion (−92.6% from 2001 peak) and NRT (−81.7% since the 2005 peak) (Statista 2021c, Statista 2021b,

Table 6.3 Proportion of current UK smokers who have never vaped, 2015–19. Source: Office for National Statistics 2020b.

Year	% who have never vaped
2015	35.8%
2016	35.4%
2017	34.1%
2018	33.7%
2019	32.3%

Table 6.4 Proportion of UK ex-smokers who have never vaped, 2015-19. Source: Office for National Statistics 2020b.

Year	% who have never vaped
2015	83.0%
2016	77.6%
2017	77.0%
2018	76.9%
2019	76.9%

Statista 2021a) while vaping soared, it is likely that some of those who quit via vaping would have been smokers who might otherwise have quit using those methods. This positive figure – however large it actually is when the additional cessation forgone from these large reductions in use of other medications is netted out – needs to be contextualised against concerns that e-cigarettes may be holding many smokers in smoking who might otherwise have quit. As we have seen, there is considerable evidence that this is occurring.

Response to Professor McNeill's letter titled "Additional Comment to the Australian Select Committee on Tobacco Harm Reduction"

Referring to our submission, where we wrote, "Relapse to smoking is very prevalent (A UK 15-month follow-up of vapers (Brose, Bowen et al. 2019) found that overall 39.6% had relapsed to smoking, with those using tank systems faring worst (45.6%))", Professor McNeill claims that this is misleading in a number of ways. She wrote:

> Rather than go into the details, I copy here the conclusions of the study (Brose, Bowen et al. 2019), but would be happy to provide further information if required: "In a group of ex-smokers who had stopped smoking for at least 2 months, relapse to smoking during a 15-month follow-up period was likely to be more common among those who at baseline vaped infrequently or used less advanced devices".

As an author on the Brose et al. paper, McNeill would know that daily vapers in the study had almost exactly the same risk of relapse back to smoking as those who had never vaped (34.5% vs 35.9%). The clear messages from that paper are that vaping does not prevent relapse and that even daily vaping is barely different from not vaping in preventing relapse.

McNeill was also an author on a recent analysis of ITC Four Country Survey data which concluded not only that "Among all W1 (baseline) daily smokers, there were no differences in discontinued smoking between daily smokers who vaped (concurrent users) and exclusive daily smokers" but that "Most ex-smokers remained abstinent from smoking, and there was no difference in relapse back to smoking between those who vaped and those who did not" (Gravely, Cummings et al. 2021).

The great English success story of vaping?

Finally, drawing on recent data from the Smoking in England database from 18 November 2021 (West, Kale et al. 2021), my colleague Matthew Peters has described what he calls the "non-sensagon" – nine facets to the supposedly Great English Success Story of Vaping and Smoking:

1. EC use has remained relatively stable since 2013 and the decline in smoking prevalence has plateaued since 2019.
2. The proportion of 18–24-year-olds who have ever smoked rose from 24% in 2019 to 33% in 2020 and 34% in 2021.
3. Cigarette smoking prevalence in 18–21-year-olds is up from 16.7% to 19.9% between 2019 and 2021.

4. EC use among recent ex-smokers has declined from a peak in 2016.
5. EC use for quitting has declined from a peak in 2016.
6. Half of EC users are current smokers (dual users).
7. Twenty percent of EC users are long-term ex-smokers (not active quitters).
8. The most common quit strategy is unassisted (ECs are the most common quitting *aid*).
9. Only 14% of vapers are using ECs for intended harm reduction.

New Zealand's dramatic decline in adult smoking and rise in vaping

Just as the writing of this book was nearing completion, data was released in New Zealand on smoking and vaping for 2020-21. An excellent summary and commentary was published on the *Public Health Expert* blog (Edwards, Ball et al. 2021). Daily smoking prevalence in 2020-21 was 9.4% and current (at least monthly) smoking prevalence was 10.9% with the authors noting, "There was a steady, though unspectacular, decline in current and daily smoking prevalence of about 0.6% per year in absolute terms from 2011/12 to 2019/20. However, from 2019/20 to 2020/21, daily smoking prevalence fell by 2.5% and current smoking prevalence by 2.8%." This fall was unprecedented.

> Use of ECs was first assessed in 2015/16; since then, the prevalence of current and daily EC use has steadily increased. The increase in EC use was much greater in 2020/21: current EC use grew from 5.3% in 2019/20 to 8.2% in 2020/21 and daily EC use from 3.5% to 6.2% over the same period. The increase in daily and current EC use between 2019/20 and 2020/21 occurred concurrently with the large reduction observed in smoking prevalence [Figure 6.5], whereas the more gradual increase in EC use between 2015/16 and 2019/20 was not associated with a substantial change in the rate of decline in smoking prevalence.

In their discussion, the blog authors emphasised that "caution is required when interpreting survey data and extrapolating trends from a single survey year". They also explored several possible explanations for this fall, other than the rise in vaping which occurred most in younger

6 Vaping to quit: the latest mass distraction

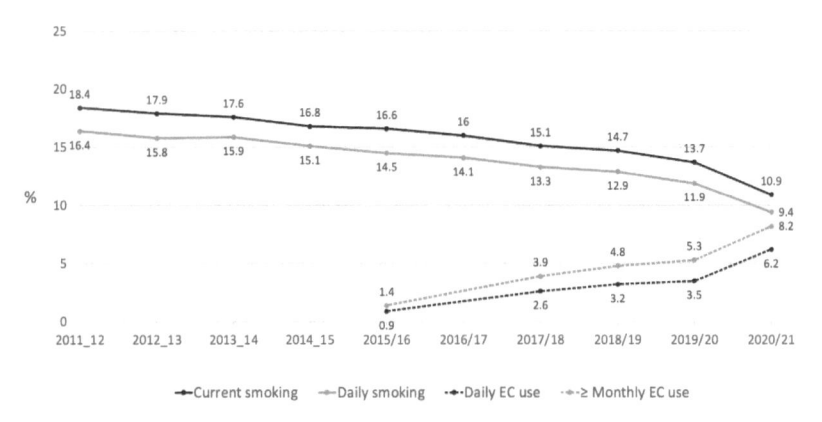

Figure 6.5 Trends in current (≥monthly) and daily smoking and e-cigarette use (NZHS 2011–12 to 2020–21) (Source: Edwards, Ball et al. 2021).

adults in whom smoking also fell the most. These were: the chance that a random variation had occurred; that COVID-19 had caused people to quit out of generalised heightened concerns for health; and that other tobacco control policies were responsible. They found each of these unlikely to be as plausible as the role of vaping.

New Zealand then, presents today as a nation where the case for vaping reducing smoking through a quitting effect seems very plausible. However, as I discussed earlier in the chapter, there is important evidence that both vaping and smoking are also rising in school-aged children in New Zealand, concerning developments which no one but those profiting from this would applaud. In Chapter 8, I'll discuss how vaping regulation policy might best ensure that smokers believing they might quit with NVPs can get access while children and those simply wanting to vape with little interest in quitting would find it harder.

Does vaping reduce smoking frequency (number of cigarettes smoked)?

Advocates for e-cigarettes also point to reduced smoking as a positive outcome from vaping. They emphasise that at the times when people are vaping they are not smoking as they otherwise would be likely to be doing. So across a day, month and year, vapers who still smoke are likely to smoke fewer cigarettes than if they did not vape. Obviously this is no-brainer evidence of harm reduction, they insist.

An early paper from the US national PATH cohort (Berry, Reynolds et al. 2019) found that daily e-cigarette smokers had 5.7 times the odds of reducing their average daily cigarette use by at least 50% compared with smokers in the cohort who did not vape. Daily vapers were also 7.9 times more likely than non-vapers to have stopped all smoking for at least 30 days. Given that many smokers take up vaping to try to quit or cut down their smoking, this almost certainly means that taking up vaping is a marker of attempting to quit. It was therefore quite predictable when comparing smokers not vaping with those who did, that a higher proportion would quit for at least a short time in the cohort who were vaping because vaping was a marker of trying to quit. Many smokers in the cohort who were not vaping were not even trying to quit. Across the time the longitudinal study was conducted, vaping was the most popular assisted method of trying to quit.

So what does the evidence say about whether *reducing* smoking, as opposed to *quitting smoking altogether*, actually reduces harm? While there is strong evidence for a causal association between disease and early uptake, amount smoked, and duration of smoking, the evidence on "reverse engineering" harm by continuing to smoke while cutting back is far from strong. We have good evidence from several large cohort studies conducted in Norway, South Korea, Scotland and the USA where smokers were followed up for several years and the health outcomes of those who reduced smoking over time compared with those who did not reduce.

A 2007 systematic review examining the health effects of reducing smoking by more than half found only "small health benefit" (Pisinger and Godtfredsen 2007). Since then, five cohorts (Tverdal and Bjartveit 2006, Song, Sung et al. 2008, Hart, Gruer et al. 2013, Inoue-Choi, Christensen et al. 2020) with a combined total of 1,011,120 people followed for up to 25 years have reported findings such as "no evidence that smokers who cut down their daily cigarette consumption by >50% reduce their risk of premature death significantly" (Tverdal and Bjartveit 2006). One of the largest, from South Korea (Song, Sung

6 Vaping to quit: the latest mass distraction

et al. 2008) found no association between smoking reduction and all cancer risk but a significant decrease in risk of lung cancer, but with the size of risk reduction "disproportionately smaller than expected". A USA cohort with 505,500 people followed for different lengths of time between 1992 and 2011 concluded, "Although reducing smoking from daily to nondaily was associated with decreased mortality risk, cessation was associated with far greater benefit. Lifelong nondaily smokers have higher mortality risks than never smokers, even among those smoking 6 to 10 cigarettes per month. Thus, all smokers should quit, regardless of how infrequently they smoke" (Inoue-Choi, Christensen et al. 2020).

An important 2018 paper considered the surge in e-cigarette use in England and whether this was reducing the number of cigarettes being smoked at the population level across the country (Beard, Brown et al. 2018). The authors concluded:

> No statistically significant associations were found between changes in use of e-cigarettes while smoking and daily cigarette consumption. Neither did we find clear evidence for an association between e-cigarette use specifically for smoking reduction and temporary abstinence, respectively, and changes in daily cigarette consumption. If use of e-cigarettes and licensed NRT while smoking acted to reduce cigarette consumption in England between 2006 and 2016, the effect was likely very small at a population level.
>
> Data from 2019 from the UK government's annual Opinions and Lifestyle Survey also show that the average number of cigarettes smoked daily by smokers who vape (8 a day) is almost identical to that by smokers who have never vaped (8.1 a day) (Office for National Statistics 2021).

These data echo comments by Robert West, former editor-in-chief of *Addiction*, on BBC Radio 4 in February 2016. At 7 min. 44 sec. West says, "Now, that raises an interesting question. If [e-cigarettes] were a game changer, if they were going to have the massive effect on, you know, everyone switching to e-cigarettes and stopping smoking, we might have expected to see a bigger effect than we've seen so far, which has actually been relatively small." At 10 min. 40 sec., he continues, "We know that most people who use e-cigarettes are continuing to smoke and when you ask them they tell you that they are mostly doing that to cut down the amount they smoke. But we also know that they are smoking, it's not really that much more different from what they would have done since they started using e-cigarettes" (Porter 2016).

7
Insights from qualitative research with unassisted quitters

Self-change research pioneers Harald Klingemann, and Mark and Linda Sobell have emphasised that "When treatments are perceived as overly intensive, demeaning and requiring unnecessarily severe changes in life-style, they lack appeal and are unlikely to be utilized", that "it needs to become common knowledge among the public that self-change is a frequent occurrence" and that "We need to develop new ways of assessing 'tacit knowledge' from various angles because 'people know more than they can say'" about pathways out of addiction (Klingemann, Sobell et al. 2010).

These three wise observations were at the heart of a three-year NHMRC study I led titled *The natural history of unassisted smoking cessation in Australia*. From knowing that unassisted smoking cessation was comparatively massively understudied compared to assisted cessation methods (Chapman and MacKenzie 2010), we were curious if qualitative researchers had shone their torches on this phenomenon and explored insights hidden among the vast numbers of ex-smokers who had quit on their own. Our work used grounded theory and an interpretive, social constructionist approach (Charmaz 1990, Charmaz 2006) to explore the factors associated with successful quitting in a sample of ex-smokers who had quit between six months and two years earlier. A social constructionist approach allowed the exploration of the subjective and complex experiences of participants to provide an account of how ex-smokers understood and made sense of the process of successful quitting that they had used.

Our research led to seven published papers (Smith and Chapman 2014, Smith, Carter et al. 2015a, Smith, Carter et al. 2015b, Smith, Chapman et al. 2015, Smith, Carter et al. 2017, Smith, Carter et al. 2018, Smith 2020) and a PhD thesis written by Andrea Smith who was employed on the grant and led the writing on all of the papers.

This chapter is an edited amalgam of two of these papers: a synthesis of the findings of all qualitative research on unassisted cessation, *The views and experiences of smokers who quit smoking unassisted. A systematic review of the qualitative evidence* (Smith, Carter et al. 2015b) and *Why do smokers try to quit without medication or counselling? A qualitative study with ex-smokers* published in *BMJ Open* (Smith, Carter et al. 2015a). I have edited both papers to concentrate on the research questions addressed, principal findings and discussion sections of the papers. Readers are referred to the papers, both published in open access, for the complete texts, tables, figures and references.

Paper 1: The views and experiences of smokers who quit unassisted. A systematic review of the qualitative evidence

Research into smoking cessation has achieved much. Researchers have identified numerous variables related to smoking cessation and relapse, including heaviness of smoking, quitting history, quit intentions, quit attempts, use of assistance, socioeconomic status, gender, age, and exposure to mass-reach interventions such as mass media campaigns, price increases and retail regulation. Behavioural scientists have developed a range of health behaviour models and constructs relevant to smoking cessation, such as the theory of planned behaviour, social cognitive theory, the transtheoretical model and the health belief model. These theories have provided constructs to smoking cessation research such as perceived behavioural control, subjective norms (Azjen 1991), outcome expectations, self-regulation (Vohs, Baumeister et al. 2017), decisional balance (Prochaska and DiClemente 1983), perceived benefits, perceived barriers and self-efficacy (Becker 1974).

The knowledge generated has informed the development of a range of pharmacological and behavioural smoking-cessation interventions.

Yet, although these interventions are somewhat efficacious, as we have seen throughout the book the majority of smokers who quit successfully do so without using them, choosing instead to quit unassisted; that is, without pharmacological or professional support (Edwards, Bondy et al. 2014, Smith, Chapman et al. 2015). Many smokers also appear to quit unplanned as a consequence of serendipitous events (West and Sohal 2006), throwing into question the predictive validity of some of these cognitive models. The enduring popularity of unassisted cessation persists even in nations advanced in tobacco control where cessation assistance such as nicotine replacement therapy (NRT) and the stop-smoking medications bupropion and varenicline are readily available and widely promoted. Yet little appears to be known about this population or this self-guided route to cessation success. In contrast, the phenomenon of self-change (also known as natural recovery) is comparatively well documented in the fields of drug and alcohol addiction (Miller and Smith 2010, Slutske 2010), and health behaviour change (for example, eating disorders, obesity and gambling) (Sobell 2007).

In our systematic review of unassisted cessation in Australia (Smith, Chapman et al. 2015) we established that the majority of contemporary cessation research is quantitative and intervention focused (Kluge 2009). While completing that review we determined that the available qualitative research was concerned primarily with evaluating smoker and ex-smoker perceptions of mass-reach interventions such as marketing or retail regulations, tax increases, graphic health warnings, smoke-free legislation or intervention acceptability from the perspective of the GP, current smoker, or third parties likely to be impacted by mass-reach interventions. Australian smoking-cessation research provided few insights into quitting from the perspective of the smoker who quits unassisted. However, our systematic review highlighted that 54% to 69% of ex-smokers quit unassisted and 41% to 58% of current smokers had attempted to quit unassisted (Smith, Chapman et al. 2015).

We consequently became interested in what the qualitative cessation literature had to say about smokers who quit unassisted. Qualitative approaches offer an opportunity to explain unexpected or anomalous findings from quantitative research and to clarify relationships identified in these studies (Dixon-Woods, Agarwal et al. 2004, Atkins, Lewin et al. 2008). By integrating individual qualitative research studies into a qualitative synthesis, new insights and understandings can be generated and a cumulative body of empirical work produced (Barnett-Page and Thomas 2009). Such syntheses have proved useful to health policy and practice (McDermott, Graham et al. 2004, Thomas and Harden 2008). By focusing our review on the views of smokers (i.e. on the people to whom the interventions are directed), we might start to better understand why many smokers continue to quit unassisted instead of using the assistance available to them. Such an understanding might help us to decide whether we should be developing better approaches to unassisted cessation or focusing our attention on directing more smokers to use the efficacious pharmacological and professional behavioural support that already exists.

In this review, we examined the qualitative literature on smokers who quit unassisted in order to answer the following research questions: (1) How much and what kind of qualitative research has explored unassisted cessation? (2) What are the views and experiences of smokers who quit unassisted? Our search strategy (see original article for full description) found just 11 eligible qualitative papers.

Research question 1: How much and what kind of qualitative research has explored unassisted cessation?

The earliest study identified was a 1977 US study investigating why smokers seeking treatment (psychotherapy) often fared no better than smokers who quit unassisted (Baer, Foreyt et al. 1977). This was followed in the late 1980s and 1990s by studies (from the US and Sweden) investigating unassisted cessation as a phenomenon in its own right (Solheim 1989, Mariezcurrena 1996, Stewart 1999), and one US study in which unassisted cessation data were reported but this was not the primary focus of the study (Thompson 1995). Subsequent to this, no qualitative studies were identified that focused on unassisted cessation *per se*: the six post-2000 studies (from Hong Kong, US, UK, Canada and Norway) had as their primary focus either cessation in general (Abdullah and Ho 2006, Nichter, Nichter et al. 2007, Bottorff,

Radsma et al. 2009, Murray, McNeill et al. 2010, Medbø, Melbye et al. 2011) or health behaviour change (Ogden and Hills 2008).

Research question 2: What are the views and experiences of smokers who quit unassisted?
The full set of concepts derived from the qualitative literature were grouped into those that included descriptive themes that have already been covered in the literature (Figure 7.1 below the line) and those concepts that included descriptive themes that provided potentially new insights into unassisted cessation (Figure 7.1 above the line). The existing quantitative smoking-cessation literature had, for example, already often reported on attitudes to assistance, reasons for quitting, strategies used to quit and reasons for relapsing. While encouraged by the consistency between the qualitative and quantitative studies, our aim was to focus on what the qualitative literature could report from the smokers' perspective about quitting unassisted that had the potential to offer new or alternative insights into the process or experience of unassisted cessation. From this perspective the most interesting themes were those that related to three concepts: (1) motivation; (2) willpower; and (3) commitment. Four further concepts (timing, decision making, ownership and the perception that quitting unassisted was a positive phenomenon) were of interest but insufficient data were available on which to base an analysis.

Although these concepts appear in the literature on smoking cessation, below we explore the meaning of these concepts as defined by smokers and ex-smokers who have quit unassisted, as well as the researchers who studied them.

Motivation. Although motivation was widely reported, it was difficult to discern exactly what motivation meant to smokers as opposed to researchers. Smokers rarely talked directly about motivation or used the word motivation to describe their quit attempt. Yet motivation was frequently included in the accounts *researchers* gave of how and why smokers quit.

That is, there appeared to be a disjunct between the way that researchers talked about motivation and the way that ex-smokers understood it. On looking at the data related to motivation it became

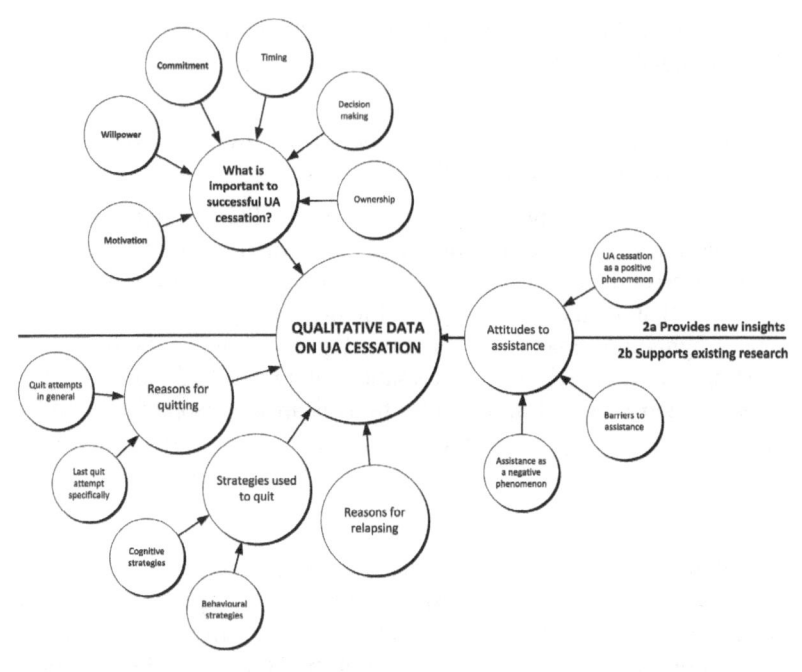

Figure 7.1 Themes and concepts derived from the 11 primary studies. Source: (Smith, Carter et al. 2015b).

clear to us that when researchers talked about motivation they were in fact talking almost exclusively about *reasons for quitting*. Typical reasons included cost, a sense of duty, health concerns, feeling out of control, feeling diminished by being a smoker, deciding the disadvantages of smoking outweighed the benefits, or expectations that life would be better once they quit. We concluded that the data on motivation reported in these 11 qualitative studies added no new insights to the data on reasons for quitting which had not already been reported in the quantitative literature.

Smokers used the word *motivation* differently: not to describe the reason they quit, but to describe what sustained them through their quit attempt. We included these data (Stewart 1999) under the concept of commitment (see below). Our main conclusion about motivation was that smokers and researchers appear to be using the word to denote different concepts.

Willpower. The concept of willpower was clearly important to smokers and often used by researchers to account for smokers' success or failure, but was rarely examined or unpacked. Willpower was reported to be a method of quitting, a strategy to counteract cravings or urges (much as NRT or counselling is regarded as a method of quitting or a way of dealing with an urge to smoke), or a personal quality or trait fundamental to quitting success. For example, although Ogden and Hill (2008) classified their participants according to whether they had "stopped smoking through willpower or a smoking course", they gave no definition or explanation of what willpower was. Similarly, Thompson (1995) reported many participants used "sheer willpower to overcome the strong urges to smoke", and Abdullah and Ho (2006) reported relapsed smokers cited "willpower and determination" as key factors for quitting success, but did not elaborate on what was meant by willpower. Stewart's 1999 study of smokers who quit unassisted attempted to understand willpower from the smokers' perspective, yet despite directly questioning smokers about willpower, Stewart could find no agreement among smokers as to what willpower was. In summing up, Stewart concluded: "it is difficult to connect a successful cessation attempt with the use of willpower without creating a tautology: one is successful if one has willpower, and one has willpower if one is successful" (Stewart 1999), capturing what is arguably still an issue in contemporary smoking-cessation research.

Commitment. Smokers' talk about commitment was nuanced and multilayered. In contrast to motivation and willpower we did not need to rely upon the researchers' interpretations to gain an insight into what commitment might mean to smokers. Smokers talked directly about being committed. To them it meant being determined, serious or resolute. Being committed was essential to their quitting success. Commitment was what differentiated a serious quit attempt from previous unsuccessful quit attempts, and was the hallmark of their final successful quit attempt.

Commitment could also be tentative or provisional. Medbø (2011) reported smokers who appeared keen to try to quit but were not necessarily committed to seeing the quit attempt through. It is possible a further level of commitment was being withheld, contingent perhaps on how difficult quitting turned out to be or on how the smoker felt about having quit once they got there. One of Stewart's participants illustrated the difference, "OK I'm going to give this a valiant attempt and if it's not going to work then I'll go back to smoking and it will be OK." The smoker is committed to trying but not necessarily committed to quitting.

Commitment could also be cumulative. Smokers talked about a point of no return, which described a point in the cessation process when they had made a firm commitment to quit, they had made a decision and they would not change their mind. Smokers described this as the point in time at which they believed there was too much invested to relapse now.

Discussion

In this review we synthesised the qualitative data reporting on the views and experiences of smokers who successfully quit unassisted (without pharmacological or professional behavioural support). The existence of only a handful of studies over more than 50 years, with no study specifically addressing unassisted cessation post-2000, indicates that up until now little research attention has been given to the lived experiences and understanding of smokers who successfully quit unassisted. As a consequence relatively little is known about smokers' perspectives on what is the most frequently used means of quitting and the way described by the majority of ex-smokers as being the most "helpful" (Hung, Dunlop et al. 2011, Newport 2013). It is widely accepted that searching qualitative literature is difficult (McDermott, Graham et al. 2004, Shaw, Booth et al. 2004). Although it is possible that relevant studies were missed, given the comprehensiveness of our search strategy, the comparative lack of studies found through searching seems likely to reflect an evidence gap, and therefore an important area for future research.

This lack of qualitative research was unexpected for two reasons. First, we were aware of a small but not insubstantial body of quantitative evidence on smokers who quit unassisted; and second, in the course of our literature search we had identified a considerable number of qualitative studies on smoking cessation. On closer examination it became clear that few of these reported specifically on smokers who quit unassisted. This supports what Kluge found in 2009; that is, the qualitative smoking-cessation research that does exist is concerned primarily with evaluating the success or acceptability of smoking cessation interventions, particularly in vulnerable populations such as adolescents or the socially disadvantaged (Kluge 2009).

Concepts central to self-quitting

Motivation was identified as a central concept in this review, but analysis of the studies showed that motivation appeared primarily in the researchers' accounts of quitting rather than in the smokers' accounts of quitting. On closer examination, the data related to motivation consisted almost entirely of reasons for quitting. Within the quantitative literature on smoking cessation, motivation is an established psychological construct which has been operationalised in numerous studies designed to determine the role of motivation in quitting success (Borland, Yong et al. 2010, Smit, Fidler et al. 2011). Motivation has been identified as critical to explaining cessation success (Nezami, Sussman et al. 2003). The lack of explicit discussion about motivation by smokers who quit unassisted in the studies included in this review is therefore interesting. Though motivation could be inferred from the smokers' accounts, it had to be done by using the variables that comprise motivation, such as reasons (motives) for quitting or the pros and cons of smoking versus quitting. Given the relative lack of data, it is difficult to conclude whether this is (1) because smokers do not talk directly about motivation, or (2) whether from the participants' perspective motivation is not the driving force behind successful unassisted cessation (either because another concept is more important or because too much time has passed since their quit attempt for them and they have forgotten how important motivation was to them).

From the studies included in this review, it appears that – at least in smokers' self-understanding – commitment might be more important than motivation as an explanation of successful unassisted cessation. The enthusiastic and explicit talk about being determined, committed or serious suggests that this concept resonates more with smokers than the concept of motivation. The overlapping and at times contradictory natures of commitment and motivation have been highlighted recently by Balmford and Borland who concluded that it may be possible to quit successfully while ambivalent, as long as the smoker remains committed in the face of ebbs and flows in motivation (Balmford, Borland et al. 2011) Further complicating the relationship, some regard commitment as a component of motivation, operationalising motivation as, for example, "determination to quit" (Segan, Borland et al. 2002) or "commitment to quit" (Kahler, Lachance et al. 2007).

The greater research interest in reasons for quitting or pros and cons of quitting (i.e. motivation) as opposed to commitment may be because motivation is simpler to measure; for example, by asking people to rate or rank reasons, costs or benefits. From a policy and practice perspective, it may also be easier to draw attention to these reasons, costs and benefits, rather than engage with commitment. For example, mass-media campaigns can remind smokers of why they should quit by pointing out the benefits to short-term and long-term health. However, this review draws attention to the importance of commitment for sustained quitting, at least from the point of view of smokers and quitters. The UK's annual Stoptober campaign in which smokers committed to being smoke-free for 28 days indicates that creative approaches to addressing commitment can be successful (Public Health England 2013).

The final concept identified, willpower, was described in terms of multiple constructs (a personal quality or trait, a method of quitting, a strategy to counteract cravings or urges), suggesting smokers and researchers may use it as a convenient or shorthand heuristic when talking about or reporting on quit success. Despite this lack of clarity, the word has persisted in the qualitative and quantitative smoking cessation literature. It could be fruitful for future research to further examine the meaning of willpower, and particularly its relationship to other more tightly defined concepts such as self-efficacy (Etter, Bergman et al. 2000), self-regulation (Vohs, Baumeister et al. 2017) and self-determination (Deci and Ryan 2010), from the perspective of both researchers and smokers.

No matter how widely available and affordable smoking-cessation assistance becomes, it is likely there will always be a significant proportion of smokers who choose to quit unassisted. It is important to understand what drives these smokers to quit this way and to better understand their route to success. Orford and colleagues working on the UK Alcohol Treatment Trial made a strong case for including the client's perspective, arguing that it is wrong to assume that clients have no perspective into their own change processes, and that we should resist the dominant "drug metaphor" which has adopted the model of an active professional applying a technique to a passive recipient (Orford, Hodgson et al. 2006). McDermott and Dobson also advocated for the need for contemporary public health policy to ground itself in the experiences of those whose lifestyles it seeks to change (McDermott, Dobson et al. 2006). As the vast majority of smokers who quit successfully continue to do so without formal help, it is likely that a better understanding of this experience, from the perspective of the smokers and ex-smokers themselves, could inform more nuanced and effective communication and support for quitting.

Conclusion

Our review identified three key concepts –motivation, willpower and commitment – circulating in smokers' and ex-smokers' accounts of quitting unassisted. Insufficient qualitative evidence currently exists to fully understand these concepts, but they do appear to be important in smokers' and ex-smokers' accounts and so worthy of research attention. A more detailed qualitative investigation of what motivation, willpower and commitment mean to smokers and ex-smokers would complement the existing body of behavioural science knowledge in tobacco control. A better understanding of these concepts from the smokers' perspective may help to explain the often puzzling popularity of quitting unassisted rather than opting to use the efficacious pharmacological or professional assistance that is available. Health practitioners could potentially use such knowledge, in combination with what we already know from population-based research into smoking cessation, to better support all smokers to quit, whether or not they wish to use assistance.

Paper 2: Why do smokers try to quit without medication or counselling? A qualitative study with ex-smokers

Summary

Objective When tobacco smokers quit, between half and two-thirds quit unassisted: that is, they do not consult their GP, use pharmacotherapy (NRT, bupropion or varenicline) or phone a quitline. We sought to understand why smokers quit unassisted.

Design This was a qualitative grounded theory study (in-depth interviews, theoretical sampling, concurrent data collection and data analysis). Full details of design, sample selection and data coding and analysis can be read in the published paper.

Participants Twenty-one Australian adult ex-smokers were studied (aged 28–68 years; nine males and 12 females) who quit unassisted within the past six months to two years. Twelve participants had previous experience of using assistance to quit; nine had never previously used assistance.

Results Along with previously identified barriers to use of cessation assistance (cost, access, lack of awareness or knowledge of assistance, including misperceptions about effectiveness or safety), our study produced new explanations of why smokers quit unassisted: (1) they prioritise lay knowledge gained directly from personal experiences and indirectly from others over professional or theoretical knowledge; (2) their evaluation of the costs and benefits of quitting unassisted versus those of using assistance favours quitting unassisted; (3) they believe quitting is their personal responsibility; and (4) they perceive quitting unassisted to be the "right" or "better" choice in terms of how this relates to their own self-identity or self-image. Deeply rooted personal and societal values such as independence, strength, autonomy and self-control appear to be influencing smokers' beliefs and decisions about quitting.

Conclusions The reasons for smokers' rejection of the conventional medication model for smoking cessation are complex and go beyond modifiable or correctable problems relating to misperceptions or treatment barriers. These findings suggest that GPs could recognise and respect smokers' reasons for rejecting assistance, validate and approve their choices, and modify brief interventions to support their preference for quitting unassisted, where preferred. Further research and translation may assist in developing such strategies for use in practice.

Introduction

Smoking-cessation researchers, advocates and healthcare practitioners have tended to emphasise that the odds of quitting successfully can be increased by using pharmacotherapies, such as NRT, bupropion and varenicline, or behavioural support such as advice from a healthcare professional or from a quitline. However, instead of using one or more of these forms of assistance, most quit attempts have always and continue to be unassisted and most long-term and recent ex-smokers quit without pharmacological or professional assistance.

Researchers have identified a number of issues relating to the choice to use assistance. They generally conclude that failure to use assistance can be explained by treatment-related issues such as cost and access, and patient-related issues such as lack of awareness or knowledge about assistance, including misperceptions about the effectiveness and safety of pharmacotherapy or concerns about addiction (Etter and Perneger 2001, Bansal, Cummings et al. 2004, Gross, Brose et al. 2008, Shiffman, Ferguson et al. 2008).

The policy and practice response to the low uptake of cessation assistance has typically focused on improving awareness of, access to and use of assistance – in particular, pharmacotherapy. NRT, bupropion and varenicline are often provided free of charge or heavily subsidised by the government or health insurance companies. NRT is on general sale in pharmacies and supermarkets, and is widely promoted through direct-to-consumer marketing. Clinical practice guidelines in the UK, USA and Australia advise clinicians to recommend NRT to all nicotine-dependent (>10 cigarettes per day) smokers. Specialist stop-smoking clinics, and dedicated telephone and online quit services provide smokers with tailored support and advice. These products and services have not had the population-wide impact that might have been expected from clinical trial results (Wakefield, Durkin et al. 2008, Zhu, Lee et al. 2012, Wakefield, Coomber et al. 2014), leading some researchers to suggest that patient-related barriers such as misperceptions about effectiveness and safety are a greater impediment than treatment-related barriers (Vogt, Hall et al. 2008). Little attention, however, has been given to how and why smokers quit unassisted. If we can explain how the process of unassisted quitting comes about and what it is about unassisted quitting that appeals to smokers, we may be better placed to support all smokers to quit, whether or not they wish to use assistance.

We conducted a qualitative study to understand why half to two-thirds of smokers choose to quit unassisted rather than use smoking-cessation assistance. Smoking-cessation researchers have highlighted the importance of gaining the smokers' perspective (DiClemente, Delahanty et al. 2010, Orleans, Mabry et al. 2010) and suggested qualitative research might provide the means of doing so (Cook-Shimanek, Burns et al. 2013). Although a number of qualitative studies have examined non-use of assistance in at-risk or disadvantaged subpopulations (Kishchuk, Tremblay et al. 2004, Bryant, Bonevski et al. 2011, Hansen and Nelson 2011), only a few have looked at smokers in general. Few studies have examined explicit self-reported reasons of why smokers do not use NRT; to our knowledge, none has examined explicit, self-reported reasons of why smokers do not use prescription smoking-cessation medication.

The two research questions guiding the study were what does quitting unassisted mean to smokers? And what factors influence smokers' decisions to quit unassisted?

Results

Our central analytical focus was the original, previously unreported categories in our analysis. When grouped, these suggested four new processes that could help explain unassisted quitting:

1. Prioritising lay knowledge.
2. Evaluating assistance against unassisted quitting.
3. Believing quitting is their personal responsibility.
4. Perceiving quitting unassisted to be the "right" or "better" choice.

The four analytical categories that explain the process and meaning of quitting unassisted, with illustrative quotes from the interviews, are shown in Table 7.1.

Prioritising lay knowledge

Many participants expressed views about assistance that were at odds with accepted knowledge in smoking cessation on the effectiveness, side effects and long-term safety of assistance. These "misperceptions" about assistance appear to arise because participants' personal experiences and lay knowledge of assistance do not tally with what they have been told about assistance by their GP, pharmacist or through direct-to-consumer marketing of NRT by pharmaceutical companies. The gulf between what smokers have personally experienced or heard from others, and what health professionals are telling them was particularly evident in participants' talk of unmet expectations of what assistance could realistically do for them. For many, the experience of using assistance had not been as expected, including not being as effective as they had believed it would be.

Participants talked of the importance of shared narratives of assistance that were predominantly negative and shared narratives of quitting unassisted that were predominantly positive. Shared stories of assistance – both personal and second-hand – were stories of failure to quit, and of unpleasant and sometimes serious side effects. In contrast, talk about quitting unassisted often featured family and friends who had managed to quit successfully on their own.

In order to resolve the tension between what is going on in "their world" and what the professional medical and healthcare worlds are endorsing, participants prioritised what they knew: either directly from their own experiences or indirectly from "trusted" sources. As a consequence, participants appeared to discount professional advice in favour of their own first-hand quitting experiences and the collective narratives of quitting successes and failures that circulated in their social groups. This lay knowledge-making based on personal and collective experiences appears to be a powerful force at play in smokers' decisions about quitting.

Table 7.1 The four analytical categories that explain the process and meaning of quitting unassisted, with illustrative quotes

Category: Prioritising lay knowledge
- Valuing personal experiences
- Being influenced by shared/collective knowledge

Participant quotes

"I've done this, I've done the gum before, it's my turn to just do it by myself with common sense and willpower." Female, 57 years old

"I've known a couple of people around town that have tried to give up with patches and that and they've gone 3 or 4 weeks and they've started smoking again and all that." Female, 52 years old

"I've got friends that have used the patches and the gum a lot. They've been unsuccessful. They've done the gum and the patches, I don't know how many times. They've spent so much money on them, and they just cannot make it work." Female, 31 years old

"Well [assistance] hadn't worked in the past and I didn't think – I'd come to the realisation that it was just in the mind, it was just a matter of willpower, it was just a matter of saying no and sticking to it." Male, 59 years old

Category: Evaluating assistance against unassisted quitting
- Weighing up the "value" assistance brings to them and their quit attempt (is it worth using assistance to quit?)
- Wanting to save money *now* (spending money to quit is irrational, especially on something that brings no "pleasure")
- Wanting to quit "instantly", be a non-smoker *now* (which assistance does not allow)
- Disliking the "inconvenience" of assistance (assistance is too complicated, too fiddly)
- Associating assistance with additional effort (e.g. adopting new, but temporary, routines)

Participant quotes

"It was a big thing that if I'm going to save money by not smoking then why should I spend money on not smoking." Male, 45 years old

7 Insights from qualitative research with unassisted quitters

"The cigarettes, that's the fun. Why would you spend $20 on non-fun?" Female, 34 years old

"I found [NRT] expensive. I thought that if you're going to get nicotine anyway at least there should be some positive reason for it." Female, 56 years old

"If I'm going to quit smoking I'm going to do it cold turkey and get it over and done with." Female, 52 years old

"I went to the GP and he said oh, you need to continue to smoke though for a couple of – what was it? It is a week? I was like oh no, but I want to stop now." Female, 34 years old

"It's too much of a hassle . . . You've got to go out and buy the thing. You've got to stick it on or chew it or unwrap it." Male, 61 years old

Category: Believing quitting is their personal responsibility

- Smoking and quitting are personal problems (and the responsibility of the individual)
- Smoking and quitting are not medical conditions
- The smoker is best placed to know how to quit, what will work

Participant quotes

"It's my problem. Not problem, I think that's a bad choice of words, but I was the one smoking." Male, 28 years old

"That's so important that you don't make an issue out of it. It is a personal – you're right. You are so right. It is a personal thing." Male, 61 years old

"Yeah, okay, I screwed up, I smoked for years, I really need to do something about this and cope with it." Female, 57 years old

"I'm not much of someone to go to a doctor unless there was, unless I thought there was a serious problem with myself I don't normally go to a doctor." Male, 45 years old

"I'm independent and I'm stubborn and that's the only way that I knew how to do it. I wasn't going to – I'm not a person to ask for help. So I don't think I would have asked for help to quit smoking." Female, 31 years old

"OK I did the Champix, I stopped for maybe – I can't remember if it was two or three months – but like it didn't work because it actually, the change sort of wasn't from within," Female, 56 years old

219

"*I think quitting cold turkey, you're going to have more chance of actually [staying] a non-smoker, if you quit cold turkey . . . because I think that you need that willpower to stay motivated to not smoke.*" Female, 31 years old

"*Because in the grand scheme of things, it's always your willpower that's going to stop you. So you might be able to use other methods to help you quit smoking, but six months down the track, you need to have that willpower to stop you doing that again.*" Female, 31 years old

"*I feel a sense of accomplishment in knowing that I did it cold turkey. Knowing that I didn't have to go to other means to do it. That I was able to use my willpower.*" Female, 31 years old

Category: Perceiving quitting unassisted to be the "right" or "better" choice

- Quitting unassisted is the "best" way to quit
- Equating quitting unassisted with being serious about quitting

Participant quotes

"*I think I just didn't want to [use assistance], I just felt that for me to do it properly I actually had to be able to do it myself.*" Female, 50 years old

"*[Taking medication] had crossed my mind, but I'm a fairly stubborn person I suppose. I don't really – I believe that I should be able to do it myself, without those sorts of things.*" Male, 31 years old

"*I think that if you're truly committed you don't need anything.*" Female, 56 years old

---

Evaluating assistance against unassisted quitting

On the whole, participants did not seem to be quitting unassisted because of a lack of awareness or knowledge about the assistance available to them. Instead participants appeared to have engaged in an evaluation of the perceived costs and benefits of using assistance compared with the costs and benefits of quitting unassisted. Factors in this cost–benefit balance related primarily to the perceived convenience of unassisted quitting (in terms of time to being "quit" and the effort required to make the quit attempt happen) and the importance of short-term financial savings. These arguments were sometimes explicit and sometimes implicit.

Participants talked about wanting to quit now, immediately. NRT and smoking-cessation medication both involve a treatment period in which the smoker is still a smoker: they cannot yet call themselves a "non-smoker". In their opinion, use of assistance essentially delays their progression to being totally quit. In contrast, going "cold turkey" provides an immediate satisfaction and instant non-smoker status. There often appeared to be a sense of urgency or a need for an immediate and complete change of status in those who opted to quit unassisted.

Using assistance was also associated with an investment of practical and logistical effort. Assistance required the adoption of new – but temporary – routines and habits. It was a middle ground or halfway house through which the smoker would have to pass. They would have to complete this "assistance" phase before being able to adopt yet another set of routines and habits to become nicotine free or drug free. These temporary routines associated with assistance included obtaining or purchasing assistance, carrying it around and remembering to use it. For some, this temporary, additional set of routines appeared simply too complex, too bothersome and too high a price to pay in terms of the inconvenience generated.

For a number of participants, spending money to quit, especially when quitting was motivated by a desire to save money, appeared counter-intuitive. For such participants, thoughts were focused on the here and now, on the short-term rather than long-term savings. Few participants appeared to regard money spent on assistance as a long-term investment in future financial savings. As a consequence, using assistance to quit was viewed as a barrier to maximising potential savings while quitting. For NRT specifically, this balancing of the pros and cons extended beyond the financial cost of cigarettes versus cost of NRT to the perceived pleasure that the financial spend was likely to provide. Spending $20 on cigarettes was reasonable because it would deliver pleasure; spending $20 on something that was going to make you miserable was not. An unwillingness to spend on NRT also appeared related to an inability to reconcile nicotine's dual role as part of the problem and the solution, and to fears of becoming addicted to NRT gums, patches or inhalers.

Believing quitting is their personal responsibility

Quitting appeared to be an intensely individual experience and one that the smoker believed only they could take charge of. Ultimately quitting was something they had to face themselves. Many participants seemed to have reached a point where they regarded smoking to be their problem and quitting to be their personal responsibility. Quitting was, therefore, not necessarily something that could be helped or facilitated by external support (be it from family, friends or health professionals).

Participants often talked about being the person best placed to know why they smoked, why they wanted to quit, and what was likely to work for them. To these participants, external help or assistance was unlikely to be useful or necessary. For many this appeared to be because they had previous experience of unsuccessful assisted quit attempts (with, for example, OTC NRT, prescription NRT, smoking-cessation medications or behavioural support) and had learnt that for them, assistance was unhelpful or solved only part of the problem. Conversely, other participants had not previously used professional or pharmacological support to quit and therefore did not see the need to do so now. Still others simply did not equate smoking with being ill, or regard smoking and quitting as medical conditions: this meant medical support was not appropriate and little benefit would be gained from involving a GP in the quit attempt. Several participants implied that a GP would be able to offer only generic or lay quitting advice that was unlikely to be relevant to them personally: in other words, from the participant's perspective, the GP could add little to the participant's own personal store of quitting experiences.

A number of participants also appeared to have an issue with adopting a substitute behaviour (i.e. NRT or smoking-cessation medication). To these participants, the use of NRT or drugs meant that they were still dependent on nicotine or another substance to deal with their need for nicotine. If they really wanted to quit and to quit for good, they needed to take that step themselves, which to them essentially precluded the use of assistance and in particular, NRT.

Perceiving quitting unassisted to be the "right" or "better" choice

In contrast to the dominant medical and health promotion discourse about quitting unassisted being undesirable or even foolhardy, many participants saw quitting unassisted as the "right" or "better" way to quit. This belief appeared to be closely associated with what participants referred to as "being serious" about quitting. It appears that underlying these beliefs may be a set of values that the participant and perhaps also Australian society, as a whole, endorses.

Participants talked, either explicitly or implicitly, about the values that were important to them in relation to their quit attempt: independence, strength, autonomy, self-control and self-reliance. These values are, broadly speaking, also reflective of values central in many western societies and cultures. It seems likely that these broadly held values were influential in shaping participants' beliefs about quitting unassisted being the right or better choice and the belief that quitting was "up to me". Quitting unassisted allowed the participant to realise a need to feel independent, in control and autonomous, something that they would not necessarily have felt if they had used assistance. Some participants even suggested that seeking help from a GP or another source such as a quitline would be tantamount to admitting failure. The independent nature of their quit attempt was seen as an important contributor to the success of that attempt.

In summary, many participants believed they had achieved something of value by quitting unassisted, and appeared to take this achievement as an indicator of the strength of their moral character. In this context, quitting unassisted was presented as a morally superior option; quitting unassisted was evidence of personal virtue. It is important to note, however, that this was rarely used as a measure of the moral worth of others. Participants rarely suggested that other smokers who used assistance to quit were morally inferior. Rather, they presented their final, unassisted quit attempt as evidence that their personal virtue had increased over time, thus bolstering their own sense of identity and self-worth.

Discussion

In this community sample of ex-smokers who had quit on their own without consulting their GP or using smoking-cessation assistance, issues of cost and access to assistance, misperceptions relating to the effectiveness and safety of pharmacotherapy, and confidence in their ability to quit on their own affected their decision to quit unassisted. This was consistent with earlier quantitative and qualitative research. However, we found that the influences on non-use of assistance were more complex, involving careful judgements about the value of knowledge, the value of different quitting strategies, the importance of taking personal responsibility and the moral significance of quitting alone. Future efforts to improve uptake of assistance may need to take some of these influences into consideration.

In an effort to understand what appears to be conflicting advice about quitting and how to quit successfully, participants appear to fall back on trusting their intuition or common sense, giving preference to their personal and shared knowledge of quitting over professional or theoretical knowledge. Lay knowledge (or lay epidemiology) has previously been used to understand how health inequalities develop in smokers (Graham 1994, Lawlor, Frankel et al. 2003, Graham 2009), to inform health promotion practices in smoking cessation (Springett, Owens et al. 2007) and to explain the range of self-exempting beliefs used by smokers to avoid quitting (Oakes, Chapman et al. 2004). Our study is the first to demonstrate how lay knowledge influences non-use of assistance when attempting to quit smoking.

Participants who quit on their own often appeared reluctant to consult their GP, primarily because they did not view smoking or quitting as an illness, reflecting what others have also reported (Levinson, Borrayo et al. 2006, Fu, Burgess et al. 2007). Our analyses show that this reluctance to consult a GP may also be because smokers perceive the GP has little to offer beyond the smoker's own lay knowledge, reflecting what others have recently reported for smoking cessation consultations in general practice in the UK (Pilnick and Coleman 2010). This reluctance to consult a GP may be reinforced if the smoker is hesitant about using pharmacotherapy or if they believe smoking is not a "doctorable" condition. Doctorable is a term coined by Heritage and Robinson (Heritage and Robinson 2006) to explain the way in which patients in the USA account for their visits to

7 Insights from qualitative research with unassisted quitters

primary care physicians and to demonstrate how patients orientate to a need to present their concerns as doctorable. Before visiting a physician, patients make a judgement as to whether they require medical help. They are aware that the physician will subsequently judge their judgement when they present at the surgery. It is conceivable that this need to present only when the individual perceives the condition to be doctorable could apply not just to smoking cessation, but to other difficult-to-change health behaviours such as losing weight or getting fit.

In addition to judgements relating to the value of lay knowledge, our study highlights how smokers make judgements about the value of different quitting strategies based on perceptions of time and effort required, convenience and cost. This process of evaluation has been reported for decisions related to the taking of other prescribed medications. Pound et al. reported that patients often weigh up the benefits of taking a medicine against the costs of doing so and are often driven by an overarching desire to minimise medicine intake (Pound, Britten et al. 2005). In the current study, this evaluation of different quitting strategies often resulted in the participant forming a negative opinion of assistance and, in particular, of NRT. Given nicotine's complicated history and transformation from an addictive, toxic and potentially harmful drug to a medically useful drug it was not surprising that many participants found it difficult to reconcile nicotine's portrayal as being part of the problem and a possible solution (Keane 2013), and as a result appeared to be resisting use of medications to assist them to quit.

Underneath the prioritising of lay knowledge and the evaluation of different quitting strategies were deep-rooted cultural values, such as independence, strength, self-reliance, self-control and autonomy, which influenced participants' views on assisted and unassisted quitting. Lay knowledge in combination with these multilayered influences led many participants to believe that quitting unassisted was the "right" or "better" way to quit, that the participant was personally responsible for their quitting and that quitting unassisted was a prerequisite for "being serious" about quitting. This key concept, being serious, is one we believe is critically important to Australian smokers and one we are exploring further in our ongoing research.

It should be noted that this study included only successful ex-smokers (quit for at least six months). Given that these individuals were interviewed in the context of a successful quit attempt, attribution theory (Weiner 1985) might provide some insight into the emergence of independence, strength, self-control and personal virtue as components of the successful unassisted quit attempt in these interviews. Attribution theory suggests a self-serving bias in attributions such that success is attributed to internal factors (such as personal virtue), and failure to external or situational factors. It might be informative to conduct some research with smokers who tried to quit on their own and failed, as well as with ex-smokers who successfully quit with assistance to explore whether concepts relating to external or internal attributions emerge for these different groups of quitters.

Implications and future research

A proportion of smokers is unlikely to choose to use assistance to quit smoking or is reluctant to do so. Too much focus on pharmacological assistance may fail this group. It may be a more productive and a potentially more patient-centred approach to acknowledge that for these smokers quitting unassisted is a valid and potentially effective option.

Evidence-based medicine and clinical practice guidelines prioritise results from randomised controlled trials and meta-analyses of RCTs. As a consequence, current smoking-cessation guidelines in the UK (National Institute for Health and Care Excellence 2018), USA (Krist, Davidson et al. 2021) and Australia (Royal Australian College of General Practitioners 2021) position pharmacotherapy as first-line therapy for those dependent on nicotine (>10 cigarettes per day). A range of government policies ensures pharmacotherapy is free or heavily subsidised, available on prescription and/or OTC, and that smokers have access to widely promoted and free quitline advice and support, and/or dedicated stop-smoking services.

As discussed in Chapter 2, RCTs are designed to evaluate the efficacy of interventions, such as medications, in carefully controlled study populations; they cannot capture and often seek to eliminate the complexities associated with patients' lived experiences. This complexity may, however, be of relevance when making decisions about how to manage patients with complicated health-related behaviours, such as smoking. By retaining and examining some of the complexity surrounding quitting smoking, we have highlighted how participants' beliefs, values and preferences can influence the decision to quit unassisted. Previous research into patient-centred care has also identified that respect for a patient's beliefs and values (McCormack and McCance 2006), needs and preferences, (Laine and Davidoff 1996), and knowledge and experience (Byrne and Long 1976) are central to delivering care that is tailored to the needs of the individual patient. Accordingly, patient-centred care for smokers may include recognising and respecting smokers' reasons for declining assistance, validating and approving their choices, and modifying brief interventions to support their preference for unassisted quitting, where preferred.

Healthcare policy does not operate in a vacuum. As our study indicates, success of any given policy is critically dependent on the broader social and cultural context. This is especially true for tobacco control given the influence of key stakeholders such as the tobacco industry. Recent research highlights how the tobacco industry capitalised on the powerful notion of personal responsibility to frame tobacco problems as a matter for individuals to solve (Mejia, Dorfman et al. 2014). To our knowledge, our analysis is the first to indicate smokers do indeed feel personally responsible for quitting. Smokers' beliefs about quitting have been heavily influenced by social and cultural ideals, some of which are highly likely to have been shaped by the tobacco industry's individual choice rhetoric. The complexity of how such rhetoric has influenced smokers has to date been unexplored.

The value placed on lay knowledge and on different quitting strategies by participants indicates that GPs, health promotion practitioners and pharmaceutical companies may be advised to be mindful of the consequences of overselling assistance and potentially unrealistically raising smokers' outcome expectations, further fuelling the apparent gulf between lay experiences and expert-derived knowledge. The low absolute efficacy rates of NRT and stop-smoking medications create a challenge: is it possible to communicate about these products without disheartening smokers or making promises that may be difficult to deliver?

Cultural values are likely to play a role in the choice to use assistance or not, and future research should explore these issues in other cultures. It would be useful to replicate this study in other cultural contexts and in countries less advanced in tobacco control to determine whether the study findings are applicable across countries, cultural dimensions and stages of the tobacco epidemic.

For those patients who do seek medical advice, GPs may need to be cognisant of the role of lay knowledge and the patient's evaluation of different quitting strategies when counselling and advising about quitting smoking. The challenge will be to support those smokers who wish to quit unassisted while avoiding stigmatisation of those smokers who want or need assistance to quit.

Conclusion

A smoker's reluctance to use assistance to quit may sometimes be difficult to understand. Through this empirical work we are now able to suggest some explanations for this behaviour.

The reasons for smokers' rejection of the conventional medical model for smoking cessation are complex and go beyond the modifiable or correctable issues relating to misperceptions or treatment barriers. Lay knowledge and contextual factors are critically important to a smoker's decision to seek or resist assistance to quit. Smokers prioritise lay knowledge, evaluate assistance against unassisted quitting, believe quitting is their personal responsibility and perceive quitting unassisted to be the right or better option.

8
Strategies for reducing smoking across populations

Psychologist Stanton Peele commenced his 1989 iconoclastic book *Diseasing of America: how we allowed recovery zealots and the treatment industry to convince us we are out of control* (Peele 1989) by summarising what he found fundamentally misleading about "disease theory" in addiction. His book contested the disease theory's contentions that:

1. An addiction exists independently of the rest of a person's life and drives all choices about the substance(s) to which a person is addicted.
2. Addiction is progressive and irreversible, so that the addiction inevitably worsens unless the person seeks medical treatment or joins a support group.
3. The addict cannot recognise the disease in the absence of education by addiction experts.
4. Addiction means the person is incapable of controlling his or her addictive behaviour without assistance.

He wrote that his book was an attempt to "oppose this nonsense by understanding its sources and contradicting disease ideology". Peele's criticisms focused entirely on the addiction treatment industry and the ways in which it disabled personal agency in those wanting to end their dependencies. Throughout this book, I've set out evidence for how this process arose and consolidated for the case of smoking.

Peele's four criticisms provide a bedrock for understanding why it is that the excessive medicalisation and commodification of smoking cessation emerged and has been sustained. But it is important to emphasise that nothing in this perspective requires any disagreement that nicotine is a highly addictive drug which ticks all the definitional boxes for a dependence-producing drug. Tobacco and vaping industry chemists know a great deal about how to fine-tune the grip of nicotine to maximise the probability of experimental users developing quickly into daily users and holding them there.

That said, disease theory has infected popular understanding of addiction – including smoking – with often ridiculous hard determinist narratives: if you are a smoker, you'll find it very hard to quit, you'll fail perhaps many times to quit, and you'd be very foolish to think that you can quit without professional help or being medicated in your efforts.

Our 2010 *PLOS Medicine* paper on the neglect of unassisted quitting research and its dissemination to smokers concluded with a plea for restoring balance in communications with smokers about smoking cessation. We wrote, "public sector communicators should be encouraged to redress the overwhelming dominance of assisted cessation in public awareness, so that some balance can be restored in smokers' minds regarding the contribution that assisted and unassisted smoking cessation approaches can make to helping them quit" (Chapman and MacKenzie 2010).

In our paper we also provided a summary of messages that should be given to smokers, but rarely are. These include:

- A serious attempt at stopping *need not* involve using NRT or other drugs, or getting professional support (note: we did not say that it *must not* involve pharmacotherapy).
- Assistance should be considered a second-line choice for those who really need help. It should not be the first-line as it is now throughout the professionalised guidance literature on quitting.
- NRT, other prescribed pharmaceuticals and professional counselling or support have helped many smokers, but are certainly not necessary for quitting.

- Along with motivational "why" messages designed to stimulate cessation attempts, smokers should be repeatedly told that going cold turkey or reducing then quitting are the methods that have been and remain most commonly used by successful ex-smokers.
- Many quit efforts are not serious attempts but little more than flaccid gestures with little conviction.
- So-called failures in quit attempts are a normal part of the natural history of cessation. For millions, they have been rehearsals for eventual success. Just because you did not succeed in an unassisted attempt doesn't mean that a later attempt will also not succeed.
- More smokers find it unexpectedly easy or moderately difficult than find it very difficult to quit.
- Many successful ex-smokers do not plan their quitting in advance and those who don't plan have greater success, probably because they have greater determination and are not distracted by largely evidence-free professional folklore about taking a staged approach to quitting.
- In a growing number of countries today, there are far more ex-smokers than smokers.

The core message I have tried to emphasise throughout this book has been that the overwhelming dominance of assisted cessation in the way that quitting has been framed over the past three decades has done a huge disservice to public understanding of how most smokers quit. Around the world, many hundreds of millions of smokers have stopped without professional or pharmacological help. In Chapter 5 we saw there is no strong evidence that while all this has been happening, today's smokers have become "hardened". If anything, the very opposite is the case.

The persistence of unassisted cessation as the most common way that most smokers have succeeded in quitting is an unequivocally positive message which, far from being suppressed or ignored, should be openly embraced by primary health care workers and public health authorities as the front-line "how to" message in all clinical encounters and public communication about cessation. It should be shouted from the rooftops of every government health department, non-government health organisation and emphasised opportunistically in media interviews about the importance of quitting.

Because of their trusted roles with patients, clinicians can play vital roles in motivating quit attempts and assisting smokers to quit. Drugs can certainly be a part of this. But what I lament is the way that unassisted cessation is mostly ignored and frequently denigrated by the professional smoking-cessation community, many of whom also have occupationally vested interests in maintaining the fiction that unassisted cessation is not a sensible or "evidence-based" way to quit. I support stepwise approaches to triaging assistance to smokers, but note that many smokers can quit unassisted and that the primary message to smokers ought not to overstate the difficulty of quitting by constantly characterising cessation as something that has virtually no chance of success when the experience of most ex-smokers abundantly shows otherwise.

In this chapter, I want to focus on what has driven so many to quit smoking since the 1950s. I will explore what lessons this holds for those working today in tobacco control, public health and government and what they should focus on more, rather than diverting energy to distracting strategies that can never deliver the large numbers necessary for driving smoking down across whole populations. Or worse, naïvely enabling strategies to flourish which risk slowing or reversing the trend away from smoking.

The melding of primary and secondary prevention

In public health, a basic approach to conceptualising preventive policies and interventions is the primary, secondary and tertiary distinction. Primary prevention involves actions taken to prevent a given health problem from ever occurring; secondary prevention is where steps are taken to identify a nascent problem early so that it might be treated early where evidence shows that early direction and treatment can improve outcomes; and tertiary prevention is activity designed to helping people better manage long-term health problems (e.g. chronic diseases, permanent impairments) to improve as much as possible their functioning, quality of life and life expectancy.

Smoking declines in populations in two ways: growth in the proportion of people who have never smoked, and increases in the proportion of smokers who quit permanently. The first is achieved by primary prevention and the second by the interplay of many factors which often work together to motivate smokers to quit (secondary prevention).

When it comes to cessation in nations which have embraced comprehensive approaches to tobacco control across several decades, there's an elephant in the room unavoidable to anyone looking at the very top line of data on progress. In such nations, ex-smokers today significantly outnumber those who smoke. In the USA since 2002, there have been more former smokers in the USA than current smokers (United States Surgeon General 2020).

Australia is another perfect example, with there being more ex-smokers than smokers in all eight national Australian Institute of Health and Welfare triennial surveys conducted between 1998 and 2019. In 1998, 25.4% of Australians aged 14 and over smoked (daily or less than daily and any form of combusted tobacco) and 25.9% were ex-smokers. By 2019 this had changed to 14.9% (2.9 million) smoking, 22.8% (4.8 million) being ex-smokers, with 13.2 million having never smoked (Australian Institute of Health and Welfare 2020h).

This 12% fall in the proportion who were ex-smokers between these 21 years is a product of smokers quitting or dying, but most importantly also because of the continual growth in the proportion of Australians who have never smoked (49.2% in 1998 and climbing to 63.1% in 2019) (Australian Institute of Health and Welfare 2020g). By definition, an ex-smoker must have once smoked. So when the size of the pool of never smokers keeps expanding, there are far fewer smokers available to contribute to the ex-smoking pool. By far the biggest contribution to increasing the proportion of people who do not smoke today (never smokers plus ex-smokers) comes from the huge primary prevention success story in reducing smoking uptake in young people. Around 60% of all smokers in Australia commenced regular smoking before the age of 18.

So in tobacco control, primary prevention has made the biggest impact by – across the years – greatly increasing the proportion of the population who have never smoked. Activities designed to motivate and help smokers to quit are secondary prevention, and around the world these too have seen cumulatively many hundreds of millions quit, particularly since the 1960s. However, it is vital to understand that many policies and initiatives often operate in both modalities. As we will see later in this chapter, consonant with what occurs with nearly all goods and services, rises in retail price such as via tobacco tax can motivate smokers to both quit or reduce daily cigarette consumption. But they can also be a factor which, along with others, deter uptake in young people on zero or very low incomes who are highly price sensitive.

Similarly, quit-smoking campaigns designed to motivate quitting in smokers are also seen by vast numbers of teenagers who don't smoke. Many of them experience the same deterrent effects that smokers experience. Instead of thinking as smokers do, "I think I'll quit," they think, "Wow, I really don't want to risk those illnesses happening to me. I won't start" (White, Tan et al. 2003).

Throughout this book, we have seen that for as long as smokers have been quitting, a substantial majority of ex-smokers made their final, successful and long-term sustained quit smoking attempt unaided. They have not swallowed, worn, chewed or inhaled any aid or received any sustained assistance from any professional therapist, counsellor or advisor. Hundreds of millions of people around the world who once smoked discovered they had the agency to end what for many was a strong addiction without recourse to assistance. And as we saw in Chapter 5, the proposition that all of these people were simply the low-hanging fruit of light smokers who were able to quit more easily – an assumption of the hardening hypothesis – is simply not borne out by the evidence.

I've laid out evidence for this phenomenon and for the efforts of commercial interests in the pharmaceutical and NVP industries to discredit it and distract smokers from industry income-subverting thoughts that they might quit without using these industries' products. Sadly, they have often been abetted in their efforts by leaders in public health and medicine, many of whom have been supported by grants and conference travel from those industries. Together, for the reasons I've set out, these interest groups have been major, industrial-strength purveyors of methods of quit-smoking mass distraction.

Big Tobacco, now also heavily invested in NVPs, sees an ideal nicotine delivery device as one which either holds smokers in smoking through dual use, or grips vapers in the other frantic nicotine self-dosing rituals we've all seen and which I described in Chapter 6. An ideal smoking-cessation product for a pharmaceutical or NVP company is not one which succeeds quickly and therefore renders continual use of such products no longer necessary. It is rather a product that doesn't work very well at all but which can be cloaked in ever-changing marketing appeals that smokers need to use it longer, try it again, use it in combination with other drugs, or use it forever. NRT in particular fits that description like a glove.

The new narrative: don't quit ... switch!

Even well before the early 1960s, the dominant narrative about smoking has been that it was something that most people who did it regretted and struggled to end. But today this narrative is being undermined by a shift from one about *quitting* smoking to one about *switching* to NVPs, to the great delight of those in the industries whose very existence rests on the widespread continuation of nicotine dependency. Today, it is common to hear interviews with people introduced as authorities in tobacco control who give a perfunctory nod to quitting before gushing forth with snakeoil-like carnival barker style claims that make vaping sound like a wonder drug and nicotine as an almost vitamin-like substance.

Some of the very worst are down-in-the-last-shower, inexperienced people who were never engaged in any substantive way with the decades of successful tobacco control that saw smoking rates continually fall; the tobacco industry treated by governments, the media and the public as the corporate pariahs they have always been (Christofides, Chapman et al. 1999); and every advocacy campaign that was ever fought to curtail their dissembling and marketing succeed with the passage of laws the industry loathed and fought. Some of these "researchers" are supported by lavish grants originating from the tobacco industry and feted with international travel support laundered through "independent" third-party slush funds.

In sidelining quitting to put the spotlight on switching, two huge and inconvenient truths have become marginalised under the weight of anecdotal evidence from cult-like vaping advocates. First, as we saw in Chapter 6, the accumulating evidence is that a majority of those who take up vaping never give up smoking but instead engage in dual use, often for many months or years. And these dual users do not reduce their exposure toxicants: they in fact get *more* than smokers who do not vape

– see Chapter 6 (Miller, Smith et al. 2020). Second, relapse to smoking rates in those who vape, including those who vape regularly, are higher than those smokers who try to quit without vaping (McMillen, Klein et al. 2019, Miller, Smith et al. 2020, Gravely, Cummings et al. 2021). Knowing this, the interests of the tobacco industry in promoting vaping are obvious (Sollenberger and Bredderman 2021).

And this is before we even touch on the alarming rise in regular nicotine use via NVPs in young people, who were on track in several nations to keep breaking all records in having the lowest smoking rates (and lowest of any nicotine use) since smoking began being monitored in national surveys.

But while all this has been happening, unassisted smoking has continued each year to deliver more net long-term ex-smokers than all other quitting methods combined. So what does the evidence show about factors which have fomented, stimulated, triggered and sustained this massive, ongoing but little appreciated and understudied phenomenon?

Attribution problems in smoking cessation research

When former or current smokers are questioned about their smoking, they are generally asked about their smoking history, their smoking frequency (how often and how many cigarettes they smoke), the number of times and the duration of their past attempts to quit, and whether they used any aids in their quit attempts and how long they persisted with these. Some studies also explore factors that quitters believe were responsible for their decision to try to quit.

As we saw in Chapters 3 and 7, for many smokers, having a method to quit (a *how*), is far less front-of-mind than having a reason to quit (the *why* of quitting). I've also emphasised that the obsession among many in tobacco control with cessation *rates* without giving equal or more weight to any cessation method's population *reach* has muzzled efforts to encourage unassisted cessation. The key to unleashing more quitting throughout a nation's smokers, then, may be to focus less on *how* to quit, and far more on motivating more smokers with a *why* to try to quit and to do this more frequently, regardless of whether these quit attempts are assisted or unassisted.

In this I'm reminded of German philosopher Friedrich Nietzsche who said that those who have a "why" to live for can endure almost any "how". So adapting Nietzsche, smokers who have deeply internalised powerful motivations for quitting will usually find a way to quit.

The vital importance of promoting quit attempts

A seminal paper from 2012 by Shu-Hong Zhu and colleagues (Zhu, Lee et al. 2012) is apposite here. The authors looked at US National Health Interview Survey population data from 1991 to 2010, to examine the key equation of *population cessation impact = effectiveness × reach*. The authors observed:

> it might seem obvious that smokers must first try to quit before they can succeed, making the importance of quit attempts self-evident. However, the field of cessation has focused so much on developing interventions to improve smokers' odds of success when they attempt to quit that it has largely neglected to investigate how to get more smokers to try to quit and to try more frequently.

In making this case, Zhu et al. noted that in both the USA and the UK, significant rises in using smoking cessation medications had not translated to higher quit rates. In the USA in 2000, 22.1% of smokers making quit attempts used medications and this increased to 31.2% by 2010. But they emphasised that there was "no corresponding incremental increase in the 3-month quit rate" and that changes in the quit rate across that time "correspond[ed] more to changes in the quit attempt rate than to changes in the use of cessation medications".

When the UK turbo-charged the promotion of medications commencing in 1999, medication use changed dramatically. From 1999 to 2001, the proportion of quit attempts that involved cessation medications leapt from 28% to 61% (West, DiMarino et al. 2005). A corresponding change in the population cessation rate was projected but not found for those years (Kotz, Fidler et al. 2011).

So what do we know about how best to motivate more smokers to make more quit attempts?

What "works" in tobacco control?

Across some 45 years of working in tobacco control, there have been countless times when I've been asked, "So, has [insert here] policy or [insert here] campaign worked?" Most asking this do not then go on to explain what they mean by "worked", but many hundreds of such conversations have taught me that they are most often wanting to know "What's the evidence that a policy or campaign causes many extra smokers to quit for good?"

The question has its roots in clinical interventions where we all have had many experiences of the desired changes after using a drug. We all know what happens when we take an analgesic for pain, get an injection before having a tooth pulled or root canal therapy, apply a fungicide on athlete's foot, or use contraceptives and avoid pregnancy. It quickly becomes very obvious when these things work!

So it's understandable that people should ask the same about a piece of tobacco control legislation or a multimillion-dollar TV campaign about smoking when "doses" of these are given to whole communities. Do these things make a difference across whole populations? For example, in the wake of Philip Morris International being ordered to pay the Australian government $50 million in legal costs over the company's failed attempt to thwart plain packaging (Donovan 2017), I was asked the question, "Has plain packaging worked?" many times. Those interested in this question can read a vast amount of research on this in *Packaging as promotion: evidence for and effects of plain packaging* (Greenhalgh and Scollo 2019).

The cauldron of proximal and distal influences

While many asking these questions demand a simple yes or no answer, the forensics of understanding how it is that people both try and succeed in quitting are far more complicated than the clinical assessment of a drug. In 1999, the late Tony McMichael, professor of epidemiology at the Australian National University, published a classic paper in the *American Journal of Epidemiology* titled "Prisoners of the proximate: Loosening the constraints on epidemiology in an age of change". He wrote about the need to understand the determinants of population health in terms that extended beyond proximate single influences and drew as well on distal influences that can often simmer and percolate for many years before manifesting in cultural and individual change (McMichael 1999).

While a smoker might nominate a particular policy, conversation with a doctor or anti-smoking campaign as being *the* reason they quit, much of what went on before provides the broad shoulders of concern that condition and carry the final, typically proximal attribution. There are synergies between all these factors and the demand to separate them all is like the demand to completely unscramble an omelette: we know that when all the ingredients are cooked together, the result can be very satisfying. But all cooks know that the final result is greater than the simple sum of each of the ingredients.

In science though, the appetite in the dining room is for all cooks to give reductionist explanations, where the goal is to pinpoint the *exact* contribution of every variable to an outcome (Shuttleworth 2008).

When they finally succeed, ex-smokers will often nominate a reason "why" they quit as they share their story with others. People will sometimes nominate a recent "straw that broke the camel's back" as the precipitating reason for the final decision to quit and their resolve to see it through. This can be a symptom they have experienced; an incident like the smoking-caused death of a friend or family member; a particularly poignant campaign advertisement that they couldn't get out of their head; the heartfelt pleading from a child or partner that they quit smoking; the sudden realisation that very few of their colleagues or friends smoke; an epiphany about being yoked by nicotine addiction when having to leave a restaurant to smoke out in a cold street with others with similar nicotine dependency; or being faced with a psychological barrier like cigarette prices going up to $35 a pack. Sometimes smokers are keen to point to several of these things clustering around *the* incident or conversation which they feel finally made them do it.

These proximal triggers can certainly stimulate quit attempts: factors easily identified, nominated by smokers aware of their influence, and sometimes easy to quantify with proxy measures like immediate boosts in calls to quitlines after known scheduling of televised quit messages (Miller, Wakefield et al. 2003).

But there are also vital distal or background factors at play, slowly and subconsciously eating away the foundations of smokers' feelings of disease invincibility or apathy and denormalising pro-smoking social environments. Smokers get fewer positive reminders about smoking and experience a growing awareness that smoking is not something that the great majority of people do anymore.

Examples of these distal factors are advertising bans, graphic warnings on packs, plain packaging, smoke-free public spaces, tobacco taxation, and the constant flow of news and campaign information about the harm from smoking. Most countries with advanced tobacco control have implemented most of these policies. Few if any smokers will say they quit smoking because tobacco advertising was banned. Thirty years ago when we fought for advertising bans, tobacco companies used to jubilantly hold such survey findings aloft, pleading with governments to keep their hands off advertising. "See, this survey shows that no one names tobacco advertising as either a reason they took up smoking or continue to do it." But does this mean that both advertising and its banning have no impacts?

The obvious question so often able to be asked about such tobacco industry protests is why, if a policy really offers no threat to tobacco sales, does the industry even worry about its introduction? Why bother spending hundreds of millions around the world to stop advertising bans, graphic health warnings on packs, plain packaging or the spread of smoke-free policies if none of these things allegedly makes any difference?

Advertising can have rapid effects, as any manufacturer or retailer can attest. But the impact of advertising bans also works in slow-burn fashion. Instead of the best efforts of advertising agencies to imbue every opportunity with memorable imagery and persuasions about the joys of smoking, in 1996 the final curtain came down forever in Australia on that long-running effort when the last outlet for tobacco sporting sponsorship ended. A child born in 1996 is 26 today in 2022. They have lived all their life never having been exposed to any form of tobacco advertising, promotion or sponsorship that can be controlled by Australian legislation.

While some smokers experienced an increased urgency to quit by the purposefully unappealing plain packs with their ghoulish (but deadly accurate) large graphic health warnings (Wakefield, Hayes et al. 2013), the primary goal for plain packs was to have whole generations grow up never having been beguiled by the designer edginess of tobacco pack branding and noting the exceptionalism of plain packaging among all other consumer goods. Tobacco is the only product where legislation mandates plain packaging (32 nations have either implemented, legislated it or announced that they will) (Canadian Cancer Society and International Status Report 2021) and out-of-sight retail display bans (Harper 2006). These thoughts ("Hmm, why does all this apply only to tobacco?") might help shake the fragile foundations of the belief that tobacco is just another of the many risks in life.

Importantly, all these factors do not act in isolation, but like a constant and unstoppable termite colony, they work often unnoticed in synergy to erode the appeal of smoking.

A day in the life of Australian smoker Mr Rex Lungs, 2022

In my 1992 *BMJ* paper "Unravelling gossamer with boxing gloves: problems in explaining the decline in smoking" (Chapman 1993), I described a day in the life of a smoker who had just quit. The smoker woke to radio news of yet more bad research news about smoking; lived with disapproving family members who had often urged him to quit because they had been educated about the risks; winced every time at the price he had to pay for a pack; was acutely aware of all the places he couldn't smoke and why those laws had been introduced; was self-conscious about the stench of stale tobacco that he carried about; and couldn't shake some of the powerful anti-smoking advertising that intruded on his TV viewing.

A smoker might well nominate just one of these influences as top-of-mind when a researcher calls, but all play a part in a comprehensive approach to reducing the world's leading cause of death, if we exclude poverty. A huge amount has changed in the day-to-day life of smokers in countries like Australia in the 38 years since that paper was published. So below, I have updated a day in the life of a smoker from 1993 to what it might be like in 2022. Let's consider a recent day in the life of an Australian smoker, Rex.

As he wakes, Rex listens to a news item on his bedside radio concerning a new report which calculated that lung cancer is still the leading cause of cancer death in Australia and that 14% of smokers will develop lung cancer, including 7.7% of those who are currently smoking only 1–5 cigarettes/day and 26.4% of those who smoke >35 cigarettes a day (compared to 1.0% in never smokers) (Weber, Sarich et al. 2021). He had heard these grim reports so often since he started smoking as a teenager, but this one sticks in his mind because he'd taken some comfort in thinking that his mere 10 cigarettes a day would not be very risky. There goes another comforting rationalisation down the drain (Chapman, Wong et al. 1993, Oakes, Chapman et al. 2004).

The night before, he had been to a football match. It seemed like aeons ago that teams played for a trophy sponsored by a brand of cigarettes (the last tobacco-sponsored sporting event ended in Australia in April 1996). Now they even sold salads and sushi as well as the usual pies, hamburgers and greasy fries at sports stadia. And even though it was an outdoor stadium he'd been to, you weren't allowed to smoke in the stands but had to go some distance behind one grandstand to a grim fenced-off "smoking area" and stand smoking with others.

As Rex sat at the breakfast table, one of his kids remarked that she could tell he'd already been out in the garden smoking because she could smell it on him. It seemed there had been dozens of these embarrassing jibes over the years. He wondered what people he worked with thought about this, but kept quiet about it. He knew his kids had lessons about smoking risks at school and felt bad that his smoking might make them worried about him dying early.

His wife, who, like the great majority of Australian women in their 40s didn't smoke, actively disliked smoking. Ever since the late 1980s when Rex's workplace had banned smoking, he had agreed to only smoke out in the garden and not in sight of their children. In making this request, it seemed to Rex that she was not really being overzealous. He had often heard scientists in the media talking about the risks of exposure to other people's tobacco smoke and it seemed it was only the tobacco companies and shouty, swivel-eyed libertarian extremists who ever tried to dispute this. Smoking had become thoroughly denormalised (Chapman and Freeman 2008).

When he smoked outside, he always felt self-conscious and embarrassed that he was setting a bad example to his kids. He really didn't want them to smoke and had recently had the thought that he had never heard any smoker ever express hope that their kids would take up smoking, at any age. He was definitely one of the 90% of smokers who regretted he'd ever started smoking (Fong, Hammond et al. 2004). He knew it was harming him. It was hideously expensive. It made him smell. He had long felt any loyalty toward smoking seeping away. Was there any product to which its loyal customers felt such loathing and ambivalence?

On the way to the train station to go to work he stopped to buy a new pack. He looked at the price board in the newsagent (there had been no cigarettes on retail display for over a decade since state government legislation forced all tobacco stock to be stored out of sight). His usual 25-stick-pack of premium cigarettes now costs $48.50 – just under $2 a cigarette – while the average 20-cigarette pack costs $35. Ten years ago, Rex used to smoke a full pack a day. At today's prices that would set him back $17,700 over a year. So he had deliberately cut down to 10 cigarettes a day. But even that was still gouging $7,080 from his wallet each year. He'd seen a travel package offer showing where, for that money, he could take his whole family of four on a week's luxury holiday to Bali, flights included, when travel resumed after COVID-19.

One of the sweeteners of pre-COVID-19 overseas travel had been that he could bring back two cartons of duty-free cigarettes, saving big money on what they would have cost him in Australia. But that too had all stopped, with duty-free being now limited to just one unopened pack.

Boarding his train, he pondered that here he was in the place where all these smoking bans started. Public transport had gone smoke-free in New South Wales way back in 1976, joined in 1987 by all domestic flights in Australia. These days there was not a single airline anywhere in the world which allowed smoking or vaping.

His daughter was soon to move interstate to attend a specialised course at a Melbourne university. She would need shared rental accommodation. As he browsed his phone for what was available, he noticed how many of the "share accommodation" listings specified that only non-smokers need apply. Indeed, as far back as 1992, 42% of share accommodation advertisements specified this requirement – a higher rate than any other quality sought by advertisers (Chapman 1992).

Smoking had been banned in all indoor workplaces in the years after all government departments banned smoking in offices in 1987.

He'd even heard that lonely hearts advertisements overwhelmingly specified that people ruled out smokers when looking for a date (Chapman, Wakefield et al. 2004). Browsing his newspaper, he saw a large advertisement from a life-insurance company offering substantially reduced rates for non-smokers.

Walking from the train and arriving at work, Rex stubbed out what would be his last cigarette until lunchtime. You hadn't been able to smoke in restaurants since 1990, and in bars and pubs since 2 July 2007. At lunchtime, Rex went with some colleagues to a nearby café for a coffee and sandwich. He noticed that even at the tables outside the café on the footpath, smoking was not allowed. At the ever-diminishing number of cafés where you could still smoke outside, he was often self-conscious about the death stares he'd get from nearby tables when he lit up. He then passed a street sign warning him that he could be fined for discarding his cigarette butt in the street – the non-biodegradability of butts made them a major pollution problem, especially in a city where stormwater ran into the picturesque harbour around which the city was built. Being very environmentally conscious, he felt quietly ashamed about his usual throw-away method of disposing of butts.

And if you were driving your own car, the police could pull you over and fine you if you were smoking in your car when you had children inside (Freeman et al. 2008). He'd been to an outdoor prog-rock concert recently, and despite it being outdoors, announcements were made from the stage about there being a sectioned-off smoking area, way back near the toilet areas.

Home that evening, Rex relaxed in front of the TV where on the news he heard a report linking smoking with yet another dreaded disease. "Was there *anything* that smoking didn't cause?" he thought to himself, reflecting on all the news reports he had heard about the subject over the years. Being a sports fan, he zapped his TV between channels showing the national soccer and basketball competitions. And there it was again: anti-smoking sponsorship messages on the sidelines and even on the players' clothing.

He'd given some thought to taking up vaping. But as an avid Twitter user, he'd noticed that so often when posts were made about vaping, they were made by those who seemed to have little interest in anything else. Their Twitter handles even described them as vapers. Their photographs often showed them vaping. Some even talked about their "vaping lifestyle" and went to vaping meet-ups. This reminded him of many stock-market obsessives, golfers, video gamers and dope smokers he tried to avoid. They were so one-dimensional. He liked wine and craft beers too. But he'd no sooner want to badge his whole identity on Twitter as a wine drinker as it would ever occur to him to proudly present himself there as a steak eater (he liked steak too). It seemed like taking up vaping ran big risks of being pulled into a kind of cult. And the massive plumes of vapour you'd see vapers billowing down the street looked very try-hard "please look at me". So vaping held little appeal.

The next day, Rex decided that he would finally quit. Over the years, he'd made several gestures to do so that lasted a few days. And again, over the next 12 months, he made a few unsuccessful attempts, one inspired by a brief warning given to him by his doctor, and another being a few weeks where he used OTC nicotine gum after prompting from his pharmacist. Eighteen months after his initial decision, he smoked what would be his last cigarette. In doing so, he joined approximately 4.8 million Australian adults who identify themselves as former smokers (Australian Institute of Health and Welfare 2020h).

Shortly after he finally stopped smoking, he was interviewed by a researcher working on the evaluation of a government media quit-smoking campaign. Rex joined those responding that they had seen the campaign; who said they strongly agreed that the campaign made them think about quitting; and who responded that "health reasons", "social unacceptability" and "cost" were the three main reasons they stopped smoking.

The researchers subsequently wrote a scientific article where they claimed that their statewide media campaign was probably a key factor responsible for a quit rate within the state which was higher than that found in other states without such campaigns. This claim was based on extrapolations made from the sample of aggregated recent quitters like Rex.

Bringing the background into the foreground

While Rex provided the researcher with what he thought were the "main" reasons he decided to finally quit, the many other influences in the typical day just described were not irrelevant. They were just not top-of-mind. We might conceptualise the most acknowledged and frequently researched factors as *foreground* foci in tobacco control evaluation research. But there are also many complex "hidden in clear sight" *background* factors that rarely if ever are even acknowledged when researchers consider population-wide movements in smoking prevalence (Chapman 1999).

Hughes et al. encapsulated well the privileging of proximal factors over distal influences in accounting for cessation when they wrote in 2012, "we doubt that exposure to media advertisements on cessation would decrease the rate of relapse [to smoking] years after they were seen, but they may still be effective, even over the long-term, because they stimulated quit attempts while the advertisements were still airing" (Hughes, Cummings et al. 2012).

This is a remarkably myopic view of the way in which we should understand behaviour change. It is dismissive of the idea that decisions we take today could have anything to do with particular and many cumulative influences we may have been exposed to in sometimes even the distant past. It suggests that we change only in response to recent stimuli. And it overly atomises the part played by single variables like a particular anti-smoking message in the consolidating awareness of a broad canvas of negativity about continuing to smoke that eventually motivates cessation. Basic educational and child development psychology take it as elementary that early influences and life experiences are pivotal in influencing broad constructs like self-esteem, confidence and resilience. So the idea that exposure to anti-smoking influences in even the deep past could come home to roost much later when a confluence of more proximal, enabling factors fomented to make this happen is hardly a radical thought.

In 1998 Melanie Wakefield and Frank Chaloupka called for more attention from those in tobacco control to the description and quantification of tobacco control "inputs" (Wakefield and Chaloupka 1998). By this, they meant that we needed far more fine-grained detail

8 Strategies for reducing smoking across populations

about all the ingredients in a nation's "black box" of tobacco control policies and actions aimed at reducing smoking. It was not good enough, for example, to just note and tick off that a nation had health warnings on packs, school anti-smoking curricula, anti-smoking media campaigns or smoke-free policies. Wakefield and Chaloupka noted that the preoccupation with outcomes in evaluation research was often accompanied by overly casual accounts of the policy and intervention variables that were assumed to be the causative factors potentially producing change. They argued for the further development of a range of indices to measure the comprehensiveness of tobacco control policies and programs.

And the reliability of claims about even seemingly black and white, uncomplicated components of tobacco control can sometimes be very poor. For example, when I wrote a situation report on Papua New Guinea for the WHO's Western Pacific Office in 1987, PNG was about to introduce bans on tobacco advertising (Roemer 1993). In 1996, Hayman reported widespread tobacco advertising was still to be seen throughout the country, including music and sporting sponsorship (Hayman 1996). And in 2011, a review described the bans as very weak with over 85% of PNG youth reporting having seen tobacco advertisements (Cussen and McCool 2011). Similarly, many nations have passed smoke-free policy legislation but far fewer, particularly in low-income nations, ever implement the legislation in any way that such policies are often fully implemented and enforced in more affluent nations. My wife was a primary school teacher for nearly 40 years. Yes, she said, there was curriculum material on smoking available to use with children. But was it actually used in the way that maths, spelling, reading, art and music were always taught and never considered optional? No.

The call to better document tobacco control actions led to instruments to try and score the comprehensiveness of tobacco control policies and programs. Examples include Levy's 2001 SimSmoke simulation model (Levy, Friend et al. 2001); Levy and others' Tobacco Control Scorecard (2004 and 2017) (Levy, Chaloupka et al. 2004, Levy, Tam et al. 2018); Joossens and Raw's 2006 Tobacco Control Scale (Joossens and Raw 2006); and the World Health Organization's more simplified six policy domains MPOWER checklist from 2008 (Song, Zhao et al. 2016).

These were all important starts. But there can be large and important gaps between what those supplying information to researchers or the WHO for its regular updates on global progress in tobacco control enter into their questionnaires, and what *actually* happens in a country. Those requesting the information are often in no position to cross check these issues, particularly for low-income nations where the currency and quality of data is often poor. Across my career I've frequently seen evidence that such requests for information land on the desks of people who are either very unaware of the difference between what is *meant* to be the case and what is *actually* the case in a country. Sometimes this misinformation is deliberate, designed to not embarrass a country in international league tables on tobacco control practice when they have implemented very little.

News media coverage of tobacco control

Importantly, Wakefield and Chaloupka (Wakefield and Chaloupka 1998) also noted the need to quantify and account for "environmental" issues such as unpaid news media coverage of tobacco issues. This truly gigantic factor cannot be overemphasised. Were it possible to quantify all media coverage of tobacco in societies with 24-hour access to a multitude of radio, television, print media, the world wide web and social media, in aggregate, this coverage would routinely and massively eclipse even the most intensive coverage gained through formal, typically very time-limited, purchased public health campaigns.

Much of this huge reportage is far from being easily dismissed as inconsequential ephemera: some of the most potent and recalled episodes in the history of tobacco control have been powerful prime-time television documentaries, prolonged episodes such as the tsunami of previously secret internal tobacco documents being released before and after the US Master Settlement Agreement (Clegg Smith, Wakefield et al. 2003) and the coverage of legal cases, such as the late Rolah McCabe's suit against British American Tobacco for promoting smoking to her when she was a teenager (Wakefield, McLeod et al. 2003). Such examples are newsworthy because they often embody time-honoured news values like injustice, corruption, predatory corporate behaviour, government incompetence, wolves in sheep's clothing, duplicity and hypocrisy (Chapman 2007).

These news subtexts inflect the meaning of news stories about smoking and thereby shape public and political understanding of something ostensibly "factual" in ways that can in turn shape individuals' understandings of the meaning of smoking and public health efforts to reduce it.

Tobacco control has long been highly newsworthy (Chapman 1989, Menashe and Siegel 1998, Champion and Chapman 2005). In 1995, 38% of all front pages of the *Sydney Morning Herald* carried at least one health story (Lupton 1995). Of these, tobacco stories ranked second after those about health services. From a journalist's perspective, tobacco control offers rich pickings that often conform with editors' notions of newsworthiness. This field is resplendent with stories of conflict, corruption, moral rectitude and reprobation. To the endless delight of the media, practically every organ of the body can be afflicted by tobacco use and tobacco's stratospheric toll on health lends itself to numerous excursions into quantification rhetoric – efforts to make statistics memorable to audiences (Potter 1991). Celebrities' efforts to quit or criticism directed at the influence of their smoking on young people are routine news events (Chapman and Leask 2001).

The media's appetite for villains finds inexhaustible sustenance in the conduct of the tobacco industry, which has long provided a low benchmark for referencing ethical low-life. If you google "just like the tobacco industry", oceans of examples of unethical conduct in a wide variety of other industries are instantly returned. At the October 2021 COP26 climate meeting in Glasgow, oil companies were likened to the tobacco industry in the way both engaged in denial about the health consequences of their products. Repeatedly casting the tobacco industry in such an unfavourable light seems likely to be associated with the community's ranking of tobacco industry representatives' trustworthiness as lower than that of a used-car salesman, the traditional low standard for ethical behaviour (Chapman 2020). This in turn strengthens the hand of governments wanting to introduce tough tobacco control legislation.

The Australian Health Minister, Nicola Roxon, is responsible for introducing plain tobacco packaging, which commenced in December

2012. When I asked her about the political conditions that allowed her to pursue this radical policy, she said she was emphatic the tobacco industry's appalling reputation as corporate pariahs was important in this decision:

> When the taskforce report came, marshalling all the evidence for various measures including plain packaging, this was when I really started to give it serious thought. I can remember one of my advisors, on my personal staff, not the bureaucrats, saying to me well, this is just a "no-brainer". Meaning, it might be new and bold, but it hit a political sweet spot too – you have good evidence, you have doctors and researchers on side, you're trying to protect kids and the only one lining up against you is the tobacco industry. With a sceptical media and pretty well informed public, fighting such a discredited industry was not as dangerous as people thought (Chapman and Freeman 2014).

That corporate bottom-dwelling reputation did not happen serendipitously. It was the result of decades of tobacco control advocacy which helped focus news media attention on the industry's nefarious activities and the ever-increasing resultant related public and cross-party political antipathy toward Big Tobacco.

There can be few more important questions for tobacco control than better understanding the complex nature of dominant forces driving regret and this antipathy to smoking and the powerful industry that seeks to perpetuate it. There are also few more perplexing questions than why the study of this messy complexity does not command the same or greater research attention as the study of discrete, easily quantified and often sponsored interventions typically generates. The research privileging of sponsored interventions and the comparative neglect of the study of ubiquitous background media "noise" about smoking, such as the examples given earlier, is probably best explained by the political imperatives for evaluation: funding agencies want to know what their campaign investment has achieved and may be less concerned about issues they feel they do not control, or for which they cannot take credit.

That said, decades of experience and evidence show that there are several undeniably foundational factors in any comprehensive national tobacco control program. I'll now look at some of the most important of these.

Health concerns

Smoking of course kills. And when ex-smokers are asked about why they quit, health concerns have always been the overwhelming reason given for quitting (for example, 92% in this longitudinal study (Hyland, Li et al. 2004), followed by cost, way back at 59%, and why 90% of smokers regret that they ever started (Fong, Hammond et al. 2004). In the vast and endlessly repetitive research literature on this question, there is typically daylight between health concerns as the first nominated reason given by smokers for quitting, and every other factor named by ex-smokers and those trying to quit.

Years of smoking can cause serious, often lethal damage to practically every part and system of the body. While many smokers subscribe to a constellation of self-exempting, rationalising beliefs designed to reduce the cognitive dissonance between what they do (smoke) and what they know (smoking is profoundly unhealthy) (Chapman, Wong et al. 1993, Oakes, Chapman et al. 2004), avoidance of frequent negative information and comments about smoking is increasingly difficult.

Yet one of the most bizarre and enduring beliefs I've heard countless times across my career in public health has been from those who say to you knowingly, "Well, it's been shown that scare tactics just don't work when you are trying to get people to change their behaviour." I reply that I find that hard to believe, given that former smokers almost invariably cite concern about health consequences as the primary reason they quit; that upward of 90% of people in some nations have been fully vaccinated against COVID-19 because they are very afraid of getting seriously ill and dying; or that the use of condoms in casual sex became very widespread after campaigns promoted it as the best way to avoid acquiring the dreaded HIV/AIDS and STDs or experiencing unwanted pregnancy. Yet many are still unconvinced, and the folk-wisdom meme of scare campaigns "not working" doggedly persists.

Many of the serious health consequences of smoking are hidden away in internal organs. Those with end-stage emphysema are not out in public doing their shopping or queuing next to you to enter a cinema. They are so disabled by their laboured breathing that they can barely walk across a room. They don't get about much and don't have a sign hanging around their necks saying, "My lungs are wrecked by years of smoking." Those who have had feet or legs amputated after gangrene from peripheral vascular disease similarly don't advertise their experience so that observers understand that this was also something caused by smoking.

So where, then, do people find out about these often hidden-away diseases and their links with smoking? They read about it all in news reports about the toll of smoking. They see forthright information campaigns on television, on graphic tobacco-pack warnings and in occasional documentaries which explain the links, people suffering these conditions voice their regret and health care workers express their anger at the tobacco industry.

Yet some have argued that setting out to worry or scare people into adopting or avoiding various behaviours like smoking is "unethical". In 2018, I looked critically at this proposition in the *American Journal of Public Health* (Chapman 2018). An edited version of that paper follows.[1]

Is using scare tactics unethical?

The efficacy and ethics of fear campaigns are enduring, almost perennial debates in public health which re-emerge with whack-a-mole frequency, eloquently chronicled by Fairchild et al (Fairchild, Bayer et al. 2018). Driven by evidence-based reasoning about motivating behaviour change and deterrence (Wakefield, Loken et al. 2010), these campaigns intentionally present disturbing images and narratives designed to arouse fear, regret and disgust.

---

[1] Reproduced from *American Journal of Public Health*, S Chapman, Is it Unethical to Use Fear in Public Health Campaigns? September 2018; 108(9): 1120–1122 with permission from The Sheridan Press on behalf of the American Public Health Association.

Smoking causes a huge range of health problems which currently cause the deaths of up to two in three long-term smokers (Banks, Joshy et al. 2015) with an annual global death toll of some eight million (Global Burden of Disease 2019 Tobacco Collaborators 2021). Some of the health problems which eventually cause death, like respiratory and cardiovascular disease, can cause smokers many years of disability and wretched quality of life. Much of the damage being caused over years of smoking is internal and non-symptomatic until disease is well advanced.

Health problems can be profoundly negative experiences unappreciated by those not living with them. Pain, immobility, disfigurement, depression, isolation and financial problems are common sequelae or consequences of disease and injury. It is beyond argument that these are outcomes which are self-evidently anticipated and experienced as adverse, undesirable and so best avoided. Efforts to prevent them are therefore, prima facie, ethically beneficent and virtuous.

Five main criticisms

Criticism of the ethics of fear messaging has taken five broad directions. First, it is often asserted that fear campaigns should be opposed because they are ineffective: they simply "don't work" very well and even worse, might backfire and perversely promote the very things they are supposed to be preventing. Fairchild et al. note that this argument persists despite the weight of evidence (Fairchild, Bayer et al. 2018). One 2015 meta-analysis of the research literature on the use of fear in health communication concluded:

> Overall, we conclude that (a) fear appeals are effective at positively influencing attitude, intentions, and behaviors; (b) there are very few circumstances under which they are not effective; and (c) there are no identified circumstances under which they backfire and lead to undesirable outcomes (Tannenbaum, Hepler et al. 2015).

The ineffectiveness argument can be valid independent of the content of failed campaigns: "positive" ineffective campaigns should also be subject to the same criticism. Yet sustained criticism of ineffective "positive" campaigns is uncommon, suggesting this criticism is enlisted to support more primary objections about fear campaigns.

Victim blaming?

Second, critics argue that such campaigns target victims, not causes of health problems, and so are soft options mounted in lieu of more politically challenging "upstream" policy reform of social determinants of health such as education, employment or income distribution, or legislative, fiscal and product safety law reforms.

However, it is difficult to recall any major prescription for prevention in the last 40 years not involving advocacy for comprehensive strategies of both policy reforms and motivational interventions. For example, tobacco control advocates target advertising bans, smoke-free policies, and tax rises as well as increased public awareness campaign financing. When governments fail to enact comprehensive approaches to prevention, supporting only public awareness campaigns, this is plainly concerning. The resultant concentration of public discourse around the importance of individualistic change instead of systemic, legislative or regulatory change in controlling health problems may lead to public perceptions that solutions are mostly contingent on what individuals do or don't do (Bonfiglioli, Smith et al. 2007). This myopic definition of health problems and their solution promotes victim blaming (Crawford 1977), where notions of individual responsibility are held to explain all health problems when any volitional component is involved.

This can be a serious criticism of failed government commitment to prevention, but is it a fair and sensible criticism of public awareness campaigns in themselves? Those making this argument draw the meritless implication that until governments are prepared to embrace the full panoply of policy and program solutions to health problems, they should not implement any individual element of such comprehensive approaches: if you cannot do everything, don't do anything.

Further, in any public health utopia where governments enacted every platform of comprehensive programs and made radical political changes addressing the social determinants of health, every health problem with a behavioural, volitional component would still require individuals to make choices to act and to be sufficiently motivated to do so. Campaigns to inform and motivate such changes will always be needed. The *reductio ad absurdum* of this objection is that attention-getting warning signs and poison labels are unethical.

Stigmatisation

Third, those who live with the diseases or practice the behaviours that are the focus of these campaigns can sometimes experience themselves as having what sociologist Erving Goffman called "spoiled identities" (Goffman 1963) and may feel criticised, devalued, rejected and stigmatised by others. The argument runs that these campaigns "ignore evidence that stigma makes life more miserable and stressful and so is likely to have direct health effects" and fail to recognise that the stigmatised health states or behaviours "travel with disadvantage" (Carter, Cribb et al. 2012).

Criticism of fear campaigns is mostly applied to health issues where personal behaviour as opposed to public health and safety is the focus. Campaigns seeking to stigmatise and shame alcohol and drug-affected driving, environmental polluters, domestic violence perpetrators, sexual predators, owners of savage dogs, or restaurant owners with unhygienic premises are rarely criticised. Some people deserve to be stigmatised, apparently.

Prisoners of structural constraints?

A fourth argument used against fear campaigns is that many personal changes in health-related behaviour are difficult, requiring physical discomfort, perseverance, sacrifice and sometimes major lifestyle change, often limited by structural impediments like poor access to safe environments, cost, and work and family constraints.

But unless one subscribes to an unyielding, hard determinist position that people have no agency and are total prisoners of social and biological determinants, the idea that individuals even in the direst of circumstances cannot make changes in their lives when motivated to do so is an extreme position, difficult to sustain. It is instructive, for example, to reflect that today in many nations, it is only a minority of the lowest socioeconomic group who still smoke.

Is it always wrong to upset people?

Perhaps the most common argument, though, is that we should always avoid messaging which might upset people. This argument has two subtexts. First, an assumption is made that how people feel about something ought to be inviolate and to challenge it is disrespectful. But we all have our views challenged often on many things, and some of those challenges motivate reflection and change, and in the process make us sometimes feel uncomfortable. Why is the goal of avoiding any communication which might make people feel uncomfortable or self-questioning, self-evidently a noble, ethical criterion in the ethical assessment of public health communication?

Here, feelings about desirable health-related practices often reflect powerfully promoted commercial agendas to normalise practices like over-consumption, poor food choices, and addiction. The notion that such agendas should be not challenged out of some misguided fear of offending those who are its victims would see the door held open even wider to those commercial forces seeking to turbo-charge the impacts of their health-damaging campaigns. If a smoker gets comfort and self-assurance from inhabiting the commercially contrived meanings of smoking promoted through tobacco advertising, should we suspend strident criticism of tobacco marketing because it might be disrespectful of smokers?

It is a perverse set of ethics that sees it as virtuous to keep powerful, life-changing information away from the community simply because it upsets some people (Chapman 1988). Should we really tip-toe around, say, vividly illustrating how deadly sunburn can be through fear of offending some of those who value tanning? While advertising that vividly portrays the carnage and misery caused by speed and intoxicated driving may upset some people who are quadriplegic, how do we balance the support for such campaigns by others now living that way and evidence that fear of public shame and personal remorse works to deter both? And if ghoulish pack-warning illustrations of tobacco-caused disease like gangrene and throat cancer render the damage of smoking far more meaningful than more genteel explanations, whose interests are served by decrying such depictions as being somehow unethically disturbing?

Some in the community do not like encountering confronting information that challenges their ignorance or complacency, but public health is not a popularity contest where an important criterion for assessing the merits of a campaign is the extent to which it is liked.

Fairchild et al.'s paper (Fairchild, Bayer et al. 2018) is a superb contribution to the public health communication field's confused thinking on fear appeals in public health and deserves wide discussion.

Recent neglect of public awareness campaigns

Australia had long been a global leader in mass-reach, hard-hitting, government-funded public awareness campaigns. Across different periods, these campaigns have been run by state health and federal departments. Quit Victoria's encyclopaedic *Tobacco in Australia* website documents all of these campaigns in great detail (Bayly, Carroll et al. 2021). In particular, between 1997 and 2001, a national campaign well funded by the federal government, *Every Cigarette is Doing You Damage*, was run. The campaign featured six see-once-and-never-forget advertisements focusing on different health consequences of smoking (Chapman, Hill et al. 1998). A whole supplement of research papers on the development, implementation and impact of this campaign was published in *Tobacco Control* in 2003 (Various authors 2003).

But while Australian governments have long been magnificent in being in the global vanguard of legislative initiatives like complete advertising bans, high tobacco tax, plain packaging and smoke-free public spaces, in recent years they have taken their minds well off the importance of significantly funding mass-reach campaigns. Figure 8.1 below shows the fall-off in federal government funding across recent years. State health departments have run many campaigns in the years since.

Australian governments were among global pioneers in funding large-scale often powerfully motivating public awareness campaigns as flagship components of comprehensive tobacco control campaigns. Regrettably, support has been desultory in the years since 2013. This has

Reported campaign expenditure tobacco, Australian Government
2010-11 to 2017-18, $m

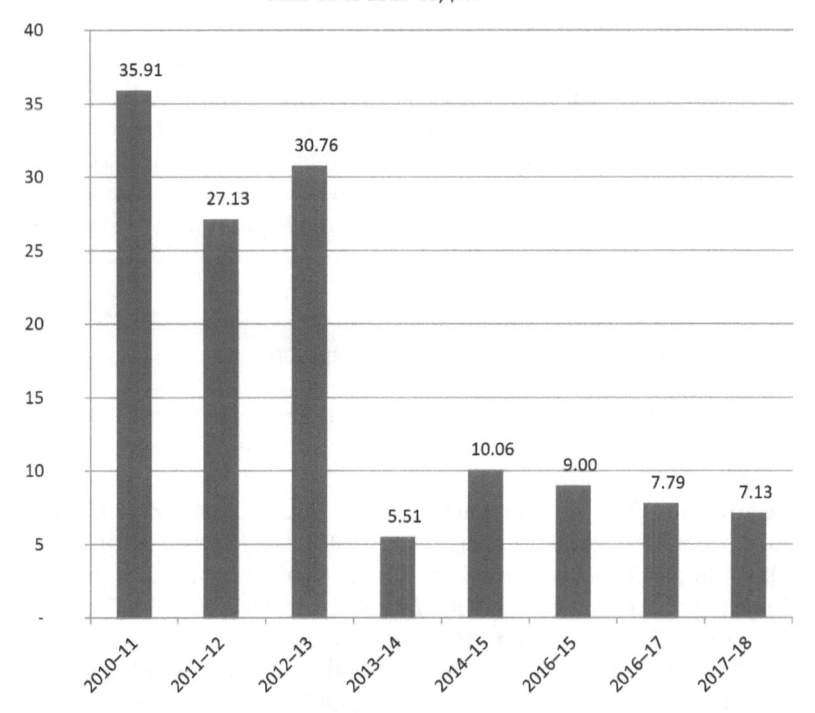

Year	$m
2010–11	35.91
2011–12	27.13
2012–13	30.76
2013–14	5.51
2014–15	10.06
2016–15	9.00
2016–17	7.79
2017–18	7.13

Figure 8.1 Annual federal government expenditure on anti-smoking advertising campaigns by financial year, adjusted for inflation to 2018 ($millions) (Source: Figure 14.3.2 in Bayly, Carroll et al. 2021).

not been because the campaigns haven't worked but almost certainly because of the confluence of two factors:

- The persistence of the erroneous view that such campaigns have achieved all they could have achieved and that remaining smokers are impervious to persuasions not to smoke (the hardening hypothesis discussed in Chapter 5).

- Most recently, the "all hands on deck" effect of COVID-19 in vacuuming almost all the attention of health authorities and seeing many health promotion staff seconded into COVID-19 related work.

If Australia is to reduce the gap between population subgroups which now have sub-10% smoking prevalence and those which sometimes have double or more those rates, re-investment in mass-reach campaigns should be at the very top of advocates' priority lists.

Tobacco taxation

There is popular cynicism that governments tax tobacco only because it is an ageless, endlessly fertile goose that just keeps laying massively lucrative golden revenue eggs. Tobacco tax including 10% added Goods and Services Tax (GST) comprised $15.744 billion (3.39%) of the $464.1 billion in total tax revenue raised by the Australian Commonwealth government in 2020-21. The government's December 2021 Mid Year Economic and Fiscal Outlook (MYEFO) also estimated that there was a significant downward trend of 9.8% likely to occur (Commonwealth of Australia 2021).

Tobacco tax certainly raises considerable revenue, but after health concerns, it is also widely regarded as the single most important factor driving down smoking, a conclusion drawn as far back as 1999 by the World Bank (The World Bank 1999). So it is a massively important win-win policy for both governments and public health. Over decades, internal tobacco industry documents have repeatedly shown their full awareness of this. Tobacco company Philip Morris (Australia) in 1983 said: "The most certain way to reduce consumption is through price" (Philip Morris Records 1983). Then again in 1985:

> Of all the concerns, there is one – taxation – which alarms us the most. While marketing restrictions and public and passive smoking do depress volume, in our experience taxation depresses it much more severely. Our concern for taxation is, therefore, central to our thinking about smoking and health. It has historically been the area to which we have devoted most

resources and for the foreseeable future, I think things will stay that way almost everywhere (Philip Morris International 1985).

And in 1993: "A high cigarette price, more than any other cigarette attribute, has the most dramatic impact on the share of the quitting population" (Schwab 1993).

In late April 2010, Australia's Rudd Labor government raised the tobacco tax unannounced and overnight by an unprecedented 25%, and at the same time announced its historic plain packaging plans, eventually implemented in December 2012. A 2010 Treasury paper modelled the likely impact of the 25% rise (Department of the Treasury 2010). They predicted that the 25% tax increase would see a decline in tobacco consumption of approximately 8% and an increase of 15% in tax revenue. But another Treasury paper from 2013 showed that this increase in fact reduced consumption of dutied tobacco products by 11% (Australian Treasury 2013).

British American Tobacco's then boss in Australia, David Crow, publicly acknowledged the impact of the tax in 2011, telling a parliamentary committee:

We saw that [tobacco tax reduces sales] last year very effectively with the increase in excise. There was a 25% increase in the excise and we saw the volumes go down by about 10.2%; there was about a 10.2% reduction in the industry last year in Australia (House of Representatives Standing Committee on Health 2011).

In 2019, Wilkinson et al. examined the impact on Australian smoking prevalence on those aged 14+ of the 2010 25% increase which was followed by annual 12.5% increases commencing in December 2013 (Wilkinson, Scollo et al. 2019). They reported that the 25% tax increase was associated with both immediate (−0.745 percentage points) and sustained reductions in smoking prevalence (monthly trend −0.023 percentage points). This was driven by reductions in the prevalence of smoking of factory-made cigarettes. However, the prevalence of smoking cheaper and (then) lower-taxed roll-your-own tobacco increased between May 2010 and November 2013. Immediate decreases in smoking and changing trends in the prevalence of smoking of roll-your-own were most evident among groups with lower socioeconomic status.

The global tobacco industry's stock line on tax-induced price rises has long been a "look-over-here" strategy where it seeks to frame the main effect of rising prices as being a stampede by smokers to buy illicit, duty-not-paid cigarettes. It has invested heavily in commissioning reports from prominent global accountancy firms to argue that tax rises drive price-sensitive smokers to purchase illicit duty-not-paid cigarettes which are much cheaper. Some of these reports have claimed as many as 1 in 6 of all cigarettes smoked in Australia are sourced from illicit trade.

Two websites, one maintained by Michelle Scollo at the Cancer Council Victoria (Scollo 2020) and one developed by the Tobacco Tactics project at the University of Bath (Tobacco Tactics 2020b) are peerless as sources of evidence and critical analysis of the often outrageous industry claims made about illicit tobacco trade, particularly in the Australian context. A 2012 review of well over 100 empirical studies of the impact of taxation on tobacco consumption concluded:

> tobacco excise taxes are a powerful tool for reducing tobacco use while at the same time providing a reliable source of government revenues. Significant increases in tobacco taxes that increase tobacco product prices encourage current tobacco users to stop using, prevent potential users from taking up tobacco use, and reduce consumption among those that continue to use, with the greatest impact on the young and the poor (Chaloupka, Yurekli et al. 2012).

A systematic review of the quality of evidence commissioned or promoted by the tobacco industry on the extent of illicit tobacco trade (ITT) identified problems with "data collection, analytical methods and presentation of results, which resulted in inflated ITT estimates or data on ITT that were presented in a misleading manner. Lack of transparency from data collection right through to presentation of findings was a key issue with insufficient information to allow replication of the findings frequently cited" (Gallagher, Evans-Reeves et al. 2019).

If illicit tobacco were as easy to obtain as the tobacco industry argues, how is it that ordinary smokers, who are increasingly drawn from less-educated population groups, can manage to find where to buy them with alleged consummate ease, while the full resources of the Australian Federal Police and tax office inspectors cannot manage to do so very often? Australia has always scored very low on indexes of corruption. It currently ranks 11th least corrupt out of 179 nations (Transparency International 2021). So suggestions that police and border force officials collude with criminals importing and distributing smuggled tobacco have little credibility.

Most amusing of all here is the duplicity of Big Tobacco's unctuous posturing about heinous tax rises encouraging smuggling and tax avoidance, when the industry uses these rises as cover to camouflage increases in its own margins. The Cancer Council Victoria's research on price changes after plain packaging reveal this. From August 2011 to February 2013, while excise duty rose 24¢ for a pack of 25 cigarettes, the tobacco companies' portion of the cigarette price (which excludes excise and GST), jumped $1.75 to $7.10 (Scollo, Bayly et al. 2015). While excise had risen 2.8% over the period, the average net price rose 27%. Philip Morris' budget brand Choice 25s rose $1.80 in this period, with only 41¢ of this being from excise and GST. Later work showed that across three years tobacco retail price increases were above the combined effects of inflation and increases in excise and customs duty (Egger, Burton et al. 2019). Moreover, there is a large body of evidence that transnational tobacco companies have had major ongoing involvement in facilitating global tobacco smuggling (Gilmore, Fooks et al. 2015, Gilmore, Gallagher et al. 2019, Tobacco Tactics 2020b).

It's often erroneously argued that those on low incomes are impervious to tobacco control measures like price rises, and suffer further deprivation with each price rise. Tobacco control is alleged to be "taking food out of children's mouths and new clothing off their backs" because of outrageous taxes. Figure 8.2 below shows the smoking status of Australians aged 14 and over in 2019 across five quintiles of social disadvantage. As can be seen, there is not a lot of difference in the proportion of ex-smokers across the quintiles.

However, these apparent similarities are due to big differences across socioeconomic quintiles in the proportions who have *ever* smoked. Instead, the "quit ratio" (the proportion of ever smokers who are former smokers) is the key indicator here (see Table 8.3 below).

8 Strategies for reducing smoking across populations

As can be seen, in 2019 some 52 % of people who ever smoked in the lowest quintile have quit, compared with nearly 73% of those who have ever smoked in the highest quintile.

Taking up smoking is much more common if you are less educated and unskilled than the obverse – a glass half empty observation. But the glass half full, more optimistic observation is that a clear majority of every socioeconomic group in Australia today have never smoked, thanks to the impact of preventive tobacco control.

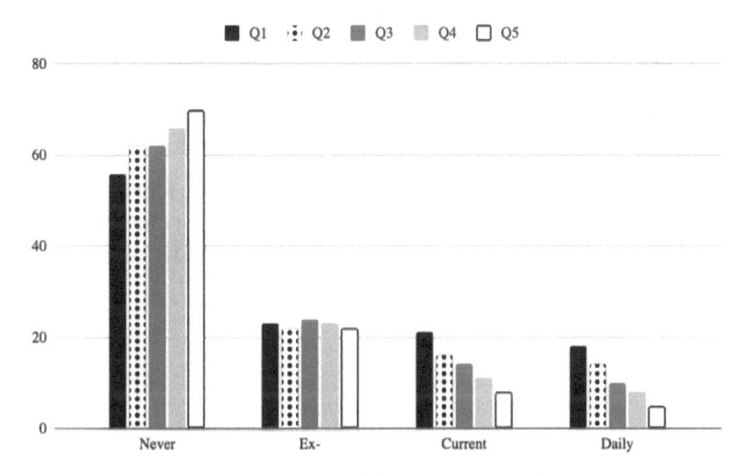

Figure 8.2 Never, ex-, current and daily smoking prevalence by five quintiles of social disadvantage (1 = highest disadvantage 5 = lowest) Australians aged 14+ 2019 (Source: Australian Institute of Health and Welfare 2020e).

Quit Smoking Weapons of Mass Distraction

Ever, Ex and Quit ratio

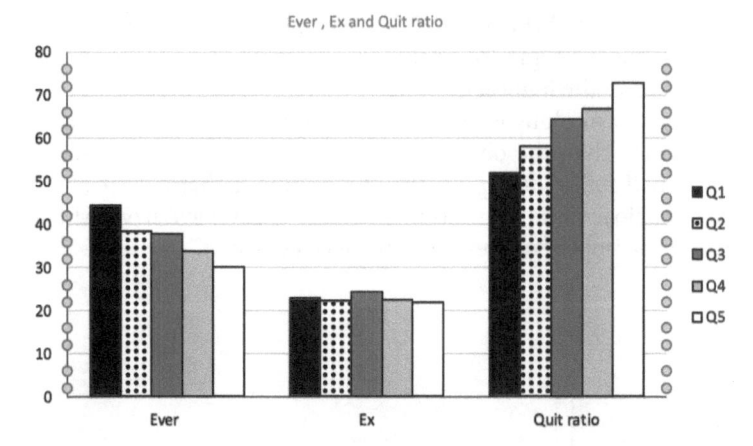

Figure 8.3 Quit ratios (proportion of ever smokers who are former smokers) by five quintiles of social disadvantage (1=highest disadvantage 5= lowest) Australians aged 14 and over, 2019 (Source: Australian Institute of Health and Welfare 2020e).

9
Controlling tobacco supply and the endgame

Comprehensive tobacco control, as embodied in the WHO's Framework Convention on Tobacco Control (FCTC), mandates a range of strategies to reduce tobacco use, including taxation, bans on tobacco advertising, labelling products with effective health warnings, regulation of contents and emissions, conducting public awareness campaigns, reducing exposure to second-hand smoke and promoting cessation (Guindon, de Beyer et al. 2003). Supply-side strategies in the FCTC include preventing illicit trade, providing economic alternatives to tobacco growers and preventing sales to minors. However, other than banning point-of-sale advertising and retail pack displays as residual forms of tobacco advertising, a supply side strategy that has only been minimally explored is the regulation and licensing of tobacco retailing and purchasing, and the introduction of retail floor prices for tobacco.

Below is an edited and updated version of a paper on these issues that I published with my colleague Becky Freeman in 2009 (Chapman and Freeman 2009).[1]

Licensing of tobacco retailers is uncommon in global tobacco control. While there are jurisdictions such as Canada, Australia, the USA and Singapore that require some form of retail licensure, the

---

1 Reproduced from *Tobacco Control*, S Chapman, B Freeman, 18, 496–501, 2009 with permission from BMJ Publishing Group Ltd.

applicable conditions are minimal and removal of licence for breaching licensing conditions is rare.

Most tobacco retail regulation and licensing are based on the objective of restricting sales to adults. Consequently, most research on retailing has focused on monitoring sales to minors and the effects of enforcement practices and threats of fines on underage sales. While threats of fines can reduce sales, there is little evidence that such reductions translate to reduced use, because of the ease with which youth can acquire cigarettes through purchases made by older friends. Even though these jurisdictions sometimes stipulate loss of licence as a penalty for multiple violations for sales to minors, there is little evidence that this is ever invoked and no research literature demonstrating the utility of this threat as a serious deterrent. This is undoubtedly why the tobacco industry has long publicly tut-tutted about the terrible problem of youth smoking and offered to work with governments to reduce youth access to tobacco. It is symbolic, empty-gesture tobacco control designed to give the industry a foot in the door of government tobacco control discussions while the companies know it will do nothing to seriously reduce youth access (Assunta and Chapman 2004, Knight and Chapman 2004).

Unlike every other facet of tobacco advertising, packaging, and retail (non) display of packs, tobacco retailing throughout the world today remains almost entirely "normalised": tobacco products can be sold by virtually any business which chooses to do so. We will now consider how regulation of tobacco retail environments might be widened from a sole concern to reduce sales to minors in the effort to further denormalise and thereby reduce tobacco use. It is based on a central concern to send an unambiguous public signal that governments regard tobacco as an exceptionally harmful product, deserving of retail sale restrictions at least as comparable to those that apply to prescribed pharmaceuticals in almost all countries.

We'll consider licensing provisions and their rationales established by governments for a range of goods and services. These restrictions are often introduced because of health considerations with parallels to the goals of tobacco control. We'll conclude that the major impediment to greater regulation of the tobacco retail environment is the historical regulatory trivialisation of tobacco products compared to assumptions

9 Controlling tobacco supply and the endgame

made about other regulated products. We argue that concerted efforts will therefore be needed to change this assumption, if tobacco products are ever to be subject to the same range of serious and enforced regulatory requirements taken for granted for many other items of commerce, particularly pharmaceutical drugs. If this was to occur, potential exists for regulatory provisions to be introduced in five broad areas of tobacco retailing in addition to restricting sales to adults:

- Restrictions on the number and location of tobacco retail outlets
- Regulation of tobacco retail displays
- Floor (minimum) price controls
- Restricting the amount of tobacco that smokers could purchase over a given time
- Loss of retail licensure following breaches of any of the conditions of licence.

We'll discuss each of these and then explore the idea that tobacco retail licences could become valued, tradable commodities in a policy environment based on the objective of limiting the number of tobacco retail outlets. Such a reduction could reduce the convenience of purchasing tobacco products and the frequency with which smokers and ex-smokers would encounter tobacco supplies in their local communities, a factor known to cue thoughts of purchase and smoking in smokers and ex-smokers (Wakefield, Germain et al. 2008).

Regulation of other goods and services

Consumers and the business sector are very familiar with the concepts of licensing and registration through a wide variety of requirements. All motor vehicle drivers and boat owners are required to be licensed and vehicles and sea craft registered. In Australia, all dogs must be registered to owners and those who wish to keep exotic animals such as reptiles must have a licence to do so. In many countries firearms can only be sold by licensed operators to those with firearm licences under very strict conditions. Food preparation and sales are also commonly subject to stringent licensing and safety inspections. In order to protect the health and safety of the public, many service professions and occupations must be licensed to legally carry out their tasks: doctors, dentists, pharmacists, electricians, plumbers, pesticide services, civil engineers, taxi drivers, and tattoo and body piercing artists are just a few examples. In this light, tobacco retailing stands out as being a curiously unregulated commercial enterprise, given the magnitude of problems arising from its commercial activity.

The licensing of purveyors of other potentially harmful products and services is based on a far wider range of concerns than simply preventing youth access, such as protecting personal and public health, safety and welfare; controlling provision and limiting availability; monitoring sales; and ensuring quality and accountability. Much licensing and regulation on a wide variety of goods and services is based on better ensuring that consumers are not harmed by the products or services they purchase.

It has often been observed that tobacco's status as a product sold with few restrictions reflects the historic, gradual emergence of knowledge of its harm and the unwillingness of governments to respond to this harm in the way they would to any newly developed product known to cause such harm, by refusing to allow such a new product onto the market. But with tobacco having no safe level of use, and 181 governments being parties to the FCTC with its central goal of reducing tobacco use, the historical laissez faire attitude toward the regulation of tobacco retailing is anachronistic and incompatible with this broad goal.

Pharmaceutical retailing as a model

The inconsistent, ramshackle and poorly enforced situation of tobacco retailer licensing across Australian states and territories today contrasts markedly with the ways in which therapeutic goods (pharmaceuticals) are retailed. There is a regulatory paradox here as the government formally acknowledges that, while tobacco products cause unparalleled harm to health, it minimally regulates their sale. By contrast, pharmaceutical products designed to *enhance* health are heavily regulated so that the possibility of harm from unlimited access is reduced.

9 Controlling tobacco supply and the endgame

Virtually every aspect of pharmaceutical retailing is subject to government regulation: from which products can be sold, to where a pharmacy can be located, which staff can dispense certain pharmaceutical categories, where products can be stored and displayed, the amount of product that can sold to each customer and what the pharmacist must communicate to customers about some dispensed products. The cost of pharmaceuticals partly reflects these regulatory costs. So how might such conditions be applied to tobacco retailing?

To sell scheduled drugs, pharmacists must have a pharmacy degree, maintain their registration and would face severe penalties, including possible imprisonment, if they were found to be selling some categories of drugs without being presented with a valid doctor's prescription.

By contrast, there are no restrictions on who can sell tobacco products, nor on where they can be sold. Accordingly, the retailing of tobacco products is ubiquitous: from all supermarkets and almost every corner store through to suburban barbers, who typically keep a few packs adjacent to gum and hair care products. The subtext of the current way tobacco products are sold is that they are in every way unexceptional, ordinary items of commerce, suitably treated in the same way that everyday grocery items are sold and undeserving of special restrictions. This view is inconsistent with the way that tobacco is regarded under many other aspects of tobacco control policy and may undermine public understanding of how seriously tobacco damages health. For example, in 1991 when tobacco advertising remained legal in Australia, a third of smokers agreed with the proposition that "If smoking was really harmful, the government would ban tobacco advertising" (Chapman, Wong et al. 1993). It is possible that the unrestricted retailing of tobacco may send a parallel message.

Following the publication of a report from a 2020 Senate committee on tobacco harm reduction convened by two political champions of "light touch" vaping regulation who were outvoted by the majority of their committee (Australian Senate 2020b), in 2021, the Australian government mandated that all nicotine liquid and NVPs would require a doctor's prescription (see later in this chapter). This policy decision was supported by the overwhelming majority of relevant professional health bodies in Australia, but implacably opposed by the three tobacco companies dominating the Australian market (each of which is heavily invested in NVPs) and a ragbag of tiny vaping lobby groups either funded directly by the industry or operating as astroturf "independent" groups with funding channelled through third parties.

Opponents of the proposal thought they were onto a winning argument by continually contrasting the open-slather, "sold everywhere" way that tobacco products have always been retailed – with restrictions on selling NVPs. Their view was that the NVP access should match that of tobacco and not be more restrictive. In effect they were arguing, "Let's repeat the same mistakes we made in allowing open slather sales and promotions with cigarettes."

But, more fundamentally, the stratospheric dangers of smoking were not fully understood for at least 40–50 years after mass consumption and the commerce that facilitated it had commenced in the first decades of the 20th century. After mechanisation of cigarette production made cigarettes as cheap as chips, it then took us 40–50 years between the 1960s and today to fight for all the policies and campaign funding that have together taken smoking down to its lowest ever levels.

Out of ignorance and under sustained pressure from the tobacco industry, the tobacco epidemic saw nations make every regulatory mistake possible when cheap, mass-produced cigarettes appeared on sale almost everywhere. Our understanding of the health risks that may be posed by NVPs is in its early infancy, given the latency periods that apply with the development of chronic disease (see Chapter 6).

It is often said that if cigarettes were invented tomorrow, and we knew now what we didn't know when they entered the market, no government in the world would permit their sale, let alone allow them to be sold in every convenience store.

With pharmaceutical products that *save* lives, treat illness and reduce severe pain, we allow only people with a four-year pharmacy degree to sell them. And only to those with a temporary licence issued by a doctor (a prescription) to use them. With cigarettes, we foolishly allow them to be sold everywhere.

Restrictions on the number and location of tobacco retailers

Numerous precedents exist for the government imposing restrictions on the number and location of various commercial activities. These restrictions are imposed for reasons including urban aesthetics, public amenity, to limit competition for certain retail activities deemed important to remain economically viable in local communities and delivered at a high standard to consumers, or (as might be argued for tobacco) to reduce the proliferation of businesses deemed less socially desirable (e.g. nightclubs which might attract large, noisy crowds in residential areas, firearms dealers, brothels, X-rated video outlets). Urban areas are often zoned residential or industrial, and from this flow restrictions on the types of business that can operate in residential zones. A person cannot decide to turn their residence into, for example, a restaurant, a brothel or a childcare centre without the permission of zoning and licensing authorities.

The arguments for reducing access to tobacco products are driven by the same core reasons for why 181 nations have ratified the WHO's FCTC: that smoking kills two in three of its long-term users (Banks, Joshy et al. 2015) – some eight million a year at present; that many other commodities which cause even a small fraction of such deaths are banned, e.g. lead in petrol and paint; asbestos in brake linings and building insulation; fireworks (Abdulwadud and Ozanne-Smith 1998); semi-automatic firearms in civilian ownership (Chapman 2013); often subject to strict regulatory control (e.g. pharmaceuticals, food additives, pesticides, and industrial and agricultural chemicals), or subject to recalls or market withdrawal (e.g. many examples of unsafe consumer goods, motor vehicles (Hemenway 2009)).

Tobacco and cigarettes have enjoyed the legacy of being sold as ordinary, largely unregulated consumer items for well over 130 years. While advertising, packaging, tax and smoke-free regulations have been widely introduced throughout the world across the last 70 years, moves to reduce and more strictly control the number of retailers and their conditions of operation are barely in their infancy.

Possible models might range from the nationalisation of tobacco retailing involving a single network of government-controlled outlets (as with alcohol in Sweden) to a model where a highly restricted number of licences based on an agreed number of tobacco retail outlets per 100,000 population could be auctioned to the highest bidder. Objections from current sellers unable to compete for such licences could be met with many precedents where major restrictions on previously open-slather retailing have been introduced in attempts to limit use.

This raises the interesting possibility that if tobacco retail licences were to be made mandatory across the country, similarly limited and the conditions pertaining to the conduct of a tobacco retail business strictly regulated, a tobacco retail licence could become a highly valued commodity promising restricted, profitable retailing access. The issuing of taxi licence plates in Australia is similarly strictly limited and prior to the advent of competition from Uber, these plates traded at prices many times higher than the value of the actual taxi itself. Retailers who risked having their retail licence revoked by breaching any condition of licence would thus risk losing a valuable asset. Provided governments acted against such breaches, this would seem a potential way of introducing large incentives to obey the law on matters, such as restricting sales to adults and enforcement of display bans.

Globally, alcohol retailing is subject to many such controls. These include: nationalisation of alcohol distribution, limiting hours and or days of sale, restrictions at community events, restricting the location, density and types of alcohol outlets, mandatory server training, and licensing and server liability. When granting liquor sales licences, community and social factors are often considered. For example, in New South Wales when applying for a liquor licence, applicants must include a National Police Certificate, a community impact statement, a scaled plan of the proposed licensed premises and a copy of the local council's development consent or approval for the proposed premises. The community impact statement summarises the results of consultation by applicants with local councils, police, health, Aboriginal representatives, community organisations and the public.

A 2021 systematic review and meta-analysis of 37 international studies looking at the relationship of tobacco retailing density and proximity to smoking prevalence concluded: "Across studies, lower levels of tobacco retailer density and decreased proximity are associated with lower tobacco use" (Lee, Kong et al. 2021).

Canadian researchers have measured the effect of tobacco outlet density around schools in Ontario and found that the "more tobacco retailers there were surrounding a school, the more likely smokers were to buy their own cigarettes and the less likely they were to get someone else to buy their cigarettes" (Leatherdale and Strath 2007). New Zealand research suggests that accessibility to retail outlets selling tobacco may not impact on national smoking rates. The researchers found that after controlling for individual-level demographic and socioeconomic variables, individuals living in neighbourhoods with the best access to supermarkets and convenience stores had higher odds of smoking compared to individuals in the worst access neighbourhoods. However, the association between smoking prevalence and neighbourhood accessibility to supermarkets and convenience stores was not apparent once other neighbourhood-level variables (deprivation and rural location) were included (Pearce, Hiscock et al. 2009). The authors suggested that restrictions on the number of tobacco outlets in residential neighbourhoods, and area-based restrictions, such as those with a high concentration of workplaces, may influence the consumption of tobacco. If tobacco retail outlets were to be limited, causing smokers to have to plan their purchases more, this may reduce "spontaneous" purchases which had not been pre-planned. If this policy was implemented in concert with price controls and limits on the number of cigarettes purchased (see both arguments below), this may reduce consumption.

Be careful what you wish for?

There are, though, several critically important concerns that need thorough investigation before such policies should be enacted. First, it seems intuitively obvious that in areas with low smoking prevalence, we would expect to find fewer tobacco retail outlets than in areas where there are more smokers. Basic due diligence about setting up a tobacco outlet would see retailers doing their homework and working out the most promising locations. Investing in establishing a tobacco business in an area with low smoking prevalence (e.g. high socioeconomic suburbs) would not be very sensible. By analogy, there are very few farm machinery shops or agricultural supply shops in cities, but plenty in rural towns.

So top-line findings of a positive association between retail outlets and smoking prevalence are likely to be highly predictable and an example of "Gosh, who'd have ever imagined!" research. The implied policy message is "if you regulate to reduce retail outlets, we'd predict this would drive down prevalence". But it might be more a case of when smoking prevalence is low or falls – perhaps because factors like rising socioeconomic status and house prices in certain suburbs – reverse causality is at play, and the lower local demand for tobacco is reflected in tobacco businesses closing or not setting up, not the other way round.

Second, 20 years ago in Australia, every suburb would have several outlets selling take-out alcohol not to be drunk on the premises, and every pub would have a takeaway section. But today almost all alcohol retailing is done by a supermarket duopoly: 76% of liquor retailing is via these two supermarkets or their liquor barn subsidiaries, with a declining 10.7% via small, typically suburban liquor stores, and the remainder sold through takeaway from pubs (Hinton 2021). These fiercely compete for the liquor market via price discounting and home delivery free for orders over $100.

Might the same not happen with reduced tobacco access policy if the outlet reduction policy was taken up? Supermarkets are already the largest tobacco retailers, with over half of all tobacco sales (Bayly & Scollo 2020). Might not this see huge concentration of tobacco retailing, leading to margins being squeezed down even further and smokers getting cheaper deals, causing an uptick in sales because of price's critical role in demand elasticity?

Parallel floor price policy (discussed below) would be essential, as would thorough vigilance of the industry's efforts to circumvent the law by all manner of marketing subterfuge.

Third, retailing (especially since COVID-19) has radically changed with online buying and home delivery, and more broadly with the drift to massive shopping centres which shoppers drive to and from. Online purchasing allows warp-speed price comparisons with reduced prices because online retailing avoids large retail shop costs. Old assumptions

9 Controlling tobacco supply and the endgame

about proximity of retailing to residence being important are looking very shaky in many locations.

Regulating tobacco retail display

Scheduled drugs which either require a doctor's prescription or which are subject to limited supply mediated and registered through a pharmacist must be stored in a part of the pharmacy designated as a dispensary. The dispensary is an area in which members of the public are not permitted to enter, and therefore are unable to handle (and potentially shoplift) drugs stored there. Many dispensaries store prescription-only drugs out of sight of customers. The same principle should apply to tobacco retailers: products should not be displayed. Research has shown that retail displays of tobacco prompt unplanned purchases and weaken resolve not to smoke (Wakefield, Germain et al. 2008, Carter, Mills et al. 2009, Carter, Phan et al. 2015). A WHO evidence brief describes the evidence underpinning display ban policy (WHO Europe 2016).

Iceland was the first nation to implement a display ban in 2001, but since then only ten other nations have followed (Australia, Canada, Croatia, Ireland, Serbia, New Zealand, Norway, Russia, Thailand and the UK) (Wikipedia 2021b). Clearly, there remains huge potential to pick up the international implementation pace of this policy.

Floor price controls

Everyone reading this will have experienced shopping for discounted prices on goods. Like all other non-luxury goods manufacturers, tobacco companies are well aware that lower prices attract purchasing and they engage in many forms of discounting to chase sales. Price controls are often reluctantly imposed by governments in free markets, with retail price competition being regarded as a sacrosanct principle of such markets. However, again there are many precedents for governments imposing minimum unit or floor price controls in situations where various national interests are invoked.

The notions of floor and ceiling prices (a price specified as the lowest or highest legal purchase price of a good or service that can be charged) exist for many commodities in agriculture, in rent control and for minimum wages. Prescribed pharmaceuticals are subject to price controls in Australia to ensure their accessibility to all who need them. In regulating retailing, governments could establish a floor price for tobacco products, below which it would be illegal to sell them. This would limit serious discounting if competition were to be further concentrated as I suggested above if policies on limiting tobacco retail outlets were pursued.

Canadian provinces led the way on floor prices with alcohol (Stockwell 2014) and in 2018 Scotland became the first nation to introduce minimum unit floor prices for alcohol (Robinson, Mackay et al. 2021). The Queensland government has legislated to restrict price discounted "happy hours" and banned hoteliers offering free drinks (Business Queensland 2019). In Sweden, all alcohol is sold via the government monopoly Systembolaget which "exists for one reason: to minimise alcohol-related problems by selling alcohol in a responsible way, without profit motive".

In the USA, as at 2011, 25 states and the District of Columbia had minimum purchase price laws that applied to cigarette sales. These laws originated to protect small businesses, not public health. Cigarette prices in these states tend not to be any higher than in states without such laws, as price discounts offered to retailers as promotional incentive programs are not used to calculate the minimum price (Tobacco Control Legal Consortium 2011). Minimum price policies will be more effective in keeping cigarette prices high if price discounting from manufacturers or wholesalers to retailers was not permitted.

Limitations on the number of cigarettes a smoker could buy

When a person is prescribed a drug by a doctor, the prescription specifies that a limited supply be released by a pharmacist. Patients requiring further supplies can then return to a doctor for a repeat prescription, allowing the doctor to determine whether further supplies are necessary; to monitor the patient's health; and if necessary, change the dose. A doctor's prescription is, in effect, a temporary licence to consume a particular drug.

With tobacco, smokers are at liberty to buy unlimited supplies. Under a policy governed by the explicit objective of reducing consumption and encouraging cessation, governments could introduce a regulation stipulating an upper weekly limit to tobacco product purchases. To facilitate this, smokers' permits or licences could be introduced incorporating a sliding scale of fees, with substantially higher fees acting as a disincentive to allow purchase of more than 15 cigarettes a day, just above the current average consumption, and a cheaper but still substantial licence allowing purchase of, say, five per day. An attractive cashback provision could be incorporated as an incentive for people wishing to permanently surrender their licence when they quit.

As discussed earlier, the great majority of smokers regret ever starting (Fong, Hammond et al. 2004), and in excess of 40% make an attempt to stop every year. I have never met a former smoker or heard one speaking in the media who regretted quitting. Many smokers are therefore likely to support such a policy in the way that many support other tobacco control policies which act as a brake and disincentive to the smoking they wished they'd never started (Edwards, Wilson et al. 2013).

In 2012, I set out the case for a smoker's licence in full in a paper in *PLOS Medicine* together with detailed exploration of objections to this idea (Chapman 2012). In summary, all adult licence holders would be issued with a swipe smart card licence calibrated to show the number of cigarettes that could be purchased in a given period, with an upper limit set to thwart anyone planning to on-sell on a large scale to unlicensed smokers. Smokers wishing to set limits to their own consumption would be free to set their own maximum number of cigarettes able to be purchased over a period. No sales would be possible without a swipe card licence, with all sales electronically reconciled against issued licences. COVID-19 rapidly accelerated global familiarity with QR code sign-ins and declarations of vaccination status. This technology could be very easily adapted to incorporate a smoker's licence (An 18-minute video explaining the concept is at https://tinyurl.com/27f2nms5).

Communities in all but the most impoverished nations have long accepted that to obtain a prescribed drug, a person must first visit a doctor, be assessed as requiring the prescribed drug, pay the doctor a fee, obtain a prescription, find a pharmacy and pay the pharmacist for the drug, sometimes subsidised by governments. I am not suggesting that smokers would have to obtain a doctor's prescription to buy tobacco, but that limitations should be placed upon the ability of smokers to acquire unlimited tobacco products, with the device of a smoker's licence acting like a de facto prescription to obtain a limited supply.

In December 2021, New Zealand became the first nation to announce adoption of the concept of the smoke-free generation. The central provision here is that from a date to be proclaimed sometime in 2022, it would be henceforth illegal for any tobacco retailer to sell tobacco products to anyone born after a particular year. Media comment suggested that this would be age 14, and that this would increase by one year on the anniversary of the 2022 proclamation. In other words, commencing sometime in 2022, anyone born later than 2008 would not legally able to ever be sold tobacco products (Ministry of Health New Zealand 2021a).

It has long been illegal in New Zealand to sell tobacco to people aged less than 18. Yet 18% of minors who are smokers report buying cigarettes (Lucas, Gurram et al. 2020). Prosecutions of shops selling to minors are uncommon to rare in most nations. So the 2021 announcement begs the question of the extent to which it would be actively implemented, given this history. The introduction of mandatory, sales-linked proof-of-age documentation via a government app with this being reconciled against retailers' tobacco stock data would go a long way to prevent retailers from ignoring the new regulation. Without such a measure, it is difficult to be optimistic that much would change in the age-old reality of many retailers being willing to ignore the law.

Loss of licensure following breaches of conditions of licence

In the states where retail tobacco licences exist, revocations of such licences are unheard of in Australia. Occasionally tobacco retailers have been fined for selling tobacco to minors, but the likelihood of this occurring is so rare that many retailers clearly reason that it is simply part of the cost of doing business with minors. In Canada, suspension of a licence can follow conviction for selling to minors, but not removal of licence. This is not the case in many jurisdictions for those repeatedly supplying alcohol to minors, where liquor suppliers can lose their licence. In the professions, doctors, lawyers and accountants are delicensed or barred from practice following successful prosecution of breaches of their professional duties. A pharmacist, for example, found to be selling restricted drugs to those without prescriptions would be subject to investigation, leading to possible prosecution and loss of registration as a pharmacist.

If retailing was concentrated in fewer outlets by the limitations I described on the number of outlets, the stakes involved in licence loss for what would then be large-scale retailers would be enormous. Selling to underage smokers would thereby be hugely disincentivised. By restricting the number of tobacco licences issued and allowing them to be tradable, loss of licence would loom as a highly significant disincentive to breach any of the conditions of licensure.

The trivialisation of tobacco retailing lies at the root of why most of the above provisions do not operate in any nation today. None of these provisions will be taken seriously by governments until tobacco retailing is radically reframed in public and political consciousness in the ways analogous with the range of absolutely normal, taken for granted controls that have long applied to pharmaceutical retailing. Concerted and imaginative effort will be needed to transform public perceptions of tobacco retailing away from its current laissez faire status as just another ordinary grocery item.

Prescription access to nicotine vaping products

From 1 October 2021 any Australian wanting to legally vape nicotine has been required to have a doctor's prescription (Therapeutic Goods Administration 2021b). The policy has been very welcomed by nearly all public health agencies, professional bodies and state health departments. Goods which require a prescription can only be retailed through pharmacists in Australia. Provision also exists for vapers to import NVPs provided the imported goods arrive in Australia with a genuine copy of the prescription in the packaged goods. If targeted or random customs inspections find unauthorised NVPs, the goods are seized and the importer fined significantly (Therapeutic Goods Administration 2021a).

The only interest groups which have been apoplectic about the policy have been all three major tobacco transnationals marketing in Australia (all have NVPs), the small number of vaping shops which are now unable to sell vapable liquids containing nicotine – as has always been the case in Australia – and want a slice of the action; convenience stores (for the same reason); a coterie of conservative backbench federal politicians; and a small rabble of vaping advocacy groups.

Why regulate NVPs?

Vaping interests have long been engaged in a global effort to rehabilitate nicotine's reputation. They are usually fine in agreeing that nicotine is addictive, but bend over backwards to promote it as being all but benign. "As risky as coffee" is a trivialising comparison commonly used. In 1976, the late addiction specialist Michael Russell wrote that "People smoke for nicotine but they die from the tar" (Russell 1976). This has become a mantra for vapers against their pet evil of nicotine regulation, rarely absent from any interview. But in fact across the 46 years since Russell wrote those words, a large research literature has emerged on concerns about nicotine's likely role as a cancer promoter (Schaal and Chellappan 2014), as a vasoconstrictor with major implications for cardiovascular disease (Kennedy, van Schalkwyk et al. 2019), as a disruptor of cognitive development (Goriounova and Mansvelder 2012) and as a possible cause of psychosis (Quigley and MacCabe 2019). I have assembled a large collection of published research on concerns about nicotine (Chapman 2019).

For these reasons, and because of the strong addictive potential of nicotine in NVPs (Jankowski, Krzystanek et al. 2019), Australia's TGA has long sensibly classified nicotine as a poison or a therapeutic substance when used in small doses (Therapeutic Goods Administration 2017).

9 Controlling tobacco supply and the endgame

Vaping advocates are fond of arguing that because nicotine is freely available in tobacco products, it follows that nicotine for vaping should enjoy at least the same, if not more accessibility and be freely sold almost anywhere. This argument has all the integrity of a chocolate teapot. Cigarettes were given their unregulated commodity status at the beginning of last century, long before the evidence accumulated about two in three long-term users dying from smoking (Banks, Joshy et al. 2015). Vaping advocates insisting that NVPs should share a regulatory level playing field with cigarette accessibility seem happy to risk repeating the Sisyphean task we have faced with tobacco of trying to reduce the damage that 120 years of non-regulation has facilitated. It's been 56 years since health warnings first appeared on tobacco packs and tobacco control commenced. The power of the tobacco industry has ensured that the legislative drag has nearly always been glacial.

Nicotine should not be exempted from regulation

Every new therapeutic substance first made available to the public is regulated in all but politically chaotic nations where almost anything can be bought over the counter in any quantity. Vaping advocates seem to believe their virtuous mission should exempt NVPs from regulation, despite their every second sentence extolling the therapeutic virtues of vaping in cessation and harm reduction, thus catapulting it straight into the ambit of therapeutic regulation.

When NRT first became available in the 1980s in gum form, in every country it was sold it was scheduled as a prescription-only drug. No one thought this was anything other than sensible and normal for a new drug. When nicotine patches, lozenges and inhaler sprays later appeared, they too were prescription-only. Over the years, as use of NRT proliferated and some ex-smokers used it for many years with only minor apparent adverse effects, NRT access was gradually liberalised through rescheduling. Approved maximum doses, however, have remained small through concerns about toxicity.

Drug scheduling can work in the opposite direction too. The very useful opiate, low-dose codeine, was available OTC in Australia in a variety of pain-relieving medications until February 2018. Following accumulating evidence of abuse and harm, it was then rescheduled to prescription-only access (Cairns, Schaffer et al. 2020).

Alex Wodak, an unswerving advocate for open access to nicotine vaping juice, has argued that "Vaping is to smoking what methadone is to street heroin" (Wodak 2020). Correct. But curiously Wodak failed to note that methadone is only available via special prescription authority, dispensed at some pharmacies and clinics. In 2020, on a census day, 53,316 persons across Australia were being treated for their opioid dependence with prescribed methadone, buprenorphine or buprenorphine-naloxone (Australian Institute of Health and Welfare 2021). Australia's new regulations will make nicotine vape juice available in much the same way, but in potentially every pharmacy.

I'm not aware of Wodak advocating for methadone to be available to whoever wants to buy it from any retailer wanting to sell it, in just the way that cigarettes can be sold. But if he does hold such views, good luck in selling that argument.

Prescribed access will greatly reduce teenage access to e-cigarettes

As discussed in Chapter 6, smoking rates in Australian teenagers have never been lower (Greenhalgh, Winstanley et al. 2019), a phenomenon also seen in other nations like the USA, Canada and the UK which, like Australia, also have had comprehensive tobacco control policies for decades. Like the tobacco industry, the business model for the vape industry (Chapman 2015), which includes all major tobacco companies, is not just about promoting its products to current adult smokers. Just as any car company which ignored young first car buyers would need its corporate head examined, all tobacco and vaping companies are well aware of the critical role that new (read "young") nicotine addicts have in their long-term commercial prospects. Reports have found 45% of US vaping retailers (Rapaport 2019) and 39% of English shops (Smithers 2016) sell to underage customers.

Vaping advocates are usually sensitive to the reception that any expressed complacency about teenage vaping will cause, and so concentrate talk about their mission on helping smokers switch. But

9 Controlling tobacco supply and the endgame

Past 30 day use of vaping products

Age group	2013	2015	2017	2019
15-19 years	3%	6%	6%	15%
20-24 years	4%	6%	6%	15%
25 years and older	—	3%	2%	3%

Figure 9.1 Past 30-day use of vaping products, by age groups, Canada 2013–19 (Source: Physicians for a Smoke-Free Canada 2020).

as the evidence about rising youth vaping uptake has accumulated and become undeniable, they fall back to, "Well, isn't it better that they vape than smoke?" As discussed in Chapter 6, successful tobacco control has succeeded in getting teenage smoking down to near rock bottom. Data released on 10 December 2021 by the Australian Bureau of Statistics for 2020–21 showed only 2% of 15–17-year-old Australians smoke (Australian Bureau of Statistics 2021a). So we are supposed to all concur that the huge, widespread problem of 2% of teenagers smoking is being kept on the leash by burgeoning rates of teenage vaping?

The wider-than-Sydney-Harbour-heads problem here is that many totally nicotine-naïve youth are now regularly – not just experimentally – vaping. In the USA "The significant rise in e-cigarette use among both student populations has resulted in overall tobacco product use increases of 38 percent among high school students and 29 percent among middle school students between 2017 and 2018, negating declines seen in the previous few years" (US Food and Drug Administration 2019).

In Canada, vaping skyrocketed in teenagers and young adults between 2017 and 2019 after being made openly accessible in 2018.

Most vaping advocates have always been careful to stress that the putative benefits of vaping are all about adult smokers who want to quit smoking. You won't hear many of these people publicly thrilling to the data I showed in Chapter 6 on the large proportion of adults who vape *and* smoke and who have no interest in quitting smoking. Nor to that on long-term ex-smokers taking up vaping. And especially to data on the huge momentum in nicotine-naïve kids taking up regular vaping.

With prescribed legal access to vapable nicotine now mandatory in Australia, two factors are currently in play which together seem likely to greatly diminish access by kids.

First, because only pharmacies are authorised to fill prescriptions, no businesses other than pharmacies are allowed to sell NVPs in Australia. In the early months of the policy, public health agencies have been reporting a steady stream of breaches of these regulations, with large fines being issued by the TGA (see Therapeutic Goods Administration 2021c, Therapeutic Goods Administration 2021a). This is a marked contrast to the rare prosecutions taken against retailers who sell cigarettes to minors.

Illegal flavoured disposable vapes being sold in convenience stores, online and at markets currently remain highly accessible. COVID has seen many health department staff seconded to other COVID-related duties, so surveillance and inspection efforts have been reduced.

Second, very few doctors would issue a NVP prescription to a child. On-sellers thinking that they could shop around doctors to get multiple prescriptions and then supply the feverish teenage demand will be easily traced via their Medicare number used in paying for their prescription.

A major Achilles heel here is that the personal importation scheme, preserved after pressure from conservative backbench MPs in 2021, needs to be urgently revoked. Those with a prescription can send a copy to an exporter in another country who can then send NVPs to the authorised personal importer. With hundreds of millions of international items arriving by post and courier into Australia every year, clearly any attempt at thoroughly screening these for unauthorised NVP imports or those with fake prescriptions will be hugely inefficient. Growing anger in the public health and school sectors over widespread access by children seems certain to increase. Inconsistencies in personal import regulations between tobacco and NVPs loom as a potent leverage point in advocacy for revoking personal NVP importation. It has been illegal since 2019 to personally import cigarettes into Australia beyond one duty-free pack carried by arriving travellers (Australian Border Force 2021). Maximum fines for unauthorised importation of NVPs currently stand at $220,000. This risk will deter many individual vapers as well as criminals intending to on-sell in bulk.

If, as most political forecasters are predicting, there is a change of government in Australia in 2022, the votes of Labor, the Greens and progressive independents will easily ensure that such a revocation will occur.

Will Australian doctors be willing to prescribe nicotine?

A weakness with this scheme is the possibility that into the future, only a few doctors will be interested in prescribing access to nicotine juice. Before the scheme was made mandatory, fewer than ten doctors out of over 122,000 registered medical practitioners across the country were said to be doing this, with an unknown but desultory number of prescriptions being issued as a result. This hugely underwhelming participation rate was largely explained by the ability of vapers and others to easily import nicotine juice, making going to a doctor to get an authority to buy nicotine from a compounding chemist uncompetitive. As this importing ability was regulated from 1 October 2021, more Australian doctors may now be willing to prescribe. But it is possible that with nicotine continuing to have what the TGA calls "unapproved product" status as a drug (Therapeutic Goods Administration 2021), many doctors will remain uninterested. Challenging legal issues may arise in the event of an adverse reaction or health problems arising from vaping nicotine which had been obtained via a prescription. It is conceivable that such patients may seek redress from doctors who issued the authority for them to use such an unapproved substance.

The end for combusted tobacco?

Throughout my career, I've been urged to support and advocate for a wide range of policies and campaigns. I have always tried to be assiduous in considering the ethical implications of any tobacco control policy. To the annoyance of some of my more "whatever it takes" colleagues, I wrote several detailed papers (Chapman 2008a, Darzi, Keown et al. 2015, Chapman 2000) that were critical of proposals that smoking should be banned in wide open spaces like parks and beaches because there is no evidence that the fleeting exposures others may experience in such contexts are harmful (Licht, Hyland et al. 2013). I support a ban on smoking inside prison buildings because the minority of prisoners who do not smoke should not be forced to be exposed to second-hand smoke for the lengthy hours that prisoners are locked in often shared cells every day. But I support prisoners being allowed to smoke in open air sections of prisons. All serious epidemiology on the harmful effects of second-hand smoke exposure has shown that it is chronic exposures in enclosed domestic and occupational settings, not fleeting exposure outdoors, that causes disease.

I also declined to join those who believe that the state should be able to instruct movie directors to censor scenes of smoking under the threat of having their movies rated R (over 18 years old), which can have major negative box-office receipt consequences (Chapman and Farrelly 2011). To me, the assumption that public health goals should be able to be used to justify intrusion into the content of cultural, artistic or cinematic expression is dangerous and redolent of the playbooks used by authoritarian political regimes. Once precedents are set, conga lines of advocates for a wide variety of censorship and restrictions on personal conduct, often passionately espoused as being for the good of society, queue up to prosecute their visions for a better society. History is full of episodes of horrendous persecution of individuals and groups who want to express their beliefs or behave in ways that meet the disapproval of others.

I have often been asked by journalists, interviewers, students and members of the public whether I support the banning of tobacco. Across a 45-year career, I have never once advocated for smoking to be banned. My reasoning here has nothing to do with my strong agreement that smoking already kills some eight million people a year and harms many more. It is rather that the acid test of the ethics of stopping people from doing various things has always been the 19th-century utilitarian philosopher John Stuart Mill's famous statement in *On Liberty* (1859): "That the only purpose for which power can be rightfully exercised over any member of a civilised community, against his will, is to prevent harm to others."

I support the right of people to end their own lives by accessing humane means of doing so. I also believe people should not be prevented from pursuing leisure or adventure activities which are dangerous to them alone, as much as we might hope that they would decide to not do these things. Obvious examples here are lone ocean sailing, mountain climbing, base-jumping and other dangerous sports. I'm happy to support some mandatory intrusions on individual liberty where there are only risks to the individual, but not to others. Examples here are compulsory seatbelts for vehicle occupants, helmets for motorcyclists and cyclists, and lifejackets for those in boats. These involve truly trivial impositions on freedom where the risk reduction benefits massively outweigh the deprivation of freedom disbenefits. The *outrageous* erosion of the freedom to not use a seat belt which might prevent a person spending the rest of their life with severe disability is such an example.

Many tobacco control policies and publicity campaigns are explicitly intended to make the choice to smoke one that is ushered through a daily obstacle course of exposures, considerations and nudges known to reduce the likelihood that someone will want to take up smoking and continue to do it.

Seriously dissuasive taxes; minimum floor prices; ghoulish, arresting graphic health warnings; banishing smoking away from exposure to others; banning all tobacco advertising (including paid product placement in movies and with social media influencers); banning misleading descriptors like "light and mild"; preventing manufacturers spicing up cigarettes with flavours that disguise what would otherwise be a far less palatable smoking experience; restricting retail purchasing to an ever-decreasing number of retail outlets and licensing smokers in the way that all users of prescribed drugs require a temporary licence to access pharmaceuticals are all policies I've been happy to advocate. Most of these are policies which have been endorsed by the 181 nations which are parties to the WHO's FCTC which came into force on 27 February 2005.

But as most of these policies play out across the world and smoking rates are at their lowest ever recorded in nations with advanced tobacco control policies, there is still an immense number of people who continue to buy tobacco products – 1.1 billion at the most recent estimate – thanks mostly to world population growth (GBD 2019 Tobacco Collaborators 2021).

So should we just continue to erode this number using the menu of policies and campaigns which have driven smoking prevalence down to record levels in nations with comprehensive tobacco control? Or is it time that tobacco control moved to the next level and treated tobacco the way that other unambiguously deadly commodities have been treated?

There is a wide-open door being held ajar here by J.S. Mill's dictum quoted earlier. When he wrote about power being exercised over "*any member* of a civilised community" to prevent harm to others, he was writing about individuals. But had Mill known that smoking could harm others chronically exposed to tobacco smoke, he may well have used smoking as an example, as ethicist Robert E. Goodin laid out in his classic 1989 analysis *The ethics of smoking*, published 130 years later, of the ethics of preventing smoking when others were exposed (Goodin 1989).

And had there been transnational tobacco corporations in the mid-19th century when Mill was writing, doing all they could to promote smoking and thwarting effective tobacco control and thereby harming millions by their daily actions, he may well have also readily agreed that industry's liberty should be very much on the table for radical constraint.

While there can be proper concerns about impositions on freedom of *individuals*, a whole different set of considerations opens up when proposed constraints on corporations' actions which harm individuals are considered.

Ever since the bad news began rolling in from the early 1950s about the inconvenient problem of the very nasty harm that smoking causes, the industry has pursued a public agenda of announcing successive generations of allegedly reduced harm products. Unfortunately, every one of these crashed as false hopes (Chapman 2016). All were primarily designed to keep nicotine-dependent customers loyal to the companies' evolving products and to dissuade people from quitting.

No industry likes seeing its longest and most loyal customers dying early. They'd far prefer that they lived to consume and be contributing cash cows for as many years as possible. There is also no industry more publicly loathed and mistrusted than the tobacco industry (Freeman, Greenhalgh et al. 2020). Against this, the harm-reduction agenda represents a trifecta of hope for Big Tobacco: it's a kind of perpetual holy grail, never reached but always sought, with the promises of seeing smokers living and consuming longer. It's also a way of enticing new generations of users into the market who each time swallow the hype about radically reduced-risk products. And it carries hope of eroding the industry's ongoing corporate pariah status (Christofides, Chapman et al. 1999), with its attendant risks of attracting sub-optimal staff indifferent to working in a killer industry (Chapman 2020). Harm reduction is a virtue-signalling cornucopia that keeps on giving.

Enter NVPs

NVPs are the latest harm-reduction debutantes. The size of the popularity wave they are riding in several nations puts these products in the league of two previous, long disgraced illusory heavyweight champions of harm reduction: filter tips and so-call light and mild cigarettes. Filters are almost universally still used today in cigarettes, but with eight million deaths a year still occurring, it's a bit like saying that arsenic is less harmful than cyanide, thanks to filters. Because of compensatory smoking, lights and milds were declared misleading and deceptive descriptors by the Australian Competition and Consumer Commission in 2005 and outlawed (Anon 2005). Tobacco companies in the USA were obliged to run court-ordered corrective advertising, including messages about the lights and milds scam (Kodjak 2017).

The rise of NVPs has been accompanied by a chorus of Big Tobacco CEOs proclaiming that they mark the beginning of the end of smoking. "Look what we are doing," they gush. "We are transforming ourselves into companies that are saving lives! We are investing billions into research, development, production and marketing of these new products."

But on the floors that house those in the executive who pull the strings for the entire companies, they know exactly how the company bread is buttered and what the future vision looks like. And for all the sloganeering about the end of smoking, that future has, as always, cigarettes right at the very front of the business model.

BAT's 2018 half-yearly report could not have been more emphatic on this from its opening paragraph, "Our strategy is *to continue to grow our combustible business* while investing in the exciting *potentially reduced risk* categories of HTP, vapour and oral. As the Group expands its portfolio in these categories, we will continue to drive sustainable growth" [my emphases] (British American Tobacco 2018).

A senior Philip Morris International spokesperson, Corey Henry, told the *New York Times* in August 2018, "As we transform our business toward a smoke-free future, we remain focused on maintaining our leadership of the combustible tobacco category outside China and the US" (Kaplan 2018).

In 2017 Altria, previously known as Philip Morris Companies, Inc., noted that Philip Morris USA candidly spoke of "making cigarettes our core product" (see https://twitter.com/SimonChapman6/status/908283373994500096).

Reduced-risk products instead of or as well as cigarettes?

In 2019, six researchers who declared that they were happy to state they worked with the tobacco industry, wrote in *Addiction*, "If the tobacco industry seeks to make money by making reduced-risk products *instead of* more risky products, we fail to see this as a menace to public health" [my emphasis] (Hughes, Fagerström et al. 2019).

Yes, I'm afraid they did fail to see the menace. Put simply, there is no evidence – apart from an incontinent river of public "trust us" declarations – of any tobacco company taking its foot off the twin business-as-usual accelerators of massively funded marketing of combustible tobacco products (chiefly cigarettes), and continuing efforts to discredit and thwart policies known to have an impact on preventing uptake and promoting cessation.

In recent years companies like BAT and Philip Morris have been relentless in seeking to dilute, delay and defeat any policy posing any threat to their tobacco sales. This is not the behaviour of an industry earnestly trying to get all its smokers to quit. Witness their massive efforts to stop Australia's historic plain-packaging legislation (Chapman and Freeman 2014). Witness their years' long efforts to stop Uruguay's graphic health warnings (Anon 2021). As recently as December 2016, BAT's lawyers wrote an appalling letter (see Herbert Smith Freehills 2016) to the Hong Kong administration trying to stop graphic health warnings going ahead. This was from a company that published in its 2016 financial results statement a call to "champion informed consumer choice" (Durante 2016).

There is a very long history of the tobacco industry, hand on heart, promising that it really wants to make cigarettes a thing of the past. These were all harm-reduction adventures of mass distraction, designed to reassure smokers that they could continue to consume the industry's tobacco products.

Phasing out cigarettes?

In a 2020 open-access paper, editors at *Tobacco Control* Elizabeth Smith and Ruth Malone articulated the most cogent case yet for tobacco control to take the gloves off and introduce radical policies which will end the sale of combustible tobacco (Smith and Malone 2020). Their argument runs like this.

In 1985, the United Nations unanimously adopted guidelines for consumer protection including that "Governments should adopt or encourage the adoption of appropriate measures … to ensure that products are safe for either intended or normally foreseeable use" (United Nations Conference on Trade and Development 1985). So when it comes to tobacco, there is arguably no other product which comes anywhere close to being the prime candidate for governments to apply such scrutiny. Smith and Malone wrote:

> All advanced nations require cars to undergo crash tests before they are sold, food manufacturers and processors are held to hygienic standards, and drugs undergo clinical trials to establish safety and effectiveness. Legal consumer products found to be hazardous are regularly pulled from the market, such as toys presenting choking hazards for children; batches of contaminated

processed food or individual components of complex goods (e.g., batteries, airbags) that work improperly. Manufacturers or retailers sometimes recall goods that appear to malfunction, even without reported injuries. For the most part, consumers assume that products offered for sale are reasonably safe.

Tobacco fails any test of consumer safety but bizarrely continues to enjoy exceptionalist status being shielded from the powers of consumer protection law. They continue:

> From the consumer protection standpoint, most people do not believe that people "need", "deserve" or "have the right to" purchase cars that are unsafe to drive, medications that poison them or food that spreads disease ... The "right to smoke" framing obscures the generally accepted ethical obligation of reputable companies to sell only products that do not cause great harm when used as intended.

So laws ensuring product safety should also apply to all tobacco products. Not just to their marketing, advertising, packaging and where they cannot be smoked in the case of combustible forms, but to the products themselves. De facto exemption of tobacco products from consumer safety laws would be like regulating civilian firearm access but deciding that dynamite and explosives were fine to be on sale to anyone who wanted to buy them.

Smith and Malone write about the "phasing out" of cigarette sales, arguing that instances of this are already happening is a very small number of US towns and cities with low smoking prevalence, driven by local governments. They suggest that these bans will in time spread to neighbouring towns or municipalities and note that similar gradual spread occurred with the rollout of smoke-free ordinances. They readily admit this will be "an arduous and lengthy process", as indeed was the smoke-free-areas chapter in tobacco control history. Smoking was first banned on trains and buses in my state of New South Wales in 1976. It took until 1 December 2006 before smoking was finally banned in pubs and bars, the so-called last bastions of freedom to ignore the occupational health and safety of bar workers.

Smith and Malone stress the importance of public health advocates continually trying to change the dominant narrative away from cigarettes being an ordinary, legal consumer product to characterise them as being an "inherently defective, unsafe product that falls into the same category as contaminated food, asbestos and lead paint. These are products that states find too hazardous to be made available to the public, and regardless of cost ... the government removes them from the marketplace." They suggest a parallel case would be comparison with the phase-out of leaded petrol: "As with tobacco, manufacturers knew for decades that leaded gasoline was hazardous and concealed that knowledge. Still, the eventual phase-out of leaded gasoline in the USA took a decade."

The comparison though is far from perfect. Leaded petrol had a ready substitute in unleaded alternatives. Similarly, calls to phase out fossil fuels always point to obvious renewable power alternatives. Incandescent bulbs rapidly disappeared with the advent of LED lighting. Records, cassettes and CDs were overtaken by MP3s and streaming. And film cameras by digital cameras and smart phones. All of these examples saw tentative consumer resistance often turn into tsunamis of uptake of the improved alternatives.

If we were confident from the hype that NVPs could indeed deliver all they promise, it would be obvious where a phase-out of tobacco could lead. Tobacco retailers would continue to profit from nicotine dependency in barely the blink of an eye, governments would see their tobacco tax receipts continue, switched to NVPs. But as we saw in Chapter 6, it is very far from clear that NVPs will indeed drive smoking down rather than sustain it through dual use and increasing relapse.

Governments derive significant revenue from tobacco tax and goods and services taxes (GST) that are added to nearly every commodity or service transaction. Many people have taken this to mean that governments have a clear interest in doing nothing that would ever kill or badly wound the goose laying these golden eggs. But this reasoning is deeply flawed. Here's why: non-smokers do not engage in daily rituals of calculating how much tax revenue their selfish acts of not smoking deprive the government in tobacco tax and then squirrel this money away in a box under their beds forever or put it through a shredder.

Instead, they use their money to purchase other goods and services. Each of these expenditures is GST inclusive, generates employment and has multiplier effects in the economy. So, if there was no smoking or vaping, there would not be a neatly packaged and easily identified bolus of tobacco tax that went directly into Treasury surrounded by dazzling neon signs calling on everyone to be grateful to Big Tobacco for their marvellous contributions to economic well-being. Instead, this money would be dissipated into many different expenditure routes, each of which – just as occurs with tobacco expenditure – generates tax, employment and economic well-being.

Moreover, as Warner and Fulton showed in a case study of what would have resulted had the state of Michigan, USA, somehow had zero tobacco consumption between 1992 and 2005, 5,600 extra jobs would have resulted (Warner and Fulton 1994). Big Tobacco has been hugely successful in spinning its story to people with low literacy in economic matters, but in fact in many nations, tobacco expenditure compares poorly in social benefit terms to expenditure on other goods and services.

It is very easy to throw the "phasing out" expression around as a sensible-sounding aspirational goal. But when we look for what would be involved in any step-by-step progression of a program of phasing out, there are scant details.

My reading of where the "phasing-out" argument rests at the moment is as follows:

1. It is unarguable that the ludicrous exceptionalist status of tobacco as a deadly product which has so far escaped serious regulation or banning as an unsafe product needs to be raised as a fundamental starting point in every global and national high-level discussion about the future of tobacco control.
2. For as long as tobacco continues to be sold as an unregulated product through virtually any retailing context, this will powerfully condition the commonly expressed view that "tobacco cannot be that harmful, because otherwise governments would ban it". Tobacco needs to be legally classified as a controlled, restricted product in all its forms.
3. Large majorities of the population, including smokers, support measures designed to make their decision to smoke a more difficult

choice. This gives strong support to "next steps" rhetoric from governments about how they might best accelerate the fall in smoking. They will be cheered on by a large proportion of the community (Gartner, Wright et al. 2021).

4. Consistent and commensurate with a formally declared status as a restricted product, tobacco access and retailing could then change. Much more restrictive regulation of tobacco retailing is an obvious candidate for a next big step. The key elements of retailing restricted products should be: licensing all retailers; introducing permanent loss of license for anyone selling to minors or breach of other licensed retailer regulations; and requiring that tobacco be sold in dedicated tobacco retail settings away from other grocery or mixed-business-style goods and only to those permitted to buy tobacco (see number 5); and requiring all retailers have electronic records to reconcile all sales with their registered inventory of tobacco stock.

5. All tobacco purchasing should be conducted through a date-of-birth-linked QR code, with capabilities to data-link purchasers with tobacco stock sold. This would ensure that all customers were over the legal age to purchase tobacco and that retailers only sold stock that had been logged onto their official stock inventories, much in the same way that pharmacists must always have fully reconcilable records of all restricted stock.

6. The evidence that NVPs are all but benign and clearly superior to other ways of quitting – including unassisted quitting – is poor and in the case of assessing any potential long-term harm, very premature. Accordingly, it would be reckless to allow NVPs to be sold in an any less restricted way than any therapeutic substance entering a market is now sold: via the authority of a doctor's prescription, as described earlier about the current Australian arrangements. Some drugs (e.g. NRT) were rescheduled as OTC access after years of monitoring for safety issues when they were prescribed. The same potential may exist for NVPs, although because there are literally many thousands of NVP apparatuses and NVP compounds, this will be much more complex than it was for NRT with its standardised formulations.

7. The overarching objective of NVP regulation should be to make approved products available under a prescription regimen *only* for adult smokers assessed as genuinely wanting to quit smoking. This will pose many challenges as NVP marketers will game the rules by incentivising doctors to provide these products to as wide a range of applicants as possible, using perfunctory assessments. Surveillance of doctors' over-prescribing here will be as important as it has been for other controlled drugs.

The endgame in chess is often the longest and slowest phase of the game. The word does not at all connote a rushed period of play just before a game ends. Much of the above will take time in the same way that all policy advances in tobacco control have taken (with rare exceptions). Where tobacco control has been taken seriously, there are now nations with national smoking prevalence below 10% (Iceland 7.3% daily and Norway 9% daily) (Australian Bureau of Statistics 2021), and subpopulations with smoking rates sometimes well below that level. In the USA only 8% of 18–24-year-olds smoke, 7.2% of Asians, 8.8% of Hispanics, 6.9% with an undergraduate education and just 4% with a graduate degree (Centers for Disease Control and Prevention 2021). In Australia 7.9% of people with a bachelors degree or higher smoke, 7.7% of those who speak a language other than English at home, and 8.2% of those in the highest socioeconomic quintile (Australian Institute of Health and Welfare 2020h). Only 8.8% of women and 8.3% of 18–24-year-olds smoke daily (Australian Bureau of Statistics 2021). In the UK, 7.3% of those with a degree smoke and 9.3% in managerial occupations (Office for National Statistics 2020a).

Tobacco control is widely regarded as the poster-child of chronic disease control in nations that have implemented comprehensive regulatory "upstream" policies which reach every smoker and potential smoker. No other non-communicable disease area – e.g. obesity, Type 2 diabetes, metabolic syndrome, sedentary lifestyles – can point to the magnitude of sustained improvements that tobacco control has caused over decades.

Throughout this book I have emphasised that far too much organised tobacco control is focused on activity that, in its net contribution to reducing smoking, is a story of the tail trying to wag the dog. The over-focus on tail wagging techniques in tobacco control

9 Controlling tobacco supply and the endgame

for the past 30 years has caused mass distraction from what is quietly going on with the dog itself. Here, there is much to both celebrate and amplify with policies and motivational campaigns that have proven track records and are detested by the tobacco industry because of that impact. Those two tests are all we really need to know in how we continue to make smoking history.

About the author

Simon Chapman AO PhD is Emeritus Professor in Public Health at the University of Sydney. Across 45 years, he has been a prominent researcher and advocate for tobacco control, gun control, wind farms and renewable energy. He was foundation deputy editor (1992–97), editor (1998–2008) and emeritus editor (since 2009) for the *British Medical Journal*'s specialist journal *Tobacco Control*. In 1997 he was awarded the World Health Organization's World No Tobacco Day Medal and in 2003 the American Cancer Society's Luther Terry Award for outstanding individual leadership in tobacco control. In 2008 he was awarded the NSW Premier's Cancer Researcher of the Year medal and in 2013 he was made an Officer in the Order of Australia for his contributions to public health, and named Australian Skeptic of the Year. He is a Fellow of the Australian Academy of Social Sciences and an honorary Fellow of the Faculty of Public Health of Royal Colleges of Physicians of the United Kingdom.

He is a life member of the Australian Consumers Association, having been a board member for 20 years and chair for four. The *Sydney Morning Herald* named him in 2008 and 2012 as one of Sydney's 100 most influential people. In 2014, he was deeply honoured when Australia's leading right-wing think tank, the Institute of Public Affairs, named him as one of 12 all-time "opponents of freedom".

His column for *The Conversation* (2015–18) has been read 3.63 million times. He blogs at simonchapman6.com and tweets @simonchapman6.

About the author

Also by Simon Chapman

Simon Chapman and Fiona Crichton (2017). *Wind turbine syndrome: a communicated disease.* Sydney: Sydney University Press.
Simon Chapman (2016). *Smoke signals: selective writing.* Sydney: Darlington Press.
Simon Chapman and Becky Freeman (2014). *Removing the emperor's clothes: Australia and tobacco plain packaging.* Sydney: Sydney University Press.
Simon Chapman (2013). *Over our dead bodies: Port Arthur and gun control.* Sydney: Sydney University Press.
Simon Chapman, Alex Barratt and Martin Stockler (2010). *Let sleeping dogs lie? What men should know before being tested for prostate cancer.* Sydney: Sydney University Press.

References

Abdullah, A.S. and W.W. Ho (2006). What Chinese adolescents think about quitting smoking: a qualitative study. *Subst Use Misuse* 41(13): 1735–43 DOI: 10.1080/10826080601006433.

Abdulwadud, O. and J. Ozanne-Smith (1998). Injuries associated with fireworks in Victoria: an epidemiological overview. *Inj Prev* 4(4): 272–75 DOI: 10.1136/ip.4.4.272

Abrams, D.B., A.L. Graham, D.T. Levy, P.L. Mabry and C.T. Orleans (2010). Boosting population quits through evidence-based cessation treatment and policy. *Am J Prev Med* 38(3 Suppl): S351–63 DOI: 10.1016/j.amepre.2009.12.011

Action on Smoking and Health (2019). *A changing landscape: stop smoking services and tobacco control in England*. London: ASH. https://ash.org.uk/wp-content/uploads/2019/03/2019-LA-Survey-Report.pdf

Action on Smoking and Health New Zealand (2021). *ASH Year 10 Snapshot Survey*. https://www.ash.org.nz/ash_year_10

Agboola, S., A. McNeill, T. Coleman and J. Leonardi Bee (2010). A systematic review of the effectiveness of smoking relapse prevention interventions for abstinent smokers. *Addiction* 105(8): 1362–80 DOI: 10.1111/j.1360-0443.2010.02996.x

Allen, M., D. Ambrose and G. Halpenny (2003). Telephone refusal rate still rising: results of the 2002 Response Rate Survey. Ontario, Canada: Marketing Research and Intelligence Association.

Alpert, H., G. Connolly and L. Biener (2012). A prospective cohort study challenging the effectiveness of population-based medical intervention for smoking cessation. *Tob Control* DOI: 10.1136/tobaccocontrol-2011-050129

American Cancer Society (2003). Cancer facts and figures 2003. http://www.cancer.org/downloads/STT/CAFF2003PWSecured.pdf

References

American Psychiatric Association (2018). What is a gambling disorder? https://www.psychiatry.org/patients-families/gambling-disorder/what-is-gambling-disorder

Amin, K. (2015). Another year, another burden for cigarette makers. *Jakarta Post*, 4 May. https://www.thejakartapost.com/news/2015/05/04/another-year-another-burden-cigarette-makers.html

Amos, A. and M. Haglund (2000). From social taboo to "torch of freedom": the marketing of cigarettes to women. *Tob Control* 9(1): 3–8 DOI: 10.1136/tc.9.1.3

Apollonio, D.E. and R.E. Malone (2010). The "we card" program: tobacco industry "youth smoking prevention" as industry self-preservation. *Am J Public Health* 100(7): 1188–201 DOI: 10.2105/AJPH.2009.169573

Assunta, M. and S. Chapman (2004). Industry sponsored youth smoking prevention programme in Malaysia: a case study in duplicity. *Tob Control* 13 Suppl 2: ii37–42 DOI: 10.1136/tc.2004.007732

Assunta, M. and E.U. Dorotheo (2016). SEATCA Tobacco Industry Interference Index: a tool for measuring implementation of WHO Framework Convention on Tobacco Control Article 5.3. *Tob Control* 25(3): 313–18 DOI: 10.1136/tobaccocontrol-2014-051934

Atkins, S., S. Lewin and H. Smith et al. (2008). Conducting a meta-ethnography of qualitative literature: lessons learnt. *BMC Med Res Methodol* 8: 21 DOI: 10.1186/1471-2288-8-21

Australian Advertising Council (2009). The Australian Effie awards: how Champix outsmarted cigarettes. Category e: Healthcare: Australian Advertising Council. https://tinyurl.com/yckucd24

Australian Associated Press (2021). Pete Evans fined $80,000 by Health Department for alleged unlawful spruiking of devices and medicines. *Guardian*, 25 May. https://tinyurl.com/yc8ynvjr

Australian Border Force (2021). Importing or bringing tobacco into Australia. https://www.abf.gov.au/importing-exporting-and-manufacturing/prohibited-goods/categories/tobacco

Australian Bureau of Statistics (2021a). Pandemic insights into Australian smokers, 2020–21. Canberra: ABS. https://www.abs.gov.au/articles/pandemic-insights-australian-smokers-2020-21

Australian Institute of Health and Welfare (2020a). *Asthma*. https://www.aihw.gov.au/reports/chronic-respiratory-conditions/asthma/contents/asthma

Australian Institute of Health and Welfare (2020b). Chapter 4: Illicit use of drugs – supplementary data tables, *National Drug Strategy Household Survey 2019*.

Canberra: AIHW. https://www.aihw.gov.au/reports-data/behaviours-risk-factors/illicit-use-of-drugs/data

Australian Institute of Health and Welfare (2020c). Table 2.3: Tobacco smoking status, people aged 14 and over, by sex, 2001 to 2019 (persons). In Chapter 2: Tobacco smoking supplementary tables, *National Drug Strategy Household Survey 2019*. Canberra: AIHW. https://www.aihw.gov.au/getmedia/77dbea6e-f071-495c-b71e-3a632237269d/aihw-phe-270.pdf.aspx?inline=true

Australian Institute of Health and Welfare (2020d). Table 2.39: Changes to smoking behaviour, smokers aged 14 and over, by sex, 2007 to 2019. In Chapter 2: Tobacco smoking supplementary tables, *National Drug Strategy Household Survey 2019*. Canberra: AIHW. https://www.aihw.gov.au/getmedia/77dbea6e-f071-495c-b71e-3a632237269d/aihw-phe-270.pdf.aspx?inline=true

Australian Institute of Health and Welfare (2020e). Table 2.58: Tobacco smoking status, people aged 14 and over, by social characteristics, 2010 to 2019. In Chapter 2: Tobacco smoking supplementary tables, *National Drug Strategy Household Survey 2019*. Canberra: AIHW. https://www.aihw.gov.au/getmedia/77dbea6e-f071-495c-b71e-3a632237269d/aihw-phe-270.pdf.aspx?inline=true

Australian Institute of Health and Welfare (2020f). *National Drug Strategy Household Survey 2019. Drug Statistics series*. Canberra: AIHW. https://www.aihw.gov.au/getmedia/77dbea6e-f071-495c-b71e-3a632237269d/aihw-phe-270.pdf.aspx?inline=true

Australian Institute of Health and Welfare (2020g). Table 2.1: Tobacco smoking status, people aged 14 and over, 1991 to 2019. *National Drug Strategy Household Survey 2019*. Canberra: AIHW. https://www.aihw.gov.au/getmedia/77dbea6e-f071-495c-b71e-3a632237269d/aihw-phe-270.pdf.aspx?inline=true

Australian Institute of Health and Welfare (2020h). Table 2.8 Tobacco smoking status, by age and sex, 2001 to 2019 (persons). In Chapter 2: Tobacco smoking supplementary tables, *National Drug Strategy Household Survey*. Canberra: AIHW https://www.aihw.gov.au/getmedia/77dbea6e-f071-495c-b71e-3a632237269d/aihw-phe-270.pdf.aspx?inline=true

Australian Institute of Health and Welfare (2021). *National Opioid Pharmacotherapy Statistics Annual Data collection*. Canberra: AIHW. https://tinyurl.com/2m4z7pm8

Australian Productivity Commission (2010). *Gambling*. Canberra: Productivity Commission. https://www.pc.gov.au/inquiries/completed/gambling-2010/report

Australian Senate (2020a). Evidence from Clive Bates to Senate Select Committee on Tobacco Harm Reduction. 19 November. https://tinyurl.com/44r9tr2s

Australian Senate (2020b). Senate Select Committee on Tobacco Harm Reduction. 19 November. https://tinyurl.com/yz6uvdnm

References

Australian Treasury (2013). Post-implementation review: 25 per cent tobacco excise increase. https://tinyurl.com/2p8f2rks

Azjen, I. (1991). The theory of planned behavior. *Organizational Behavior and Human Decision Processes* 50: 170–211 DOI: 10.1016/0749-5978(91)90020-T

Baer, P.E., J.P. Foreyt and S. Wright (1977). Self-directed termination of excessive cigarette use among untreated smokers. *J Behav Therapy Exp Psychiatry* 8(1): 71–74 DOI: 10.1016/0005-7916(77)90108-2

Baillie, A.J., R.P. Mattick and W. Hall (1995). Quitting smoking: estimation by meta-analysis of the rate of unaided smoking cessation. *Aust J Public Health* 19(2): 129–31 DOI: 10.1111/j.1753-6405.1995.tb00361.x

Bala, M.M., E. A. Akl and X. Sun et al. (2013). Randomized trials published in higher vs lower impact journals differ in design, conduct, and analysis. *J Clin Epidemiol* 66(3): 286–95 DOI: 10.1016/j.jclinepi.2012.10.005

Balfour, D.J.K., N.L. Benowitz and S.M. Colby et al. (2021). Balancing consideration of the risks and benefits of e-cigarettes. *Am J Public Health* 111(9): 1661–72 DOI: 10.2105/AJPH.2021.306416

Balmford, J., R. Borland, D. Hammond and K. Cummings (2011). Adherence to and reasons for premature discontinuation from stop-smoking medications: data from the ITC Four-Country Survey. *Nicotine Tob Res* 13(2): 94–102 DOI: 10.1093/ntr/ntq215

Bals, R., J. Boyd and S. Esposito et al. (2019). Electronic cigarettes: a task force report from the European Respiratory Society. *Eur Respir J* 53(2) DOI: 10.1183/13993003.01151-2018

Bankhead, C., J.K. Aronson and D. Nunan (2017). Attrition bias. In *Catalogue of Bias Collaboration*. https://catalogofbias.org/biases/attrition-bias/

Banks, E., K. Beckwith and G. Joshy (2020). *Summary report on use of e-cigarettes and relation to tobacco smoking uptake and cessation, relevant to the Australian context.* Canberra: Australian National University. https://tinyurl.com/h2a4hm57

Banks, E., G. Joshy and M. F. Weber et al. (2015). Tobacco smoking and all-cause mortality in a large Australian cohort study: findings from a mature epidemic with current low smoking prevalence. *BMC Med* 13: 38 DOI: 10.1186/s12916-015-0281-z

Bansal, M.A., K. Cummings, A. Hyland and G. Giovino (2004). Stop-smoking medications: who uses them, who misuses them, and who is misinformed about them? *Nicotine Tob Res* 6(Suppl 3): S303–S10 DOI: 10.1080/14622200412331320707

Barker Bausell, R.B. (2007). *Snake oil science: the truth about complementary and alternative medicine.* Oxford: Oxford University Press.

Barnett-Page, E. and J. Thomas (2009). Methods for the synthesis of qualitative research: a critical review. *BMC Med Res Methodol* 9: 59 DOI: 10.1186/1471-2288-9-59

Barrington-Trimis, J.L., R. Urman and K. Berhane et al. (2016). E-cigarettes and future cigarette use. *Pediatrics* 138(1) DOI: 10.1542/peds.2016-0379

Bauld, L., K. Bell, L. McCullough, L. Richardson and L. Greaves (2010). The effectiveness of NHS smoking cessation services: a systematic review. *J Pub Health* 32(1): 71–82 DOI: 0.1093/pubmed/fdp074

Bauld, L., K.A. Boyd and A.H. Briggs et al. (2011). One-year outcomes and a cost-effectiveness analysis for smokers accessing group-based and pharmacy-led cessation services. *Nicotine Tob Res* 13(2): 135–45 DOI: 10.1093/ntr/ntq222

Bauld, L., T. Coleman, C. Adams, E. Pound and J. Ferguson (2005). Delivering the English smoking treatment services. *Addiction* 100: 19–27 DOI: 10.1111/j.1360-0443.2005.01024.x

Baumeister, R.F. and K.D. Vohs (eds) (2017). *Handbook of self-regulation: Research, theory, and applications.* New York: Guildford Press.

Bayly, M., T. Carroll, T. Cotter and K. Purcell (2021). 14.3 Public education campaigns to discourage smoking: the Australian experience. In Greenhalgh, E.M., M.M. Scollo and M.H. Winstanley (eds) *Tobacco in Australia: facts and issues.* Melbourne: Cancer Council Victoria. https://tinyurl.com/2p97sr64

Bayly, M. and M. Scollo (2020). 10.5 Retailing of tobacco products in Australia. In Greenhalgh, E.M., M.M. Scollo and M.H. Winstanley (eds) *Tobacco in Australia: facts and issues.* Melbourne: Cancer Council Victoria. https://www.tobaccoinaustralia.org.au/chapter-10-tobacco-industry/10-5-retailing-of-tobacco-products-in-australia

BBC News (2014). Nutt: e-cigs "greatest health advance" since vaccines. https://www.bbc.com/news/av/health-26036064

Beard, E., J. Brown, S. Michie and R. West (2018). Is prevalence of e-cigarette and nicotine replacement therapy use among smokers associated with average cigarette consumption in England? A time-series analysis. *BMJ Open* 8(6): e016046 DOI: 10.1136/bmjopen-2017-016046

Beard, E., R. West, S. Michie and J. Brown (2016). Association between electronic cigarette use and changes in quit attempts, success of quit attempts, use of smoking cessation pharmacotherapy, and use of stop smoking services in England: time series analysis of population trends. *BMJ* 354: i4645 DOI: 10.1136/bmj.i4645

Beard, E., R. West, S. Michie and J. Brown (2020). Association of prevalence of electronic cigarette use with smoking cessation and cigarette consumption in

References

England: a time-series analysis between 2006 and 2017. *Addiction* 115(5): 961–74 DOI: 10.1111/add.14851

Becker M.H. (1974). *The Health Belief Model and personal health behaviour.* Thorofare, New Jersey: Charles B. Slack.

Benmarhnia, T., J.P. Pierce and E. Leas et al. (2018). Can e-cigarettes and pharmaceutical aids increase smoking cessation and reduce cigarette consumption? Findings from a nationally representative cohort of American smokers. *Am J Epidemiol* 187(11): 2397–404 DOI: 10.1093/aje/kwy129

Berry, K.M., L. Reynolds and J. Collins et al. (2019). E-cigarette initiation and associated changes in smoking cessation and reduction: the Population Assessment of Tobacco and Health Study, 2013–2015. *Tob Control* 28(1): 42–49 DOI: 10.1136/tobaccocontrol-2017-054108

Berthelot, J.M., B. Le Goff and Y. Maugars (2011). The Hawthorne effect: stronger than the placebo effect? *Joint Bone Spine* 78(4):335–336 DOI: 10.1016/j.jbspin.2011.06.001

Biener, L., C.A. Garrett and E.A. Gilpin et al. (2004). Consequences of declining survey response rates for smoking prevalence estimates. *Am J Prev Med* 27(3): 254–57 DOI: 10.1016/j.amepre.2004.05.006.

Biernacki, P. (1986). *Pathways from heroin addiction: recovery without treatment.* Philadelphia: Temple University Press.

Biernacki, P. and D. Waldorf (1981). Snowball sampling: problems and techniques of chain referral sampling. *Sociological Methods and Research*(10): 141–63 DOI: 10.1177/004912418101000205.

Bitton, A. and N. Eyal (2011). Too poor to treat? The complex ethics of cost-effective tobacco policy in the developing world. *Public Health Ethics* DOI: 10.1093/phe/phr014

Bittoun, R. and J.C. Clarke (1985). Experiences with a large-scale smoking cessation clinic. *Australian Drug/Alcohol Review* 4: 165–68 DOI: 10.1080/09595238580000251

Bommele, J., G.E. Nagelhout and M. Kleinjan et al. (2016). Prevalence of hardcore smoking in the Netherlands between 2001 and 2012: a test of the hardening hypothesis. *BMC Public Health* 16:754 DOI: 10.1186/s12889-016-3434-x

Bonfiglioli, C.M., B. Smith, L. King, S. Chapman and S. Holding (2007). Choice and voice: obesity debates in television news. *Med J Aust* 187(8): 442–45 DOI: 10.5694/j.1326-5377.2007.tb01354.x

Borland, R., L. Li and P. Driezen et al. (2012). Cessation assistance reported by smokers in 15 countries participating in the International Tobacco Control (ITC) policy evaluation surveys. *Addiction* 107(1): 197–205 DOI: 10.1111/j.1360-0443.2011.03636.x

Borland, R., T. Partos and K. Cummings (2012a). Systematic biases in cross-sectional community studies may underestimate the effectiveness of stop-smoking medications. *Nicotine Tob Res* 14(12): 1483–87 DOI: 10.1093/ntr/nts002

Borland, R., T. Partos, H-H. Yong, K. Cummings and A. Hyland (2012b). How much unsuccessful quitting activity is going on among adult smokers? Data from the International Tobacco Control four country cohort survey. *Addiction* 107(3): 673–82 DOI: 10.1111/j.1360-0443.2011.03685.x

Borland, R., H-H. Yong and J. Balmford et al. (2010). Motivational factors predict quit attempts but not maintenance of smoking cessation: findings from the International Tobacco Control Four Country project. *Nicotine Tob Res* 12 Suppl: S4–11 DOI: 10.1093/ntr/ntq050

Bottorff, J.L., J. Radsma, M. Kelly and J.L. Oliffe (2009). Fathers' narratives of reducing and quitting smoking. *Sociol Health Illn* 31(2): 185–200 DOI: 10.1111/j.1467-9566.2008.01126.x

Brady, W. (1949). Dr Brady says: silver nitrate solution aids smoker quit. *Detroit Free Press*, 29 April. https://www.newspapers.com/clip/36306712/detroit-free-press/

Brandt, A.M. (2007). *The cigarette century*. New York: Basic Books.

Brantmark, B., P. Ohlin and H. Westling (1973). Nicotine-containing chewing gum as an anti-smoking aid. *Psychopharmacologia* 31(3): 191–200 DOI: 10.1007/BF00422509

British American Tobacco (2018). British American Tobacco P.L.C. half-year report to 30 June 2018. https://www.bat.com/group/sites/UK__9D9KCY.nsf/vwPagesWebLive/DOB2ZP4L

Britton, J. (2009). In defence of helping people to stop smoking. *Lancet* 373(9665): 703–05 DOI: 10.1016/S0140-6736(09)60417-7

Brose, L.S., J. Bowen, A. McNeill and T. Partos (2019). Associations between vaping and relapse to smoking: preliminary findings from a longitudinal survey in the UK. *Harm Reduct J* 16(1): 76 DOI: 10.1186/s12954-019-0344-0

Brouwer, A.F., J. Jeon and J. Hirschtick et al. (2020). Transitions between cigarette, ends and dual use in adults in the PATH study (waves 1–4): multistate transition modelling accounting for complex survey design. *Tob Control* DOI: 10.1136/tobaccocontrol-2020-055967

Brown, J., L. Shahab and R. West (2020). Public Submission 195 to the Senate Select Committee on Tobacco Harm Reduction, "additional comment to the Australian Select Committee on Tobacco Harm Reduction". https://tinyurl.com/5au7st65

References

Bryant, J., B. Bonevski and C. Paul (2011). A survey of smoking prevalence and interest in quitting among social and community service organisation clients in Australia: a unique opportunity for reaching the disadvantaged. *BMC Public Health* 11: 827 DOI: 10.1186/1471-2458-11-827

Buchanan, T., C.A. Magee, E.O. Igwe and P.J. Kelly (2021). Is the Australian smoking population hardening? *Addict Behav* 112: 106575 DOI: 10.1016/j.addbeh.2020.106575

Business Queensland (2019). Advertising alcohol prices and deals outside of licensed venues. https://tinyurl.com/ykvd954m

Butt, Y.M., M. Smith and H. Tazelaar et al. (2019). Pathology of vaping-associated lung injury. *N Engl J Med* 381(18): 1780–81 DOI: 10.1056/NEJMc1913069

Byrne, P. and B. Long (1976). *Doctors talking to patients: a study of the verbal behaviour of general practitioners consulting in their surgeries*. London: HMSO.

Byrne, S., E. Brindal and G. Williams et al. (2018). E-cigarettes, smoking and health: a literature review update. Canberra: CSIRO. https://tinyurl.com/4axrzrzh

Cahill, K. and T. Lancaster (2014). Workplace interventions for smoking cessation. *Cochrane Database Syst Rev*(2): CD003440 DOI: 10.1002/14651858.CD003440.pub4

Cahya, G.H. (2018). Big tobacco spurns ad bans. *Jakarta Post*, 24 November. https://bit.ly/3GkON7a

Cairns, R., A.L. Schaffer, J.A. Brown, S.A. Pearson and N.A. Buckley (2020). Codeine use and harms in Australia: evaluating the effects of re-scheduling. *Addiction* 115(3): 451–59 DOI: 10.1111/add.14798.

Calabria, B., L. Degenhardt and C. Briegleb et al. (2010). Systematic review of prospective studies investigating "remission" from amphetamine, cannabis, cocaine or opioid dependence. *Addict Behav* 35(8): 741–49 DOI: 10.1016/j.addbeh.2010.03.019.

Campaign for Tobacco Free Kids (2014). Nine e-juice flavors that sound just like kids' favorite treats. *Tobacco Unfiltered*. https://www.tobaccofreekids.org/blog/2014_06_11_ecigarettes

Canadian Cancer Society (2021). *Cigarette Package Health Warnings: International Status Report*, October, 7th edn. https://tinyurl.com/469eabvj.

Cancer Council Victoria (2020). Our history: the 1970s. https://www.cancervic.org.au/about/our-history/history-1970s

Cancer Institute NSW (2009). *New South Wales Smoking and Health Survey 2009*. Sydney: CINSW. https://tinyurl.com/ycyp485h

Cancer Institute NSW (2011). *New South Wales Smoking and Health Survey 2011*. Sydney: CINSW.

Carter, O.B., B.W. Mills and R.J. Donovan (2009). The effect of retail cigarette pack displays on unplanned purchases: results from immediate postpurchase interviews. *Tob Control* 18(3): 218–21 DOI: 10.1136/tc.2008.027870

Carter, O.B., T. Phan and B.W. Mills (2015). Impact of a point-of-sale tobacco display ban on smokers' spontaneous purchases: comparisons from postpurchase interviews before and after the ban in Western Australia. *Tob Control* 24(e1): e81–86 DOI: 10.1136/tobaccocontrol-2013-050991

Carter, S.M., A. Cribb and J.P. Allegrante (2012). How to think about health promotion ethics. *Pub Health Rev* 3(1): 1–24. https://publichealthreviews.biomedcentral.com/track/pdf/10.1007/BF03391661.pdf

Caruana, D. (2020). Burning issues: the global state of tobacco harm reduction (GSTHR) 2020. *Vaping Post*, 5 November. https://tinyurl.com/vxf87h9j

CEIC Data (2022). Indonesia Monthly Earnings. https://www.ceicdata.com/en/indicator/indonesia/monthly-earnings

Centers for Disease Control and Prevention (2021). Current cigarette smoking among US adults aged 18 years and older. https://tinyurl.com/3u3jkcm4

Chaiton, M., L. Diemert and J.E. Cohen et al. (2016). Estimating the number of quit attempts it takes to quit smoking successfully in a longitudinal cohort of smokers. *BMJ Open* 6(6): e011045 DOI: 10.1136/bmjopen-2016-011045

Chaiton, M.O., J. Cohen, P. McDonald and S. Bondy (2007). The Heaviness of Smoking Index as a predictor of smoking cessation in Canada. *Addict Behav* 32(5): 1031–42 DOI: 10.1016/j.addbeh.2006.07.008

Chaloupka, F.J., A. Yurekli and G.T. Fong (2012). Tobacco taxes as a tobacco control strategy. *Tob Control* 21(2): 172–80 DOI: 10.1136/tobaccocontrol-2011-050417

Champion, D. and S. Chapman (2005). Framing pub smoking bans: an analysis of Australian print news media coverage, March 1996 – March 2003. *J Epidemiol Community Health* 59(8): 679–84 DOI: 10.1136/jech.2005.035915

Chan, B.S., A. Kiss, N. McIntosh, V. Sheppeard and A.H. Dawson (2021). E-cigarette or vaping product use-associated lung injury in an adolescent. *Med J Aust* 215(7): 313–14 e1 DOI: 10.5694/mja2.51244

Chapman, S. (1980). A David and Goliath story: tobacco advertising and self-regulation in Australia. *BMJ* 281(6249): 1187–90 DOI: 10.1136/bmj.281.6249.1187

Chapman, S. (1985). Stop smoking clinics: a case for their abandonment. *Lancet* 1(8434): 918–20 DOI: 10.1016/s0140-6736(85)91685-x

Chapman, S. (1986). *The natural history of smoking cessation: how and why people stop smoking*. London: National Health and Medical Research Council,

References

Australia and The Health Education Council, London. https://tinyurl.com/2p9yus42

Chapman, S. (1988). For debate: the means/ends problem in health promotion. *Med J Aust* 149(5): 256–60 DOI: 10.5694/j.1326-5377.1988.tb120598.x

Chapman, S. (1989). The news on smoking: newspaper coverage of smoking and health in Australia, 1987–88. *Am J Public Health* 79(10): 1419–21 DOI: 10.2105/ajph.79.10.1419

Chapman, S. (1992). Shared accommodation: non-smokers wanted. *Tob Control* 1: 248.

Chapman, S. (1993). Unravelling gossamer with boxing gloves: problems in explaining the decline in smoking. *BMJ* 307(6901): 429–32 DOI: 10.1136/bmj.307.6901.429

Chapman, S. (1999). The news on tobacco control: time to bring the background into the foreground. *Tob Control* 8(3): 237–39 DOI: 10.1136/tc.8.3.237

Chapman, S. (2000). Banning smoking outdoors is seldom ethically justifiable. *Tob Control* 9(1): 95–97 DOI: 10.1136/tc.9.1.95

Chapman, S. (2003a). "It is possible he is a kind of nut": how the tobacco industry quietly promoted Dr William Whitby. *Tob Control* 12 Suppl 3: iii 4–6 DOI: 10.1136/tc.12.suppl_3.iii4

Chapman, S. (2003b). "We are anxious to remain anonymous": the use of third party scientific and medical consultants by the Australian tobacco industry, 1969 to 1979. *Tob Control* 12 Suppl 3: iii 31–7 DOI: 10.1136/tc.12.suppl_3.iii31

Chapman S. (2007). *Public health advocacy and tobacco control: making smoking history*. Oxford: Blackwell.

Chapman, S. (2008a). Going too far? Exploring the limits of smoking regulations. *William Mitchell Law Rev* 34(4): 1605–29. https://tinyurl.com/23mhvfk2

Chapman, S. (2008b). Questionable inflated estimate of smoking prevalence among mentally ill persons in Australia. *Aust N Z J Psychiatry* 42(7): 646–48 DOI: 10.1080/00048670802653372

Chapman, S. (2009). The inverse impact law of smoking cessation. *Lancet* 373(9665): 701–03 DOI: 10.1016/S0140-6736(09)60416-5

Chapman, S. (2012). The case for a smoker's license. *PLOS Med* 9(11): e1001342 DOI: 10.1371/journal.pmed.1001342

Chapman, S. (2013). *Over our dead bodies: Port Arthur and the fight for gun law reform*. Sydney: Sydney University Press.

Chapman, S. (2015). The future of electronic cigarette growth depends on youth uptake. *Med J Aust* 202(9): 467–68 DOI: 10.5694/mja15.00304

Chapman, S. (2016). The failed history of tobacco harm reduction. *Conversation*, 30 August. https://theconversation.com/the-failed-history-of-tobacco-harm-reduction-64561

Chapman, S. (2018). Is it unethical to use fear in public health campaigns? *Am J Public Health* 108(9): 1120–22 DOI: 10.2105/AJPH.2018.304630

Chapman, S. (2019). As "safe as drinking coffee"? Research spoiling the e-cigarette rehabilitation of nicotine party. *Simon Chapman AO*, 21 March. https://tinyurl.com/yck8uuww

Chapman S. (2020). Want to work for a pariah industry? Big tobacco fears it is unable to attract top staff. *Simon Chapman AO*, 15 February. https://tinyurl.com/2p8nre37

Chapman, S. (2020a). Evidence to Senate Committee on Tobacco Harm Reduction, 19 November. *Senate Committee on Harm Reduction.* https://tinyurl.com/3h7he9r2

Chapman, S. (2020b). Quit smoking ads from Australia and England, early 1980s. *YouTube.* https://www.youtube.com/watch?v=8wwrTtHRf-Y&t=76s

Chapman, S. (2021). Vaping advocates say the darndest things: (3) Australia's prescribed vaping model "privileges big tobacco". *Simon Chapman AO*, 15 February. https://tinyurl.com/3bk86hhp

Chapman, S., D. Bareham and W. Maziak (2019). The gateway effect of e-cigarettes: reflections on main criticisms. *Nicotine Tob Res* 21(5): 695–98 DOI: 10.1093/ntr/nty067

Chapman, S. and S.M. Carter (2003). "Avoid health warnings on all tobacco products for just as long as we can": a history of Australian tobacco industry efforts to avoid, delay and dilute health warnings on cigarettes. *Tob Control* 12 Suppl 3: iii13–22 DOI: 10.1136/tc.12.suppl_3.iii13

Chapman, S., M. Daube and M. Peters (2020). Public Submission 195 to the Senate Select Committee on Tobacco Harm Reduction. https://tinyurl.com/5au7st65

Chapman, S. and M.C. Farrelly (2011). Four arguments against the adult-rating of movies with smoking scenes. *PLOS Med* 8(8): e1001078 DOI: 10.1371/journal.pmed.1001078

Chapman, S. and B. Freeman (2008). Markers of the denormalisation of smoking and the tobacco industry. *Tob Control* 17(1): 25–31 DOI: 10.1136/tc.2007.021386

Chapman, S. and B. Freeman (2009). Regulating the tobacco retail environment: beyond reducing sales to minors. *Tob Control* 18(6): 496–501 DOI: 10.1136/tc.2009.031724

Chapman, S. and B. Freeman (2014). *Removing the emperor's clothes: Australia and tobacco plain packaging.* Sydney: Sydney University Press

References

Chapman, S., S. Haddad and D. Sindhusake (1997). Do work-place smoking bans cause smokers to smoke "harder"? Results from a naturalistic observational study. *Addiction* 92(5): 607–10 DOI: 10.1111/j.1360-0443.1997.tb02918.x

Chapman, S., A. Haynes and G. Derrick et al. (2014). Reaching "an audience that you would never dream of speaking to": influential public health researchers' views on the role of news media in influencing policy and public understanding. *J Health Commun* 19(2): 260–73 DOI: 10.1080/10810730.2013.811327

Chapman, S., S. Holding and J. Ellerm et al. (2009). The content and structure of Australian television reportage on health and medicine, 2005–2009: parameters to guide health workers. *Med J Aust* 191(11–12): 620–24 DOI: 10.5694/j.1326-5377.2009.tb03354.x

Chapman S. and J.A. Leask (2001). Paid celebrity endorsement in health promotion: a case study from Australia. *Health Promot Int* 16(4): 333–38 DOI 10.1093/heapro/16.4.333

Chapman, S. and R. MacKenzie (2010). The global research neglect of unassisted smoking cessation: causes and consequences. *PLOS Medicine* 7(2): e1000216 DOI: 10.1371/journal.pmed.1000216

Chapman, S. and R. MacKenzie (2012). Can it be ethical to apply limited resources in low-income countries to ineffective, low-reach smoking cessation strategies? A reply to Bitton and Eyal. *Public Health Ethics* 5(1): 29–37 DOI: 10.1093/phe/phr035

Chapman, S. and R. MacKenzie (2013). There's nothing that succeeds like failure: discerning the woods from the trees in smoking cessation debates. *Nicotine Tob Res* 15(3): 750–51 DOI: 10.1093/ntr/nts237

Chapman, S. and W. Smith (1994). Deception among quit smoking lottery entrants. *Am J Health Promot* 8(5): 328–30 DOI: 10.4278/0890-1171-8.5.328

Chapman, S., W. Smith, G. Mowbray, C. Hugo and G. Egger (1993). Quit and win smoking cessation contests: how should effectiveness be evaluated? *Prev Med* 22(3): 423–32 DOI: 10.1006/pmed.1993.1035

Chapman, S. and M.A. Wakefield (2013). Large-scale unassisted smoking cessation over 50 years: lessons from history for endgame planning in tobacco control. *Tob Control* 22(Suppl 1): i33–i35 DOI: 10.1136/tobaccocontrol-2012-050767

Chapman, S., M. Wakefield and S. Durkin (2004). Smoking status of 132,176 people advertising on a dating website: are smokers more "desperate and dateless"? *Med J Aust* 181(11–12): 672–74 DOI: 10.5694/j.1326-5377.2004.tb06519.x

Chapman, S., W.L. Wong and W. Smith (1993). Self-exempting beliefs about smoking and health: differences between smokers and ex-smokers. *Am J Public Health* 83(2): 215–19 DOI: 10.2105/ajph.83.2.215

Charmaz, K. (1990). 'Discovering' chronic illness: using grounded theory. *Soc Sci Med* 30: 1161–72 DOI: 10.1016/0277-9536(90)90256-r

Charmaz, K. (2006). *Constructing grounded theory: a practical guide through qualitative analysis.* London: SAGE Publications Ltd.

Chen, K. and D.B. Kandel (1998). Predictors of cessation of marijuana use: an event history analysis. *Drug Alcohol Depend* 50(2): 109–21 DOI: 10.1016/s0376-8716(98)00021-0

Chen, R., J.P. Pierce and E.C. Leas et al. (2020). Use of electronic cigarettes to aid long-term smoking cessation in the United States: prospective evidence from the PATH cohort study. *Am J Epidemiol* 189(12): 1529–37 DOI: 10.1093/aje/kwaa161

Chiang, P.P. and S. Chapman (2006). Do pharmacy staff recommend evidenced-based smoking cessation products? A pseudo patron study. *J Clin Pharm Ther* 31(3): 205–09 DOI: 10.1111/j.1365-2710.2006.00649.x

CHOICE magazine (1961). Australian-made cigarettes: a preliminary report. *Choice: The Journal of the Australian Consumers' Association Ltd* 11(2): 36–43.

Christensen, C.H., J. Chang and B. Rostron (2021). Biomarkers of inflammation and oxidative stress among adult former smoker, current e-cigarette users-results from Wave 1 PATH study. *Cancer Epidemiol Biomarkers Prev* DOI: 10.1158/1055-9965.EPI-21-0140

Christofides, N., S. Chapman and A. Dominello (1999). The new pariahs: discourse on the tobacco industry in the Sydney press, 1993–97. *Aust N Z J Public Health* 23(3): 233–39 DOI: 10.1111/j.1467-842x.1999.tb01248.x

Chun, L.F., F. Moazed, C. Calfee, M. Matthay and J. Gotts (2017). Pulmonary toxicity of e-cigarettes. *Am J Physiol Lung Cell Mol Physiol* 313(2): L193–L206 DOI: 10.1152/ajplung.00071.2017

Cision (2021). Health Canada announces new restrictions to prevent youth vaping. Health Canada News Release, 18 June. https://tinyurl.com/3sjd2t4m

Clegg Smith, K.M., M. Wakefield and M. Nichter (2003). Press coverage of public expenditure of Master Settlement Agreement funds: how are non-tobacco control related expenditures represented? *Tob Control* 12(3): 257–63 DOI: 10.1136/tc.12.3.257

ClinCalc (2021). The top 300 of 2021. https://clincalc.com/DrugStats/Top300Drugs.aspx

Cochrane Collaboration (2020). Cochrane tobacco addiction. https://tobacco.cochrane.org/our-reviews

References

Cochrane Community (2020). Cochrane's revised conflict of interest policy for Cochrane library content will take effect in October 2020. https://tinyurl.com/36us5fsk

Cohen, G., J. Schroeder and R. Newson et al. (2015). Does health intervention research have real world policy and practice impacts: testing a new impact assessment tool. *Health Res Policy Syst* 13: 3 DOI: 10.1186/1478-4505-13-3

Cohen, S., E. Lichtenstein and J. Prochaska et al. (1989). Debunking myths about self-quitting: evidence from 10 prospective studies of persons who attempt to quit smoking by themselves. *Am Psychol* 44(11): 1355–65. DOI: 10.1037//0003-066x.44.11.1355

Coleman, B., B. Rostron and S.E. Johnson et al. (2019). Transitions in electronic cigarette use among adults in the Population Assessment of Tobacco and Health (PATH) study, Waves 1 and 2 (2013–2015). *Tob Control* 28(1): 50–59 DOI: 10.1136/tobaccocontrol-2017-054174

Colgrove, J., R. Bayer and K.E. Bachynski (2011). Nowhere left to hide? The banishment of smoking from public spaces. *N Engl J Med* 364(25): 2375–77 DOI: 10.1056/NEJMp1104637

Commonwealth of Australia (2021) Mid-year economic and fiscal outlook 2021–22. 11 January. https://budget.gov.au/2021-22/content/myefo/download/myefo-2021-22.pdf

Conrad, P. (1992). Medicalization and social control. *Ann Rev Sociology* 18: 228–39 https://www.jstor.org/stable/2083452

Cook-Shimanek, M., E.K. Burns and A.H. Levinson (2013). Medicinal nicotine nonuse: smokers' rationales for past behavior and intentions to try medicinal nicotine in a future quit attempt. *Nicotine Tob Res* 15(11): 1926–33 DOI: 10.1093/ntr/ntt085

Cooper, J., R. Borland and H.-H. Yong (2011). Australian smokers increasingly use help to quit, but number of attempts remains stable: findings from the International Tobacco Control study 2002–09. *Aust N Z J Public Health* 35(4): 368–76 DOI: 0.1111/j.1753-6405.2011.00733.x

Cooper, J., R. Borland and H.-H. Yong et al. (2010). To what extent do smokers make spontaneous quit attempts and what are the implications for smoking cessation maintenance? Findings from the International Tobacco Control four country survey. *Nicotine Tob Res* 12: S51–S57 DOI: 10.1093/Ntr/Ntq052

Crawford, R. (1977). You are dangerous to your health: the ideology and politics of victim blaming. *Int J Health Serv* 7(4): 663–80 DOI: 10.2190/YU77-T7B1-EN9X-G0PN

Crystal (2020). Reviews. *Lazer Iz.* https://lazer-iz.com/reviews/

Cummings, K.M. and A. Hyland (2005). Impact of nicotine replacement therapy on smoking behavior. *Annu Rev Public Health* 26: 583–99 DOI: 10.1146/annurev.publhealth.26.021304.144501

Cummins, S.E., L. Bailey, S. Campbell, C. Koon-Kirby and S. H. Zhu (2007). Tobacco cessation quitlines in north America: a descriptive study. *Tob Control* 16(Suppl 1): i9–i15 DOI: 10.1136/tc.2007.020370

Currie, L., S. Keogan, P. Campbell, M. Gunning, Z. Kabir and L. Clancy (2010). An evaluation of the range and availability of intensive smoking-cessation services in Ireland. *Ir J Med Sci* 179(2): 225–31 DOI: 10.1007/s11845-009-0356-y

Curry, S.J., A. Sporer, O. Pugach, R. Campbell and S. Emery (2007). Use of tobacco cessation treatments among young adult smokers: 2005 National Health Interview survey. *Am J Public Health* 97(8): 1464–69 DOI: 10.2105/AJPH.2006.103788

Cussen, A. and J. McCool (2011). Tobacco promotion in the Pacific: the current state of tobacco promotion bans and options for accelerating progress. *Asia Pac J Public Health* 23(1): 70–78 DOI: 10.1177/1010539510390925

Dai, H. and A.M. Leventhal (2019). Association of electronic cigarette vaping and subsequent smoking relapse among former smokers. *Drug Alcohol Depend* 199: 10–17 DOI: 10.1016/j.drugalcdep.2019.01.043

Daily Sabah (2021). Turkey's Sabancı to hand down Philip Morris shares to parent company. 7 October. https://tinyurl.com/4bjcr4c7

Danaher, B.G. (1977). Rapid smoking and self-control in the modification of smoking behavior. *J Consult Clin Psychol* 45(6): 1068–75 DOI: 10.1037//0022-006x.45.6.1068

Darzi, A., O. P. Keown and S. Chapman (2015). Is a smoking ban in UK parks and outdoor spaces a good idea? *BMJ* 350: h958 DOI: 10.1136/bmj.h958

De Angelis, C., J. M. Drazen and F. A. Frizelle et al. (2004). Clinical trial registration: a statement from the International Committee of Medical Journal Editors. *Ann Intern Med* 141(6): 477–78 DOI: 10.7326/0003-4819-141-6-200409210-00109

De Leon, J. and F.J. Diaz (2005). A meta-analysis of worldwide studies demonstrates an association between schizophrenia and tobacco smoking behaviors. *Schizophr Res* 76(2–3): 136–57 DOI: 10.1016/j.schres.2005.02.010

Deci, E.L. and R.M. Ryan (2010). *Self-determination*. Hoboken, NJ: John Wiley & Sons Inc.

Department of the Treasury (2010). Issues in tobacco taxation. https://tinyurl.com/3shxr28a

Deyo, R. A. and D.L. Patrick (2005). *Hope or hype: the obsession with medical advances and the high cost of false promises*. New York: AMACOM.

References

Dickinson, J.A., J. Wiggers, S.R. Leeder and R.W. Sanson-Fisher (1989). General practitioners' detection of patients' smoking status. *Med J Aust* 150(8): 420–22, 425–26 DOI: 10.5694/j.1326-5377.1989.tb136560.x

DiClemente, C.C., J.C. Delahanty and R.M. Fiedler (2010). The journey to the end of smoking: a personal and population perspective. *Am J Prev Med* 38(3, Supplement): S418–S28 DOI: 10.1016/j.amepre.2009.12.010

Dixon-Woods, M., S. Agarwal, B. Young, D. Jones and A. Sutton (2004). Integrative approaches to qualitative and quantitative evidence. London: Health Development Agency. https://tinyurl.com/ys27bze7

Doll, R. and A.B. Hill (1950). Smoking and carcinoma of the lung: preliminary report. *BMJ* 2(4682): 739–48 DOI: 10.1136/bmj.2.4682.739

Doll, R., R. Peto, J. Boreham and I. Sutherland (2005). Mortality from cancer in relation to smoking: 50 years observations on British doctors. *Br J Cancer* 92(3): 426–29 DOI: 10.1038/sj.bjc.6602359

Donovan, S. (2017). Philip Morris ordered to pay Australia's costs in plain packaging case. The World Today, *ABC News*, 10 July. https://tinyurl.com/adyj38ej

Doran, C.M., L. Valenti, M. Robinson, H. Britt and R. Mattick (2006). Smoking status of Australian general practice patients and their attempts to quit. *Addict Behav* 31(5): 758–66 DOI: 10.1016/j.addbeh.2005.05.054

Doron, G. (1979). *The smoking paradox: public relations and the tobacco industry*. Cambridge, MA: Abt Books.

Dunlop, S., T. Cotter, D. Perez and M. Wakefield (2013). Televised antismoking advertising: effects of level and duration of exposure. *Am J Public Health* 103(8): e66–73 DOI: 10.2105/AJPH.2012.301079

Dunn, A.G., E. Coiera, K.D. Mandl and F.T. Bourgeois (2016). Conflict of interest disclosure in biomedical research: a review of current practices, biases, and the role of public registries in improving transparency. *Res Integr Peer Rev* (1) DOI: 10.1186/s41073-016-0006-7

Durante, N. (2016). Preliminary results 2016. London: BAT https://www.bat.com/latestresults#

Durante, N. (2018). Analyst briefing. London: BAT https://tinyurl.com/2p94y7u3

Dutra, L.M. and S.A. Glantz (2017). E-cigarettes and national adolescent cigarette use: 2004–2014. *Pediatrics* 139(2) DOI: 10.1542/peds.2016-2450

Dwan, K., C. Gamble, P.R. Williamson, J.J. Kirkham and Reporting Bias Group (2013). Systematic review of the empirical evidence of study publication bias and outcome reporting bias: an updated review. *PLOS One* 8(7): e66844 DOI: 10.1371/journal.pone.0066844

Dyer, C. (2018). Boss who made £7.9m from selling fake cancer cure is jailed for 15 months. *BMJ* 363: k5042 DOI: 10.1136/bmj.k5042

Editors of Eur Respir J (2021). Retraction notice for: "Characteristics and risk factors for COVID-19 diagnosis and adverse outcomes in Mexico: an analysis of 89,756 laboratory-confirmed COVID-19 cases". T.V. Giannouchos, R.A. Sussman, J.M. Mier, K. Poulas and K. Farsalinos. *Eur Respir J* 57:2002144, https://erj.ersjournals.com/content/erj/57/3/2002144.full.pdf

Edwards, R., J. Ball, J. Hoek, N. Wilson and A. Waa (2021). Key findings on smoking and e-cigarette use prevalence and trends in the 2020/21 NZ Health Survey. *Public Health Expert.* https://tinyurl.com/2xndwwze

Edwards, R., N. Wilson, J. Peace, D. Weerasekera, G.W. Thomson and H. Gifford (2013). Support for a tobacco endgame and increased regulation of the tobacco industry among New Zealand smokers: results from a National Survey. *Tob Control* 22(e1): e86–93 DOI: 10.1136/tobaccocontrol-2011-050324

Edwards, S.A., S.J. Bondy, R.C. Callaghan and R.E. Mann (2014). Prevalence of unassisted quit attempts in population-based studies: a systematic review of the literature. *Addict Behav* 39(3): 512–19 DOI: 10.1016/j.addbeh.2013.10.036

Egger, G., W. Fitzgerald and G. Frape et al (1983). Results of large scale media antismoking campaign in Australia: North Coast "Quit. For Life" programme. *Br Med J (Clin Res Ed)* 287(6399): 1125–28 DOI: 10.1136/bmj.287.6399.1125

Egger, M. and G.D. Smith (1998). Bias in location and selection of studies. *BMJ* 316(7124): 61–66 DOI: 10.1136/bmj.316.7124.61

Egger, S., S. Burton, R. Ireland and S.C. Walsberger (2019). Observed retail price of Australia's market-leading cigarette brand before and up to 3 years after the implementation of plain packaging. *Tob Control* 28(e2): e86–e91 DOI: 10.1136/tobaccocontrol-2018-054577

Eisenger, R. (1972). Psychosocial predictors of smoking behavior change. *Soc Sci Med* 6: 137–44. DOI: 10.1016/0037-7856(72)90013-3

Eissenberg, T., A. Bhatnagar and S. Chapman et al (2020). Invalidity of an oft-cited estimate of the relative harms of electronic cigarettes. *Am J Public Health* 110(2): 161–62 DOI: 10.2105/AJPH.2019.305424

El Dib, R., E.A. Suzumura and E.A. Akl et al (2017). Electronic nicotine delivery systems and/or electronic non-nicotine delivery systems for tobacco smoking cessation or reduction: a systematic review and meta-analysis. *BMJ Open* 7(2): e012680 DOI: 10.1136/bmjopen-2016-012680

Etter, J-F., M.M. Bergman and T.V. Perneger (2000). On quitting smoking: development of two scales measuring the use of self-change strategies in current and former smokers (SCS-CS and SCS-FS). *Addict Behav* 25(4): 523–38 DOI: 10.1016/s0306-4603(00)00068-x

Etter, J-F. M. Burri and J. Stapleton (2007). The impact of pharmaceutical company funding on results of randomized trials of nicotine replacement therapy for

References

smoking cessation: a meta-analysis. *Addiction* 102(5): 815–22 DOI: 10.1111/j.1360-0443.2007.01822.x

Etter, J.-F. and T.V. Perneger (2001). Attitudes toward nicotine replacement therapy in smokers and ex-smokers in the general public. *Clin Pharmacol Ther* 69(3): 175-83 DOI: 10.1067/mcp.2001.113722

Etter, J.-F. and J.A. Stapleton (2006). Nicotine replacement therapy for long-term smoking cessation: a meta-analysis. *Tob Control* 15(4) DOI 10.1136/Tc.2005.015487

EurekAlert! (2020). Chemicals in e-cigarettes mix together to form new, unexpectedly toxic compounds. News Releases, 2 September. https://www.eurekalert.org/news-releases/842083

European Public Health Association (2018). Facts and fiction on e-cigs. https://eupha.org/repository/advocacy/EUPHA_facts_and_fiction_on_e-cigs.pdf

Ewen, S. (1976). *Captains of consciousness: advertising and the social roots of consumer culture*. New York: McGraw-Hill.

Fagerström, K. and H. Furberg (2008). A comparison of the Fagerström test for nicotine dependence and smoking prevalence across countries. *Addiction* 103(5): 841–45 DOI: 10.1111/j.1360-0443.2008.02190.x

Fairchild, A., R. Bayer and S. Green (2018). The two faces of fear: a history of hard-hitting public health campaigns against tobacco and aids. *Am J Public Health* 108(9): 1180–86 DOI: 10.2105/AJPH.2018.304516

Farsalinos, K.E., K. Poulas, V. Voudris and J. Le Houezec (2016). Electronic cigarette use in the European Union: analysis of a representative sample of 27,460 Europeans from 28 countries. *Addiction* 111(11): 2032–40 DOI: 10.1111/add.13506

Farsalinos, K.E., G. Romagna, D. Tsiapras, S. Kyrzopoulos and V. Voudris (2014). Characteristics, perceived side effects and benefits of electronic cigarette use: a worldwide survey of more than 19,000 consumers. *Int J Environ Res Public Health* 11(4): 4356–73 DOI: 10.3390/ijerph110404356

Feliu, A., F.T. Filippidis and L. Joossens et al (2019). Impact of tobacco control policies on smoking prevalence and quit ratios in 27 European Union countries from 2006 to 2014. *Tob Control* 28(1): 101–09 DOI: 10.1136/tobaccocontrol-2017-054119

Ferguson, J., L. Bauld, J. Chesterman and K. Judge (2005). The English smoking treatment services: one-year outcomes. *Addiction* 100 Suppl 2: 59–69 DOI: 10.1111/j.1360-0443.2005.01028.x

Ferguson, J., G. Docherty and L. Bauld et al (2012). Effect of offering different levels of support and free nicotine replacement therapy via an English national telephone quitline: randomised controlled trial. *BMJ* 344: e1696 DOI: 10.1136/bmj.e1696

Ferguson, S.G., S. Shiffman, J.G. Gitchell, M.A. Sembower and R. West (2009). Unplanned quit attempts: results from a US sample of smokers and ex-smokers. *Nicotine Tob Res* 11(7): 827–32 DOI: 10.1093/ntr/ntp072

Fernandez, E., A. Lugo and L. Clancy et al (2015). Smoking dependence in 18 European countries: hard to maintain the hardening hypothesis. *Prev Med* 81: 314–19 DOI: 10.1016/j.ypmed.2015.09.023

Filippidis, F.T., A.A. Laverty, U. Mons, C. Jimenez-Ruiz and C.I. Vardavas (2019). Changes in smoking cessation assistance in the European Union between 2012 and 2017: pharmacotherapy versus counselling versus e-cigarettes. *Tob Control* 28(1): 95–100 DOI: 10.1136/tobaccocontrol-2017-054117

Fiore, M.C., T. Novotny and J. Pierce et al (1990). Methods used to quit smoking in the United States: do cessation programs help? *JAMA* 263(20): 2760–65 DOI: 10.1001/jama.1990.03440200064024

Flavor and Extracts Manufacturing Association (FEMA) (2021). The safety, assessment and regulatory authority to use flavors: focus on e-cigarettes. https://www.femaflavor.org/node/24344

Fong, G.T., D. Hammond and F. Laux et al (2004). The near-universal experience of regret among smokers in four countries: findings from the International Tobacco Control Policy Evaluation Survey. *Nicotine Tob Res* 6 Suppl 3: S341–51 DOI: 10.1080/14622200412331320743

Fortune Business Insights (2021). Nicotine replacement therapy (NRT) market size, share and COVID-19 impact analysis, by type (gums, patches, lozenges, inhalers, and others), by distribution channel (hospital pharmacy, retail pharmacy, and online pharmacy) and regional forecast, 2021–2028. Report ID FBI103362. https://tinyurl.com/2p88autw

Francey, N. and S. Chapman (2000). "Operation Berkshire": the international tobacco companies' conspiracy. *BMJ* 321(7257): 371–74 DOI: 10.1136/bmj.321.7257.371

Freeman, B., S. Chapman and P. Storey (2008) Banning smoking in cars carrying children: an analytical history of a public health advocacy campaign. *Aust N Z J Public Health* 32(1): 60–65 DOI: 10.1111/j.1753-6405.2008.00167.x

Freeman, B., E.M. Greenhalgh and M. Winstanley (2020). 10.17 Public attitudes to the tobacco industry. *Tobacco in Australia: facts and issues.* https://tinyurl.com/28d7zkz9

Fu, S.S., D. Burgess and M. van Ryn et al (2007). Views on smoking cessation methods in ethnic minority communities: a qualitative investigation. *Prev Med* 44(3): 235–40 DOI: 10.1016/j.ypmed.2006.11.002

References

Gallagher, A.W.A., K.A. Evans-Reeves, J.L. Hatchard and A.B. Gilmore (2019). Tobacco industry data on illicit tobacco trade: a systematic review of existing assessments. *Tob Control* 28(3): 334–45 DOI: 10.1136/tobaccocontrol-2018-054295

Gartner, C.E., A. Wright, M. Hefler, A. Perusco and J. Hoek (2021). It is time for governments to support retailers in the transition to a smoke-free society. *Med J Aust* 215(10): 446–48 DOI: 10.5694/mja2.51312

Global Burden of Disease 2019 Tobacco Collaborators (2021). Spatial, temporal, and demographic patterns in prevalence of smoking tobacco use and attributable disease burden in 204 countries and territories, 1990–2019: a systematic analysis from the Global Burden of Disease study 2019. *Lancet* 397(10292): 2337–60 DOI: 10.1016/S0140-6736(21)01169-7

Gendall, P. and J. Hoek (2021). Role of flavours in vaping uptake and cessation among New Zealand smokers and non-smokers: a cross-sectional study. *Tob Control* 30(1): 108–10 DOI: 10.1136/tobaccocontrol-2019-055469

Ghosh, A., R.C. Coakley and T. Mascenik et al. (2018). Chronic e-cigarette exposure alters the human bronchial epithelial proteome. *Am J Respir Crit Care Med* 198(1): 67–76 DOI: 10.1164/rccm.201710-2033OC

Gillum, R.F., S. Santibanez, G. Bennett and M. Donahue (2009). Associations of prayer, mind-body therapy, and smoking cessation in a national survey. *Psychol Rep* 105(2): 593–604 DOI: 10.2466/PR0.105.2.593-604

Gilmore, A.B., G. Fooks, J. Drope, S.A. Bialous and R.R. Jackson (2015). Exposing and addressing tobacco industry conduct in low-income and middle-income countries. *Lancet* 385(9972): 1029–43 DOI: 10.1016/S0140-6736(15)60312-9

Gilmore, A.B., A.W.A. Gallagher and A. Rowell (2019). Tobacco industry's elaborate attempts to control a global track and trace system and fundamentally undermine the illicit trade protocol. *Tob Control* 28(2): 127–40 DOI: 10.1136/tobaccocontrol-2017-054191

Gilpin, E. and J.P. Pierce (1994). Measuring smoking cessation: problems with recall in the 1990 California Tobacco Survey. *Cancer Epidemiol Biomarkers Prev* 3(7): 613–17 https://cebp.aacrjournals.org/content/3/7/613.long

Glasser, A.M., M. Vojjala and J. Cantrell et al. (2021). Patterns of e-cigarette use and subsequent cigarette smoking cessation over 2 years (2013/2014–2015/2016) in the Population Assessment of Tobacco and Health study. *Nicotine Tob Res* 23(4): 669–77 DOI: 10.1093/ntr/ntaa182

GlaxoSmithKline (2009). Path2Quit. https://tinyurl.com/2d7b8bv3

Gmel, G., M. Wicki, S. Marmet and J. Studler (2020). E-cigarette use for smoking reduction and cessation in a four-year follow-up study among young Swiss men: some may benefit, but they are few. https://www.researchsquare.com/article/rs-52878/v1

Godfrey, C., S. Parrott, T. Coleman and E. Pouniewicz (2005). The cost-effectiveness of the English smoking treatment services: evidence from practice. *Addiction* 100 Suppl 2: 70–83
DOI: 10.1111/j.1360-0443.2005.01071.x
Goffman, E. (1963). *Stigma: notes on the management of spoiled identity*. Englewood Cliffs, NJ: Prentice Hall.
Goldberg, J.O. and J. Van Exan (2008). Longitudinal rates of smoking in a schizophrenia sample. *Tob Control* 17(4): 271–75
DOI: 10.1136/tc.2008.024810
Goniewicz, M.L., D.M. Smith and K.C. Edwards et al. (2018). Comparison of nicotine and toxicant exposure in users of electronic cigarettes and combustible cigarettes. *JAMA Netw Open* 1(8): e185937
DOI: 10.1001/jamanetworkopen.2018.5937
Goodin, R.E. (1989). The ethics of smoking. *Ethics* 99(3): 574–624
https://www.jstor.org/stable/2380869
Goot, M. and K.S. Inglis (2014). Mayer, Henry (1919–1990). *Australian Dictionary of Biography*. http://adb.anu.edu.au/biography/mayer-henry-17251
Goriounova, N.A. and H.D. Mansvelder (2012). Short- and long-term consequences of nicotine exposure during adolescence for prefrontal cortex neuronal network function. *Cold Spring Harb Perspect Med* 2(12): a012120
DOI: 10.1101/cshperspect.a012120
Gornall, J. (2015). Public Health England's troubled trail. *BMJ* 351: h5826
DOI: 10.1136/bmj.h5826
Government of Canada (2021). Nicotine concentration in vaping products regulations: SOR/2021-123. https://gazette.gc.ca/rp-pr/p2/2021/2021-06-23/html/sor-dors123-eng.html
Grabovac, I., M. Oberndorfer, J. Fischer, W. Wiesinger, S. Haider and T.E. Dorner (2021). Effectiveness of electronic cigarettes in smoking cessation: a systematic review and meta-analysis. *Nicotine Tob Res* 23(4): 625–34
DOI: 10.1093/ntr/ntaa181
Graham, H. (1994). Gender and class as dimensions of smoking behaviour in Britain: insights from a survey of mothers. *Soc Sci Med* 38(5): 691–98
DOI: 10.1016/0277-9536(94)90459-6
Graham, H. (2009). Women and smoking: understanding socioeconomic influences. *Drug Alcohol Depend* 104 Suppl 1: S11–6
DOI: 10.1016/j.drugalcdep.2009.02.009
Graham, S. and R.W. Gibson (1971). Cessation of patterned behavior: withdrawal from smoking. *Soc Sci Med* 5: 319–37 DOI: 10.1016/0037-7856(71)90033-3
Grand View Research (2021). E cigarette and vape market size, share and trends analysis report by distribution channel (online, retail), by product

References

(disposable, rechargeable), by component, by region, and segment forecasts, 2021–2028. https://tinyurl.com/348se4nk

Gravely, S., K.M. Cummings and D. Hammond et al. (2021). Self-reported quit aids and assistance used by smokers at their most recent quit attempt: findings from the 2020 International Tobacco Control Four Country Smoking and Vaping Survey. *Nicotine Tob Res* DOI: 10.1093/ntr/ntab068

Gravely, S., G Meng, K.M. Cummings and A. Hyland et al. (2020). Changes in Smoking and Vaping over 18 Months among Smokers and Recent Ex-Smokers: Longitudinal Findings from the 2016 and 2018 ITC Four Country Smoking and Vaping Surveys. *International Journal of Environmental Research and Public Health* DOI: 10.3390/ijerph17197084

Gray, N.J. and D.J. Hill (1975). Patterns of tobacco smoking in Australia. *Med J Aust* 22: 819–22. https://pubmed.ncbi.nlm.nih.gov/1207580/

Greene, N.M., E.M. Taylor, S.H. Gage and M.R Munafò (2010). Industry funding and placebo quit rate in clinical trials of nicotine replacement therapy: a commentary on Etter et al. (2007). *Addiction* 105(12): 2217–18; author reply 19 DOI: 10.1111/j.1360-0443.2010.03155.x

Greenhalgh, E.M., E. Dean, S. Stillman and C. Ford (2021) 7.16 Pharmacoptherapies for smoking cessation. In Greenhalgh, E.M., M.M. Scollo and M.H. Winstanley (eds) *Tobacco in Australia: facts and issues*. Melbourne: Cancer Council Victoria. https://www.tobaccoinaustralia.org.au/chapter-7-cessation/7-16-pharmacotherapy

Greenhalgh, E.M. and M.M. Scollo (2019). 11A.9 Real-world research on the effects of plain packaging. In Greenhalgh, E.M., M.M. Scollo and M.H. Winstanley (eds) *Tobacco in Australia: facts and issues*. Melbourne: Cancer Council Victoria. https://tinyurl.com/3xuvrndr

Greenhalgh, E.M. and M.H. Winstanley (2019). 1.6 Prevalence of smoking: teenagers. In Greenhalgh, E.M., M.M. Scollo and M.H. Winstanley (eds) *Tobacco in Australia: facts and issues*. Melbourne: Cancer Council Victoria. https://tinyurl.com/4f8xmauf

Gross, B., L. Brose and A. Schumann et al. (2008). Reasons for not using smoking cessation aids. *BMC Public Health* 8(1): 129 DOI: 10.1186/1471-2458-8-129

Guindon, G.E., J. de Beyer and S. Galbraith (2003). Framework Convention on Tobacco Control: progress and implications for health and the environment. *Environ Health Perspect* 111(5): A262–63 DOI: 10.1289/ehp.111-a262

Hajek, P., A. Phillips-Waller and D. Przulj et al. (2019). A randomized trial of e-cigarettes versus nicotine-replacement therapy. *N Engl J Med* 380(7): 629–37 DOI: 10.1056/NEJMoa1808779

Halpern, M.T., R. Shikiar, A.M. Rentz and Z.M. Khan (2001). Impact of smoking status on workplace absenteeism and productivity. *Tob Control* 10(3):233–38 DOI: 10.1136/tc.10.3.233

Hansen, E.C. and M.R. Nelson (2011). How cardiac patients describe the role of their doctors in smoking cessation: a qualitative study. *Aust J Primary Health* 17(3): 268–73 DOI: 10.1071/PY10082

Hansen, J. (2021). Vaping: how tobacco companies are drawing in vapers as teen use soars. *Saturday Telegraph*, 14 June.

Harper, T. (2006). Why the tobacco industry fears point of sale display bans. *Tob Control* 15(3): 270–71 DOI: 10.1136/tc.2006.015875

Hart, C., L. Gruer and L. Bauld (2013). Does smoking reduction in midlife reduce mortality risk? Results of 2 long-term prospective cohort studies of men and women in Scotland. *Am J Epidemiol* 178(5): 770–79 DOI: 10.1093/aje/kwt038

Hart, J.T. (1971). The inverse care law. *Lancet* 1(7696): 405–12 DOI: 10.1016/s0140-6736(71)92410-x

Hartmann-Boyce, J., S.C. Chepkin, W. Ye, C. Bullen and T. Lancaster (2018). Nicotine replacement therapy versus control for smoking cessation. *Cochrane Database Syst Rev* 5: CD000146 DOI: 10.1002/14651858.CD000146.pub5

Hartmann-Boyce, J., J. Livingstone-Banks and J.M. Ordóñez-Mena et al. (2021). Behavioural interventions for smoking cessation: an overview and network meta-analysis. *Cochrane Database Syst Rev* 1: CD013229. https://www.ncbi.nlm.nih.gov/pubmed/33411338

Hartmann-Boyce, J., H. McRobbie and N. Lindson et al. (2021). Electronic cigarettes for smoking cessation. *Cochrane Database Syst Rev* Issue 4. DOI: 10.1002/14651858.CD010216.pub5

Hatsukami, D.K., L. Stead and P.C. Gupta (2008). Tobacco addiction. *Lancet* 371(9629): 2027–38 DOI: 10.1016/S0140-6736(08)60871-5

Hawkins, J., W. Hollingworth and R. Campbell (2010). Long-term smoking relapse: a study using the British Household Panel Survey. *Nicotine Tob Res* 12(12): 1228–35 DOI: 10.1093/Ntr/Ntq175

Hayman, M. (1996). Scenes from Papua New Guinea: tobacco advertising or no tobacco advertising? *Tob Control* 5: 229–30 DOI: 10.2307/20207207

Haynes, A.S., G.E. Derrick and S. Chapman et al. (2011). From "our world" to the "real world": exploring the views and behaviour of policy-influential Australian public health researchers. *Soc Sci Med* 72(7): 1047–55 DOI: 10.1016/j.socscimed.2011.02.004

Haynes, A.S., G.E. Derrick and S. Redman et al. (2012). Identifying trustworthy experts: how do policymakers find and assess public health researchers worth consulting or collaborating with? *PLOS One* 7(3): e32665 DOI: 10.1371/journal.pone.0032665

References

Haynes, A.S., J.A. Gillespie and G.E. Derrick et al. (2011). Galvanizers, guides, champions, and shields: the many ways that policymakers use public health researchers. *Milbank Q* 89(4): 564-98 DOI: 10.1111/j.1468-0009.2011.00643.x

Heenan, E.M. (2006). *Ellis, executor of the estate of Paul Steven Cotton (dec) v. the State of South Australia & ors* [2006] WASC 270.

Hemenway, D. (2009). *While we were sleeping: success stories in injury and violence prevention.* Berkeley, CA: University of California Press.

Hendlin, Y.H., M. Vora, J. Elias and P.M. Ling (2019). Financial conflicts of interest and stance on tobacco harm reduction: a systematic review. *Am J Public Health* 109(7): e1-e8 DOI: 10.2105/AJPH.2019.305106

Henningfield, J., J. Pankow and B. Garrett (2004). Ammonia and other chemical base tobacco additives and cigarette nicotine delivery: issues and research needs. *Nicotine Tob Res* 6(2): 199-205 DOI: 10.1080/1462220042000202472

Herbert Smith Freehills (2016). Response of British American Tobacco company (Hong Kong) Limited to the government's request for comment's on the proposal to increase the size of health warnings for packets and retail containers of cigarettes to 85%. https://tinyurl.com/5h287tww

Heritage, J. and J. Robinson (2006). Accounting for the visit: giving reasons for seeking medical care. In Maynard, D.W. and J. Heritage, J. (eds) *Communication in medical care: interaction between primary care physicians and patients.* Cambridge: Cambridge University Press: 45-85.

Heydari, G., F. Talischi and N. Mojgani et al (2012). Status and costs of smoking cessation in countries of the eastern Mediterrancan region. *East Mediterr Health J* 18(11): 1102-06 DOI: 10.26719/2012.18.11.1102

Hickman, L. (2013). E-cigarettes: health revolution or fresh pack of trouble? *Guardian*, 5 June. https://tinyurl.com/mtu4uxn3

Hill, D., S. Chapman and R. Donovan (1998) The return of scare tactics. *Tob Control* 7(1): 5-8 DOI: 10.1136/tc.7.1.5

Hilts, P.J. (1994). Is nicotine addictive? It depends on whose criteria you use. *New York Times*, 2 August. https://tinyurl.com/2p8n9btz

Hinton, T. (2021). Market share in alcohol retail in Australia in 2020, by store type. https://tinyurl.com/mpcjrx2n

Holmes, T.J. (1923). *'Secret recipes', compiled by the wardmaster.* https://collections.museumsvictoria.com.au/items/1806632

Hopewell, S., K. Loudon, M.J. Clarke, A.D. Oxman and K. Dickersin (2009). Publication bias in clinical trials due to statistical significance or direction of trial results. *Cochrane Database Syst Rev*(1): MR000006 DOI: 10.1002/14651858.MR000006.pub3

Horn, D. (1972). Determinants of change. In Richardson, R.G. (ed) *The Second World Conference on Smoking and Health*. London: Pittman Medical.

Horn, D. (1978). Who is quitting – and why. In Schwartz, J.L. (ed) *Progress in smoking cessation: proceedings of International Conference on Smoking Cessation*. New York: American Cancer Society.

Horwitz, A.V. and J.C. Wakefield (2007). *The loss of sadness: how psychiatry transformed normal sorrow into depressive disorder.* New York: Oxford University Press.

House of Representatives Standing Committee on Health, Aged Care and Sport (2011). Official committee Hansard. Tobacco Plain Packaging Bill 2011, Trade Marks Amendment (Tobacco Plain Packaging) Bill 2011 *House of Representatives. Standing Committee on Health and Ageing.* https://tinyurl.com/2rfdts55

House of Representatives Standing Committee on Health, Aged Care and Sport (2017). *Inquiry into the use and marketing of electronic cigarettes and personal vaporisers in Australia.* Submissions. https://tinyurl.com/2uprnkxv

Hsu, G., J.Y. Sun and S.H. Zhu (2018). Evolution of electronic cigarette brands from 2013–2014 to 2016–2017: analysis of brand websites. *J Med Internet Res* 20(3): e80 DOI: 10.2196/jmir.8550

Hughes, H. (2020). Transcript of evidence, 13 November. Select Committee on Tobacco Harm Reduction. https://tinyurl.com/8kh4p26u

Hughes, J., K.M. Cummings, J. Foulds, S. Shiffman and R. West (2012). Effectiveness of nicotine replacement therapy: a rebuttal. *Addiction* 107: 1527–28 DOI: 10.1111/j.1360-0443.2012.03925.x

Hughes, J.R. (2020). An update on hardening: a qualitative review. *Nicotine Tob Res* 22(6): 867–71 DOI: 10.1093/ntr/ntz042

Hughes, J.R., K.O. Fagerström and J.E. Henningfield et al. (2019). Why we work with the tobacco industry. *Addiction* 114(2): 374–75 DOI: 10.1111/add.14461

Hughes, J.R., D.K. Hatsukami, J.E. Mitchell and L.A. Dahlgren (1986). Prevalence of smoking among psychiatric outpatients. *Am J Psychiatry* 143(8): 993–97 DOI: 10.1176/ajp.143.8.993

Hughes, J.R., J. Keely and S. Naud (2004). Shape of the relapse curve and long-term abstinence among untreated smokers. *Addiction* 99(1): 29–38 DOI: 10.1111/j.1360-0443.2004.00540.x

Hughes, J.R., E.N. Peters and S. Naud (2011). Effectiveness of over-the-counter nicotine replacement therapy: a qualitative review of nonrandomized trials. *Nicotine Tob Res* 13(7): 512–22 DOI: 10.1093/ntr/ntr055

Hughes, J.R., S.I. Rennard, J.R. Fingar, S.K. Talbot, P.W Callas and K. Fagerström (2011). Efficacy of varenicline to prompt quit attempts in smokers not currently trying to quit: a randomized placebo-controlled trial. *Nicotine Tob Res* 13(10): 955–64 DOI: 10.1093/ntr/ntr103

Hung, W.T., S.M. Dunlop, D. Perez and T. Cotter (2011). Use and perceived helpfulness of smoking cessation methods: results from a population survey of recent quitters. *BMC Public Health* 11: 592–600
DOI: 10.1186/1471-2458-11-592

Hunt, G. (2020). Four times as many people trying to quit smoking during COVID-19. Department of Health Media Release, 1 June.
https://tinyurl.com/mrxnrc6z

Hyland, A., B.K. Ambrose and K.P. Conway et al. (2017). Design and methods of the Population Assessment of Tobacco and Health (PATH) study. *Tob Control* 26(4): 371–78 DOI: 10.1136/tobaccocontrol-2016-052934

Hyland, A., Q. Li, J.E. Bauer, G.A. Giovino, C. Steger and K.M. Cummings (2004). Predictors of cessation in a cohort of current and former smokers followed over 13 years. *Nicotine Tob Res* 6 Suppl 3: S363–9
DOI: 10.1080/14622200412331320761

Illich, I. (1975). The medicalization of life. *J Med Ethics* 1(2): 73–77
DOI: 10.1136/jme.1.2.73

Inoue-Choi, M., C.H. Christensen and B.L. Rostron et al. (2020). Dose-response association of low-intensity and nondaily smoking with mortality in the United States. *JAMA Netw Open* 3(6): e206436
DOI: 10.1001/jamanetworkopen.2020.6436

Jankowski, G.S. and H. Frith (2021). Psychology's medicalization of male baldness. *J Health Psychol*: 13591053211024724 DOI: 10.1177/13591053211024724

Jankowski, M., M. Krzystanek and J.E. Zejda et al. (2019). E-cigarettes are more addictive than traditional cigarettes: a study in highly educated young people. *Int J Environ Res Public Health* 16(13) DOI: 10.3390/ijerph16132279

Jiang, S., T. Yang and C. Bullen et al. (2021). Real-world unassisted quit success and related contextual factors: a population-based study of Chinese male smokers. *Tob Control* 30(5): 498–504
DOI: 10.1136/tobaccocontrol-2019-055594

Jiang, Y., T. Elton-Marshall, G.T. Fong and Q. Li (2010). Quitting smoking in China: findings from the ITC China survey. *Tob Control* 19 Suppl 2: i12–7
DOI: 10.1136/tc.2009.031179

Johns Hopkins University (2021). Johns Hopkins finds thousands of unknown chemicals in e-cigarettes. News Releases, 6 October.
https://tinyurl.com/hpkeahja

Joossens, L. and M. Raw (2006). The Tobacco Control Scale: a new scale to measure country activity. *Tob Control* 15(3): 247–53
DOI: 10.1136/tc.2005.015347

Jordt, S.-E., A.I. Caceres, H. Erythropel, J.B. Zimmerman, T. Dewinter and S. Jabba (2020). Flavor-solvent reaction products in electronic cigarette liquids activate respiratory irritant receptors and elicit cytotoxic metabolic responses in airway epithelial cell. *Eur Respir J* 56(4384) DOI: 10.1183/13993003.congress-2020.4384

Jorenby, D.E., J.T. Hays and N.A. Rigotti et al (2006). Efficacy of varenicline, an alpha4beta2 nicotinic acetylcholine receptor partial agonist, vs placebo or sustained-release bupropion for smoking cessation: a randomized controlled trial. *JAMA* 296(1): 56–63 DOI: 10.1001/jama.296.1.56

Judge, K.. L. Bauld, J. Chesterman and J. Ferguson (2005). The English smoking treatment services: short-term outcomes. *Addiction* 100: 46–58 DOI: 10.1111/j.1360-0443.2005.01027.x

Kahler, C.W., H.R. Lachance, D.R. Strong, S.E. Ramsey, P.M. Monti and R.A. Brown (2007). The Commitment to Quitting Smoking Scale: initial validation in a smoking cessation trial for heavy social drinkers. *Addict Behav* 32(10): 2420–24 DOI: 10.1016/j.addbeh.2007.04.002

Kaplan, S. (2018). Big tobacco's global seach on social media. *New York Times*, 24 August. https://www.nytimes.com/2018/08/24/health/tobacco-social-media-smoking.html

Kary, T. and C. Gretler (2020). Tobacco companies tried to profit off virus, lawmaker group says. Bloomberg, 22 December. https://tinyurl.com/54m94c2e

Kasza, K.A., K.C. Edwards and H.L. Kimmel et al. (2021) Association of e-cigarette use with discontinuation of cigarette smoking among adult smokers who were initially never planning to quit. *JAMA Netw Open* 4(12): e2140880 DOI: 10.1001/jamanetworkopen.2021.40880

Kasza, K.A., A.J. Hyland and R. Borland et al. (2013). Effectiveness of stop-smoking medications: findings from the International Tobacco Control (ITC) Four Country Survey. *Addiction* 108(1): 193–202 DOI: 10.1111/j.1360-0443.2012.04009.x

Keane, H. (2013). Making smokers different with nicotine: NRT and quitting. *Int J Drug Policy* 24(3): 189–95 DOI: 10.1016/j.drugpo.2013.01.011

Keith, R. and A. Bhatnagar (2021). Cardiorespiratory and immunologic effects of electronic cigarettes. *Curr Addict Rep*: 1–11 DOI: 10.1007/s40429-021-00359-7

Kelly, B.C. and M. Vuolo (2018). Trajectories of marijuana use and the transition to adulthood. *Soc Sci Res* 73: 175–88 DOI: 10.1016/j.ssresearch.2018.03.006

Kennedy, C. and H. Hartig (2019). Response rates in telephone surveys have resumed their decline. *Pew Research Center Fact Tank*, 27 February. https://tinyurl.com/ym2mrxen

References

Kennedy, C.D., M.C.I, van Schalkwyk, M. McKee and C. Pisinger (2019). The cardiovascular effects of electronic cigarettes: a systematic review of experimental studies. *Prev Med* 127: 105770 DOI: 10.1016/j.ypmed.2019.105770

Kennedy, S. (2019). The burning question: why does PMI continue to sell cigarettes in Indonesia? *Philip Morris International*, 17 September. https://tinyurl.com/5638kf4f

Khouja, J.N., S.F. Suddell, S.E. Peters, A.E. Taylor and M.R. Munafo (2020). Is e-cigarette use in non-smoking young adults associated with later smoking? A systematic review and meta-analysis. *Tob Control* (30)1: 8–15 DOI: 10.1136/tobaccocontrol-2019-055433

King, A. (1913). *The cigarette habit: a scientific cure*. Kingswood, Surrey: The World's Work.

King, L.A., R.S. Newson and G.E. Cohen et al. (2015). Tracking funded health intervention research. *Med J Aust* 203(4): 184e 1–4 DOI: 10.5694/mja14.01540

Kishchuk, N., M. Tremblay, J. Lapierre, B. Heneman and J. O'Loughlin (2004). Qualitative investigation of young smokers' and ex-smokers' views on smoking cessation methods. *Nicotine Tob Res* 6(3): 491–500 DOI: 10.1080/14622200410001696565

Klein, R. (1993). *Cigarettes are sublime*. Durham, NC: Duke University Press.

Klingemann, H., M.B. Sobell and L.C. Sobell (2010). Continuities and changes in self-change research. *Addiction* 105(9): 1510–18 DOI: 10.1111/j.1360-0443.2009.02770.x

Kluge, A. (2009). A qualitative inquiry into smoking cessation: lessons learned from smokers. *Graduate School*. Atlanta: Emory University. https://tinyurl.com/bdeff84m

Knight, J. and S. Chapman (2004). "A phony way to show sincerity, as we all well know": tobacco industry lobbying against tobacco control in Hong Kong. *Tob Control* 13 Suppl 2: ii13–21 DOI: 10.1136/tc.2004.007641

Kodjak, A. (2017). In ads, tobacco companies admit they made cigarettes more addictive. *National Public Radio*, 27 November. https://tinyurl.com/65en6n6s

Kompier, M.A. (2006). The "Hawthorne effect" is a myth, but what keeps the story going? *Scand J Work Environ Health* 32(5): 402–12 DOI: 10.5271/sjweh.1036

Kotz, D., J. Brown and R. West (2014). "Real-world" effectiveness of smoking cessation treatments: a population study. *Addiction* 109(3): 491–99 DOI: 10.1111/add.12429

Kotz, D., J.A. Fidler and R. West (2011). Did the introduction of varenicline in England substitute for or add to the use of other smoking cessation medications? *Nicotine Tob Res* 13(9): 793–99 DOI: 10.1093/ntr/ntr075

Krasnegor, N.A. (1979). Cigarette smoking as a dependence process. *Research Monograph Series 23*. Rockville, MD: National Institute on Drug Abuse.

Krist, A.H., K.W. Davidson and C.M. Mangione et al. (2021). Interventions for tobacco smoking cessation in adults, including pregnant persons: US Preventive Services Task Force recommendation statement. *JAMA* 325(3): 265–79 DOI: 10.1001/jama.2020.25019

Kuipers, M.A.G., E. Beard, R. West and J. Brown (2018). Associations between tobacco control mass media campaign expenditure and smoking prevalence and quitting in England: a time series analysis. *Tob Control* 27(4): 455–62 DOI: 10.1136/tobaccocontrol-2017-053662

Laine, C. and F. Davidoff, (1996). Patient-centered medicine: a professional evolution. *JAMA* 275(2): 152–56 DOI: 10.1001/jama.1996.03530260066035

Landman, A., P.M. Ling and S.A. Glantz (2002). Tobacco industry youth smoking prevention programs: protecting the industry and hurting tobacco control. *Am J Public Health* 92(6): 917–30 DOI: 10.2105/ajph.92.6.917

Lane, C. (2007). *Shyness: how normal behavior became a sickness*. New Haven: Yale University Press.

Larabie, L.C. (2005). To what extent do smokers plan quit attempts? *Tob Control* 14(6): 425–28 DOI: 10.1136/tc.2005.013615

Lasser, K., J.W. Boyd, S. Woolhandler, D.U. Himmelstein, D. McCormick and D.H. Bor (2000). Smoking and mental illness: a population-based prevalence study. *JAMA* 284(20): 2606–10 DOI: 10.1001/jama.284.20.2606

Lawlor, D.A., S. Frankel, M. Shaw, S. Ebrahim and G.D. Smith (2003). Smoking and ill health: does lay epidemiology explain the failure of smoking cessation programs among deprived populations? *Am J Public Health* 93(2): 266–70 DOI: 10.2105/ajph.93.2.266

Lawrence, D., J. Hafekost, P. Hull. F. Mitrou and S.R. Zubrick (2013). Smoking, mental illness and socioeconomic disadvantage: analysis of the Australian National Survey of Mental Health and Wellbeing. *BMC Public Health* 13: 462 DOI: 10.1186/1471-2458-13-462

Layden, J.E., I. Ghinai and I. Pray et al. (2020). Pulmonary illness related to e-cigarette use in Illinois and Wisconsin: final report. *N Engl J Med* 382(10): 903–16 DOI: 10.1056/NEJMoa1911614

Le Fanu, J. (2018). Mass medicalisation is an iatrogenic catastrophe. *BMJ* 361: k2794 DOI: 10.1136/bmj.k2794

Le Strat, Y., J. Rehm and B. Le Foll (2011). How generalisable to community samples are clinical trial results for treatment of nicotine dependence: a comparison of common eligibility criteria with respondents of a large representative general population survey. *Tob Control* 20(5): 338–43 DOI: 10.1136/tc.2010.038703

References

Leas, E.C., J.P. Pierce and T. Benmarhnia et al. (2018). Effectiveness of pharmaceutical smoking cessation aids in a nationally representative cohort of American smokers. *J Natl Cancer Inst* 110(6): 581–87 DOI: 10.1093/jnci/djx240

Leatherdale, S.T. and J.M. Strath (2007). Tobacco retailer density surrounding schools and cigarette access behaviors among underage smoking students. *Ann Behav Med* 33(1): 105–11 DOI: 10.1207/s15324796abm3301_12

Lee, C.W. and J. Kahende (2007). Factors associated with successful smoking cessation in the United States, 2000. *Am J Public Health* 97(8): 1503–09 DOI: 10.2105/AJPH.2005.083527

Lee, D.J., L.E. Fleming and K.E. McCollister et al. (2007). Healthcare provider smoking cessation advice among US worker groups. *Tob Control* 16(5): 325–28 DOI: 10.1136/tc.2006.019117

Lee, J.G.L., A.Y. Kong and K.B. Sewell et al. (2021). Associations of tobacco retailer density and proximity with adult tobacco use behaviours and health outcomes: a meta-analysis. *Tob Control* DOI: 10.1136/tobaccocontrol-2021-056717

Lemere, F. (1953). What happens to alcoholics? *Am J Psychiatry* 109: 674–76 DOI: 10.1176/ajp.109.9.674

Lendvai, B. and E.S. Vizi (2008). Nonsynaptic chemical transmission through nicotinic acetylcholine receptors. *Physiol Rev* 88(2): 333–49 DOI: 10.1152/physrev.00040.2006

Lennox, A.S. and R.J. Taylor (1994). Factors associated with outcome in unaided smoking cessation, and a comparison of those who have never tried to stop with those who have. *Br J Gen Pract* 44(383): 245–50.

Leonard, K.E. and G.G. Homish (2005). Changes in marijuana use over the transition into marriage. *J Drug Issues* 35(2): 409–29 DOI: 10.1177/002204260503500209

Levinson, A.H., E.A. Borrayo, P. Espinoza, E.T. Flores and E.J Pérez-Stable (2006). An exploration of Latino smokers and the use of pharmaceutical aids. *Am J Prev Med* 31(2): 167–71 DOI: 10.1016/j.amepre.2006.03.022

Levy, D.T., F. Chaloupka and J. Gitchell (2004). The effects of tobacco control policies on smoking rates: a tobacco control scorecard. *J Public Health Manag Pract* 10(4): 338–53 DOI: 10.1097/00124784-200407000-00011

Levy, D.T., K. Friend, H. Holder and M. Carmona (2001). Effect of policies directed at youth access to smoking: results from the SimSmoke computer simulation model. *Tob Control* 10(2): 108–16 DOI: 10.1136/tc.10.2.108

Levy, D.T., A.L. Graham, P.L. Mabry, D.B. Abrams and C.T. Orleans (2010). Modeling the impact of smoking-cessation treatment policies on quit rates. *Am J Prev Med* 38(3 Suppl): S364–72 DOI: 10.1016/j.amepre.2009.11.016

Levy, D.T., P.L. Mabry, A.L. Graham, C.T. Orleans and D.B. Abrams (2010). Exploring scenarios to dramatically reduce smoking prevalence: a simulation model of the three-part cessation process. *Am J Public Heath* 100(7): 1253–55 DOI: 10.2105/AJPH.2009.166785

Levy, D.T., P.L. Mabry, A.L. Graham, C.T. Orleans and D.B Abrams (2010). Reaching healthy people 2010 by 2013: a SimSmoke simulation. *Am J Prev Med* 38(3 Suppl): S373–81 DOI: 10.1016/j.amepre.2009.11.018

Levy, D.T., J. Tam, C. Kuo, G.T. Fong and F. Chaloupka (2018). The impact of implementing tobacco control policies: the 2017 Tobacco Control Policy Scorecard. *J Public Health Manag Pract* 24(5): 448–57 DOI: 10.1097/PHH.0000000000000780

Licht, A.S., A. Hyland, M.J. Travers and S. Chapman (2013). Secondhand smoke exposure levels in outdoor hospitality venues: a qualitative and quantitative review of the research literature. *Tob Control* 22(3): 172–79 DOI: 10.1136/tobaccocontrol-2012-050493

Lichtenstein, E. and R.E. Glasgow (1992). Smoking cessation: what have we learned over the past decade? *J Consult Clin Psychol* 60(4): 518–27 DOI: 10.1037//0022-006x.60.4.518

Lindson, N. and P. Aveyard (2011). An updated meta-analysis of nicotine preloading for smoking cessation: investigating mediators of the effect. *Psychopharmacol* 214(3): 579–92 DOI: 10.1007/s00213-010-2069-3

Long, A. (1975). "What does 'hazard' mean?": a survey of Sydney schoolchildren. *Med J Aust* 2(5): 175–77 DOI: 10.5694/j.1326-5377.1975.tb99496.x

Lucas, N., N. Gurram and T. Thimasarn-Anwar (2020). Smoking and vaping behaviours among 14 and 15-year-olds: results from the 2018 Youth Insights Survey. Wellington: Health Promotion Agency/Te Hiringa Hauora Research and Evaluation Unit. https://tinyurl.com/54h5ee7p

Lupton, D. (1995). Medical and health stories on the *Sydney Morning Herald*'s front page. *Aust J Public Health* 19(5): 501–08 DOI: 10.1111/j.1753-6405.1995.tb00418.x

Mackenzie, C. (1957). *Sublime tobacco.* London: Chatto & Windus.

Mandel, L.L., S.A. Bialous and S.A. Glantz (2006). Avoiding "truth": tobacco industry promotion of life skills training. *J Adolesc Health* 39(6): 868–79 DOI: 10.1016/j.jadohealth.2006.06.010

Mariezcurrena, R. (1994). Recovery from addictions without treatment: literature review. *Cognitive Behaviour Therapy* 23(3–4): 131–54 DOI: 10.1080/16506079409455971

Mariezcurrena, R. (1996). Recovery from addictions without treatment: an interview study. *Cognitive Behaviour Therapy* 25(2): 57–85 DOI: 10.1080/16506079609456012

References

Marsh, A. and J. Matheson (1983). Smoking behaviour and attitudes: an enquiry carried out on behalf of the Department of Health and Social Security. Office of Population Censuses and Surveys, Social Survey Division. London: HMSO. https://www.industrydocuments.ucsf.edu/tobacco/docs/#id=mldl0004

Martin, E.M., P.N. Clapp and M.E. Rebuli (2016). E-cigarette use results in suppression of immune and inflammatory-response genes in nasal epithelial cells similar to cigarette smoke. *Am J Physiol-Lung Cell Molec Physiol* 311(1): L135–L44 DOI: 10.1152/ajplung.00170.2016

Mathews, R., W.D. Hall and C.E. Gartner (2010). Is there evidence of "hardening" among Australian smokers between 1997 and 2007? Analyses of the Australian National Surveys of Mental Health and Well-being. *Aust N Z J Psychiatry* 44(12): 1132–36 DOI: 10.3109/00048674.2010.520116

Mattick, R. and A. Baillie (eds) (1992) An outline for approaches to smoking cessation: quality assurance in the treatment of drug dependence project. *National Campaign Against Drug Abuse Monograph Series No. 19.* Canberra: Australian Government Publishing Service.

Maziak, W. and Z. Ben Taleb (2017). Eurobarometer survey and e-cigarettes: unsubstantiated claims. *Addiction* 112(3): 545 DOI: 10.1111/add.13586

McCormack, B. and T.V. McCance (2006). Development of a framework for person-centred nursing. *J Adv Nurs* 56(5): 472–79 DOI: 10.1111/j.1365-2648.2006.04042.x

McDaniel, P.A., E.A. Lown and R.E. Malone (2017). "It doesn't seem to make sense for a company that sells cigarettes to help smokers stop using them": a case study of Philip Morris's involvement in smoking cessation. *PLOS One* 12(8): e0183961 DOI: 10.1371/journal.pone.0183961

McDermott, E., H. Graham and V. Hamilton (2004). Experiences of being a teenage mother in the UK: a report of a systematic review of qualitative studies. Glasgow: Social and Public Health Services Unit, University of Glasgow. https://tinyurl.com/22etpz9r

McDermott, L.J., A.J. Dobson and N. Owen (2006). From partying to parenthood: young women's perceptions of cigarette smoking across life transitions. *Health Ed Res* 21(3): 428–39 DOI: 10.1093/her/cyl041

McDonald, C.F., S. Jones and L. Beckert et al. (2020). Electronic cigarettes: a position statement from the Thoracic Society of Australia and New Zealand. *Respirol* 25(10): 1082–89 DOI: 10.1111/resp.13904

McKie, J. and J. Richardson (2003). The rule of rescue. *Soc Sci Med* 56(12): 2407–19 DOI: 10.1016/s0277-9536(02)00244-7

McMichael, A.J. (1999). Prisoners of the proximate: loosening the constraints on epidemiology in an age of change. *Am J Epidemiol* 149(10): 887–97 DOI: 10.1093/oxfordjournals.aje.a009732

McMillen, R., J.D. Klein, K. Wilson, J.P. Winickoff and S. Tanski (2019). E-cigarette use and future cigarette initiation among never smokers and relapse among former smokers in the PATH study. *Public Health Rep* 134(5): 528–36 DOI: 10.1177/0033354919864369

McNeill, A. (2020). Public Submission 195 to the Senate Select Committee on Harm reduction, "additional comment to the Australian Select Committee on Tobacco Harm Reduction". https://tinyurl.com/3h7he9r2

McNeill, A., L.S. Brose, R. Calder, L. Bauld and D. Robson (2020). *Vaping in England: 2020 evidence update summary*. London: Public Health England. https://tinyurl.com/4tw8tr52

McNeill, A., M. Raw, J. Whybrow and P. Bailey (2005). A national strategy for smoking cessation treatment in England. *Addiction* 100: 1–11 DOI: 10.1111/j.1360-0443.2005.01022.x

Medbø, A., H. Melbye and C.E. Rudebeck (2011). "I did not intend to stop. I just could not stand cigarettes any more": a qualitative interview study of smoking cessation among the elderly. *BMC Fam Pract* 12: 42 DOI: 10.1186/1471-2296-12-42

Mejia, P., L. Dorfman and A. Cheyne et al. (2014). The origins of personal responsibility rhetoric in news coverage of the tobacco industry. *Am J Public Health* 104(6): 1048–51 DOI: 10.2105/AJPH.2013.301754

Mellor, R., K. Lancaster and A. Ritter (2019). Systematic review of untreated remission from alcohol problems: estimation lies in the eye of the beholder. *J Subst Abuse Treat* 102: 60–72 DOI: 10.1016/j.jsat.2019.04.004

Menashe, C.L. and M. Siegel (1998). The power of a frame: an analysis of newspaper coverage of tobacco issues—United States, 1985–1996. *J Health Commun* 3(4): 307–25 DOI: 10.1080/108107398127139

Mersha, A.G., M, Kennedy, P. Eftekhari and G.S. Gould (2021). Predictors of adherence to smoking cessation medications among current and ex-smokers in Australia: findings from a national cross-sectional survey. *Int J Environ Res Public Health* 18(22): 12225 DOI: https://doi.org/10.3390/ijerph182212225

Mild, light descriptions axed. (2005). *Sydney Morning Herald,* 8 November. https://www.smh.com.au/national/mild-light-cigarette-descriptions-axed-20051108-gdmebd.html

Miller, C.L., M. Wakefield and L. Roberts (2003). Uptake and effectiveness of the Australian telephone quitline service in the context of a mass media campaign. *Tob Control* 12 Suppl 2: ii53–58 https://tobaccocontrol.bmj.com/content/tobaccocontrol/12/suppl_2/ii53.full.pdf

References

Miller, C.R., D.M. Smith and M.L. Goniewicz (2020). Changes in nicotine product use among dual users of tobacco and electronic cigarettes: findings from the Population Assessment of Tobacco and Health (PATH) study, 2013–2015. *Subst Use Misuse* 55(6): 909–13 DOI: 10.1080/10826084.2019.1710211

Miller, P.M. and J.P. Smith (2010). What do marshmallows and golf tell us about natural recovery research? *Addiction* 105: 1521–22 DOI: 10.1111/j.1360-0443.2010.03034.x

Milne, E. (2005). NHS smoking cessation services and smoking prevalence: observational study. *BMJ* 330(7494): 760 DOI: 10.1136/bmj.38407.755521.F7

Ministry of Health New Zealand (2021a). Aotearoa aspires to be world's first smokefree nation with launch of smokefree action plan. https://tinyurl.com/2wpb3res

Ministry of Health New Zealand (2021b). Vaping information for all industry. https://tinyurl.com/mpax9mme

MMWR (1997). Cigarette smoking among adults: United States, 1995. *MMWR – Morbidity and Mortality Weekly Report* 46(51): 1217–20. https://www.cdc.gov/mmwr/preview/mmwrhtml/00050525.htm

Mooney, M., D. White and D. Hatsukami (2004). The blind spot in the nicotine replacement therapy literature: assessment of the double-blind in clinical trials. *Addict Behav* 29(4): 673–84 DOI: 10.1016/j.addbeh.2004.02.010S0306460304000176

Morphett, K., D. Fraser and R. Borland et al. (2021). A pragmatic randomised comparative trial of e-cigarettes and other nicotine products for quitting or long-term substitution in smokers. *Nicotine Tob Res* DOI: 10.1093/ntr/ntab266

Moynihan, R. and A. Cassells (2005). *Selling sickness: how drug companies are turning us all into patients*. Sydney: Allen & Unwin.

Murray, R.L., S.A. Lewis, T. Coleman, J. Britton and A. McNeill (2010). Unplanned attempts to quit smoking: a qualitative exploration. *Addiction* 105(7): 1299–302 DOI: 10.1111/j.1360-0443.2010.02980.x

Ndawula, J. (2004). Carrots can help you quit smoking. *NewVision*. https://www.newvision.co.ug/news/1093021/carrots-help-quit-smoking

National Academies of Science Engineering and Medicine (2018). Public health consequences of e-cigarettes: conclusions by outcome. https://www.nap.edu/resource/24952/012318ecigaretteConclusionsbyOutcome.pdf

National Cancer Institute (2000). *Population based smoking cessation: proceedings of a conference on what works to influence cessation in the general population*. US Department of Health and Human Services, Public Health Service,

National Institutes of Health, National Cancer Institute. http://cancercontrol.cancer.gov/tcrb/monographs/12/entire_monograph-12.pdf

National Health and Medical Research Council (1957). *Report of the NHMRC's 43rd session*. NHMRC.

National Health and Medical Research Council (2019). Payment of participants in research: information for researchers, HRECs and other ethics review bodies. Canberra: NHMRC. https://tinyurl.com/mrdcebxh

National Health Service Digital (2020). Statistics on smoking, England 2020: Part 3 – affordability and expenditure on tobacco. https://tinyurl.com/2p96v8nn

National Health Service Digital (2020) Statistics on smoking, England 2020. https://tinyurl.com/m6ncd98v

National Institute for Health Care Excellence UK (2018). Stop smoking interventions and services. https://www.nice.org.uk/guidance/ng92/chapter/recommendations

National Institute for Health Innovation (2013). Professor David Nutt discusses e-cigarettes. *YouTube*. https://www.youtube.com/channel/UC7BAPQv_mJcc_qrQdNWCsRA

National Statistics (2012). Statistics on smoking in England, 2012. https://files.digital.nhs.uk/publicationimport/pub07xxx/pub07019/smok-eng-2012-rep.pdf

Neuman, M.D., A. Bitton and S.A. Glantz (2005). Tobacco industry influence on the definition of tobacco related disorders by the American Psychiatric Association. *Tob Control* 14(5): 328–37 DOI: 10.1136/tc.2004.010512

Newport, F. (2013). Most US smokers want to quit, have tried multiple times: former smokers say best way to quit is just to stop "cold turkey". https://news.gallup.com/poll/163763/smokers-quit-tried-multiple-times.aspx

Newson, R., L. King and L. Rychetnik et al. (2015). A mixed methods study of the factors that influence whether intervention research has policy and practice impacts: perceptions of Australian researchers. *BMJ Open* 5(7): e008153 DOI: 10.1136/bmjopen-2015-008153

Nezami, E., S. Sussman and M.-A. Pentz (2003). Motivation in tobacco use cessation research. *Substance Use & Misuse* 38(1): 25–50 DOI 10.1081/JA-120016564

Nguyen, T.N. and S. Chapman (2005). The fate of papers rejected from tobacco control. *Tob Control* 14: 293. DOI: 10.1081/JA-120016564

NHS Digital (2017). Statistics on smoking, England – 2017 [PAS]. https://digital.nhs.uk/data-and-information/publications/statistical/statistics-on-smoking/statistics-on-smoking-england-2017-pas

References

Niaura, R., J.T. Hayes and D.E. Jorenby et al. (2008). The efficacy and safety of varenicline for smoking cessation using a flexible dosing strategy in adult smokers: a randomized controlled trial. *Curr Med Res Opin* 24(7): 1931–41 DOI: 10.1185/03007990802177523

Nichter, M., M. Nichter and M. Muramoto et al. (2007). Smoking among low-income pregnant women: an ethnographic analysis. *Health Educ Behav* 34(5): 748–64 DOI: 10.1177/1090198106290397

Notley, C., S. Gentry and S. Cox et al. (2021). Youth use of e-liquid flavours: a systematic review exploring patterns of use of e liquid flavours and associations with continued vaping, tobacco smoking uptake, or cessation. *Addiction* DOI: 10.1111/add.15723

Nutt, D.J., L.D. Phillips and D. Balfour et al. (2014). Estimating the harms of nicotine-containing products using the MCDA approach. *Eur Addict Res* 20(5): 218–25 DOI: 10.1159/000360220

O'Brien, D., J. Long, C. Lee, A. McCarthy and J. Quigley (2020). Electronic cigarette use and tobacco cigarette smoking initiation in adolescents: an evidence review. Dublin: Health Research Board (Ireland). https://tinyurl.com/2p9b8bwm

Oakes, W., S. Chapman, R. Borland, J. Balmford and L. Trotter (2004). "Bulletproof skeptics in life's jungle": which self-exempting beliefs about smoking most predict lack of progression towards quitting? *Prev Med* 39(4): 776–82 DOI: 10.1016/j.ypmed.2004.03.001

Ochsner, A. (1971). Bronchogenic carcinoma, a largely preventable lesion assuming epidemic proportions. *Chest* 59(4): 358–59 DOI: 10.1378/chest.59.4.358

Office for National Statistics (2020a). Adult smoking habits in the UK: 2019. https://tinyurl.com/mrxkeyaj

Office for National Statistics (2020b). Data set: e-cigarette use in Great Britain. https://tinyurl.com/56vht3vn

Office for National Statistics (2021). Opinions and lifestyle survey (QMI): Smoking. https://tinyurl.com/257ub525

Ogden, J. and L. Hills (2008). Understanding sustained behavior change: the role of life crises and the process of reinvention. *Health (London)* 12(4): 419–37 DOI: 10.1177/1363459308094417

Onakpoya, I.J., C.J Heneghan and J.K. Aronson (2016). Post-marketing withdrawal of 462 medicinal products because of adverse drug reactions: a systematic review of the world literature. *BMC Med* 14: 10 DOI: 10.1186/s12916-016-0553-2

Orford, J. (1985). *Excessive appetites: a psychological view of addictions*. Chichester: John Wiley & Sons.

Orford, J., R. Hodgson, and A. Copello et al. (2006). The clients' perspective on change during treatment for an alcohol problem: qualitative analysis of follow-up interviews in the UK alcohol treatment trial. *Addiction* 101(1): 60–68 DOI: 10.1111/j.1360-0443.2005.01291.x

Orleans, C.T., P.L. Mabry and D.B. Abrams (2010). Increasing tobacco cessation in America: a consumer demand perspective. *Am J Prev Med* 38: S303–S06 DOI: 10.1016/j.amepre.2010.01.013

Osibogun, O., Z. Bursac, M. McKee, T. Li and W. Maziak (2020). Cessation outcomes in adult dual users of e-cigarettes and cigarettes: the Population Assessment of Tobacco and Health cohort study, USA, 2013-2016. *Int J Public Health* 65(6): 923–36 DOI: 10.1007/s00038-020-01436-w

Owen, N. and M.J. Davies (1990). Smokers' preferences for assistance with cessation. *Prev Med* 19(4): 424–31 DOI: 10.1016/0091-7435(90)90040-q

Parssinen, T. (2017). How Americans learned about the dangers of cigarette smoking. *ATINER Conference Presentation Series No: HUM2017-0002*. Athens. https://www.atiner.gr/presentations/HUM2017-0002.pdf

Paul, C.L., F. Tzelepis, R.A. Walsh and R. Turner (2007). Pharmacists on the front line in providing support for nicotine replacement therapy and bupropion purchasers. *Drug Alcohol Rev* 26(4): 429–33 DOI: 10.1080/09595230701373966

Pearce, J., R. Hiscock, G. Moon and R. Barnett (2009). The neighbourhood effects of geographical access to tobacco retailers on individual smoking behaviour. *J Epidemiol Community Health* 63(1): 69–77 DOI: 10.1136/jech.2007.070656

Pechacek, T., H.A. Lando, F. Nothwehr and E. Lichtenstein (1994). Quit and win: a community-wide approach to smoking cessation. *Tob Control* 3: 236–41 DOI: 10.1006/pmed.2001.0883

Peele, S. (1989). *Diseasing of America: how we allowed recovery zealots and the treatment industry to convince us we are out of control.* Lexington: Lexington Books.

Persoskie, A. and W.L. Nelson (2013). Just blowing smoke? Social desirability and reporting of intentions to quit smoking. *Nicotine Tob Res* 15(12): 2088–93 DOI: 10.1093/ntr/ntt101

Peters, M.J. (2020). Electronic cigarettes: tumultuous times. *Respirol* 25(6): 570–71 DOI: 10.1111/resp.13725

Peto, R. and A.D. Lopez (2001). Future worldwide health effects of current smoking patterns. In Pearson, C.E., C.E. Koop and M.R. Schwarz (eds), *Critical issues in global health*. San Francisco: Wiley (Jossey-Bass): 154–61.

Philip Morris International (1985). The perspective of PM International on smoking and health issues. Ness Motley Law Firm Documents: University of

References

California San Francisco. https://www.industrydocuments.ucsf.edu/docs/pxpb0040

Philip Morris International (2021). How cigarettes are made. https://www.pmi.com/investor-relations/overview/how-cigarettes-are-made

Philip Morris Records (1983). Status report on anti-industry activities in Australia 830415. Master Settlement Agreement. University of California, San Francisco. https://www.industrydocuments.ucsf.edu/tobacco/docs/#id=mmhn0127

Philip Morris v. Uruguay (2021). *Wikipedia* https://en.wikipedia.org/wiki/Philip_Morris_v._Uruguay

Physicians for a Smoke-Free Canada (2020) Tobacco in Canada. Addressing knowledge gaps important to tobacco regulation environmental scan – Winter 2019–2020 http://smoke-free.ca/SUAP/2020/environmental%20scan%20fall-winter%202019.pdf

Pierce, J.P., T. Benmarhnia and R. Chen et al. (2020). Role of e-cigarettes and pharmacotherapy during attempts to quit cigarette smoking: the PATH Study 2013–16. *PLOS One* 15(9): e0237938 DOI: 10.1371/journal.pone.0237938

Pierce, J.P., S.E. Cummins, M.M. White, A. Humphrey and K. Messer (2012). Quitlines and nicotine replacement for smoking cessation: do we need to change policy? *Ann Rev Public Health* 33: 341–56 DOI: 10.1146/annurev-publhealth-031811-124624

Pierce, J.P., T. Dwyer, G. Frape, S. Chapman, A. Chamberlain and N. Burke (1986). Evaluation of the Sydney "Quit. For Life" anti-smoking campaign: Part 1 – Achievement of intermediate goals. *Med J Aust* 144(7): 341–44.

Pierce, M. and G. Chiarenza (n.d.). 33 famous guitarists: their first guitar and how they learned to play. *Equipboard*. https://equipboard.com/posts/33-famous-guitarists-their-first-guitar-how-they-learned-to-play

Pilnick, A. and T. Coleman (2010). "Do your best for me": the difficulties of finding a clinically effective endpoint in smoking cessation consultations in primary care. *Health (London)* 14(1): 57–74 DOI: 10.1177/1363459309347489

Pine-Abata, H., A. McNeill, R. Murray, A. Bitton, N. Rigotti and M. Raw (2013). A survey of tobacco dependence treatment services in 121 countries. *Addiction* 108(8): 1476–84 DOI: 10.1111/add.12172

Pinney, J.M. (1995). Review of the current status of smoking cessation in the USA: assumptions and realities. *Tob Control* Autumn: S10–S14 https://tobaccocontrol.bmj.com/content/4/Suppl_2/S10

Pisinger, C., N. Godtfredsen and A.M. Bender (2019). A conflict of interest is strongly associated with tobacco industry-favourable results, indicating no

harm of e-cigarettes. *Prev Med* 119: 124–31
DOI: 10.1016/j.ypmed.2018.12.011
Pisinger, C. and N.S. Godtfredsen (2007). Is there a health benefit of reduced tobacco consumption? A systematic review. *Nicotine Tob Res* 9(6): 631–46
DOI: 10.1080/14622200701365327
Pollard, M.S., J.S. Tucker, K. de la Haye, H.D. Green and D.P. Kennedy (2014). A prospective study of marijuana use change and cessation among adolescents. *Drug Alcohol Depend* 144: 134–40 DOI: 10.1016/j.drugalcdep.2014.08.019
Polosa, R., F. Cibella and P. Caponnetto et al. (2017). Health impact of e-cigarettes: a prospective 3.5-year study of regular daily users who have never smoked. *Sci Rep* 7(1): 13825 DOI: 10.1038/s41598-017-14043-2
Porter, B. (2021). Tips and tricks to improve survey response rate. https://www.surveymonkey.com/curiosity/improve-survey-response-rate/
Porter, M. (2016). E-cigarettes, Asherman's syndrome, rugby. *Inside Health*. https://www.bbc.co.uk/programmes/b070dq8h
Potter, J. (1991). Quantification rhetoric. Cancer on television. *Discourse and Society* 2(3): 333–65 https://tinyurl.com/58mkuhtu
Pound, P., N. Britten and M. Morgan et al. (2005). Resisting medicines: a synthesis of qualitative studies of medicine taking. *Soc Sci Med* 61(1): 133–55
DOI: 10.1016/j.socscimed.2004.11.063
Primack, B.A., S. Soneji, M. Stoolmiller, M.J. Fine and J.D. Sargent (2015). Progression to traditional cigarette smoking after electronic cigarette use among US adolescents and young adults. *JAMA Pediatr* 169(11): 1018–23
DOI: 10.1001/jamapediatrics.2015.1742
Prochaska, J.J. and N.L. Benowitz (2019). Current advances in research in treatment and recovery: nicotine addiction. *Sci Adv* 5(10): eaay9763
DOI: 10.1126/sciadv.aay9763
Prochaska, J.O. and W.F. Velicer (1997). The transtheoretical model of health behavior change. *Am J Health Prom* 12(1):38–48
DOI: 10.4278/0890-1171-12.1.38
Prochaska, J.O. and C.C. DiClemente (1983). Stages and processes of self-change of smoking: toward an integrative model of change. *J Consult Clin Psychol* 51(3):390 DOI: 10.1037/0022-006X.51.3.390
Przulj, D., L. Wehbe, H. McRobbie and P. Hajek (2019). Progressive nicotine patch dosing prior to quitting smoking: feasibility, safety and effects during the pre-quit and post-quit periods. *Addiction* 114(3): 515–22
DOI: 10.1111/add.14483
Public Health England (2013). Stoptober challenge reaches new high as country's biggest mass quit attempt. https://www.gov.uk/government/news/stoptober-challenge-reaches-new-high-as-countrys-biggest-mass-quit-attempt

References

Public Health England (2017). Switch. *YouTube*.
https://www.youtube.com/watch?v=qljBzXmTqjE
Public Health England (2019). Health matters. Stopping smoking: What works?
https://bit.ly/3MLnzIZ
Qiu, D., T. Chen, T. Lin and F. Song (2020). Smoking cessation and related factors in middle-aged and older Chinese adults: evidence from a longitudinal study. *PLOS One* DOI: 10.1371/journal.pone.0240806
Quigley, H. and J.H. MacCabe (2019). The relationship between nicotine and psychosis. *Ther Adv Psychopharmacol* 9: 2045125319859969
DOI: 10.1177/2045125319859969.
Quigley, J., H. Kennelly and C. Lee et al (2020). Electronic cigarettes and smoking cessation: an evidence review. Dublin, Ireland: Health Research Board. https://tinyurl.com/2v8rkehp
Rahmani, N., S. Veldhuizen, B. Wong, P. Selby and L. Zawertailo (2021). The effectiveness of nicotine replacement therapy in light versus heavier smokers. *Nicotine Tob Res* DOI: 10.1093/ntr/ntab096
Ranney, L. (2019). Flavored e-cigarettes sweetly lure kids into vaping and also mislead them to dismiss danger, studies suggest. *Conversation*, 16 September. https://tinyurl.com/4jefctax
Rapaport, L. (2019). Tobacco, vape shops sell more to minors than other retailers. *Reuters*, 26 June. https://tinyurl.com/2p895ca7
Raupach, T., R. West and J. Brown (2013). The most "successful" method for failing to quit smoking is unassisted cessation. *Nicotine Tob Res* 15: 748–49
DOI: 10.1093/ntr/nts164
Rayner, J.A., P. Pyett and J. Astbury (2010). The medicalisation of "tall" girls: a discourse analysis of medical literature on the use of synthetic oestrogen to reduce female height. *Soc Sci Med* 71(6): 1076–83
DOI: 10.1016/j.socscimed.2010.06.026
Redfield, R.R., S.M. Hahn and N.E. Sharpless (2020). Redoubling efforts to help Americans quit smoking: federal initiatives to tackle the country's longest-running epidemic. *N Engl J Med* 383(17): 1606–09
DOI: 10.1056/NEJMp2003255
Renaud, M. (1975). On the structural constraints to state intervention in health. *Int J Health Serv* 5(4): 559–71 DOI: 10.2190/YRMC-J8L8-LB62-W9NA
Retail display ban. (2021) *Wikipedia*.
https://en.wikipedia.org/wiki/Tobacco_display_ban
Reuters staff. (2018). New Zealand court gives Philip Morris nod to sell heated tobacco product. *Reuters*, 28 March.
https://www.reuters.com/article/us-newzealand-pmi-idUSKBN1H333X

Riemsma, R.P., J. Pattenden and C. Bridle et al. (2003). Systematic review of the effectiveness of stage based interventions to promote smoking cessation. *BMJ* 326(7400): 1175–77 DOI: 10.1136/bmj.326.7400.1175

Robins, L.N., D.H. Davis and D.N. Nurco (1974). How permanent was Vietnam drug addiction? *Am J Public Health* 64 Suppl 12: 38–43 DOI: 10.2105/ajph.64.12_suppl.38

Robinson, M., D. Mackay, L. Giles, J. Lewsey, E. Richardson and C. Beeston (2021). Evaluating the impact of minimum unit pricing (MUP) on off-trade alcohol sales in Scotland: an interrupted time-series study. *Addiction* 116(10): 2697–707 DOI: 10.1111/add.15478

Rodda, S., D.I. Lubman, K. Letage (2012). Problem gambling: aetiology, identification, management. *Australian Family Physician* 41(7): 725–29 DOI: 10.3316/informit.737687573851487

Roemer, R. (1993). *Legislative action to combat the world tobacco epidemic.* 2nd edn. Geneva: WHO.

Roher, E. (2007). What would Baden-Powell do? *BBC News*, 27 July. http://news.bbc.co.uk/2/hi/uk_news/magazine/6918066.stm

Roizen, R., D. Cahalan and P. Shanks (1978). Spontaneous remission among untreated problem drinkers. In D.B. Kandel (ed.) *Longitudinal research on drug use: empirical findings and methodological issues.* Washington: Hemisphere.

Rothwell, P.M. (2005). External validity of randomised controlled trials: "To whom do the results of this trial apply?" *Lancet* 365(9453): 82–93 DOI: 10.1016/S0140-6736(04)17670-8

Royal Australian College of General Practitioners (2021). Supporting smoking cessation: a guide for health professionals. Sydney: RACGP. https://tinyurl.com/3efxudmv

Rudie, M. and L. Bailey (2018). Results from the 2017 NAQC annual survey of quitlines. North American Quitline Consortium. https://cdn.ymaws.com/www.naquitline.org/resource/resmgr/research/FULLSLIDESFY17.pdf

Russell, M.A. (1976). Low-tar medium-nicotine cigarettes: a new approach to safer smoking. *BMJ* 1(6023): 1430–3 DOI: 10.1136/bmj.1.6023.1430

Russell, M.A., C. Wilson, C. Taylor and C.D. Baker (1979). Effect of general practitioners' advice against smoking. *BMJ* 2(6184): 231–5 DOI: 10.1136/bmj.2.6184.231

Russo, E. (2005). Follow the money: the politics of embryonic stem cell research. *PLOS Biol* 3(7): e234 DOI: 10.1371/journal.pbio.0030234

Rychetnik, L., M. Frommer, P. Hawe and A. Shiell (2002). Criteria for evaluating evidence on public health interventions. *J Epidemiol Community Health* 56(2): 119–27 DOI: 10.1136/jech.56.2.119

References

Sami, M., C. Notley, C. Kouimtsidis, M. Lynskey and S. Bhattacharyya (2019). Psychotic-like experiences with cannabis use predict cannabis cessation and desire to quit: a cannabis discontinuation hypothesis. *Psychol Med* 49(1): 103–12 DOI: 10.1017/S0033291718000569

Saunders, W. and P. Kershaw (1979). Spontaneous remission from alcoholism: a community study. *Br J Addiction* 74: 251–68 DOI: 10.1111/j.1360-0443.1979.tb01346.x

Schaal, C. and S.P. Chellappan (2014). Nicotine-mediated cell proliferation and tumor progression in smoking-related cancers. *Mol Cancer Res* 12(1): 14–23 DOI: 10.1158/1541-7786.MCR-13-0541

Schachter, S. (1982). Recidivism and self-cure of smoking and obesity. *Am Psychologist* 37(4): 436–44 DOI: 10.1037//0003-066x.37.4.436

Schnoll, R.A., J.A. Epstein and R. Niaura et al. (2008). Can the blind see? Participant guess about treatment arm assignment may influence outcome in a clinical trial of bupropion for smoking cessation. *J Substance Abuse Treatment* 34(2): 234–41 DOI: 10.1016/j.jsat.2007.04.004

Schulenberg, J.E., A.C. Merline, L.D. Johnston, P.M. O'Malley, J.G. Bachman and V.B. Laetz (2005). Trajectories of marijuana use during the transition to adulthood: the big picture based on national panel data. *J Drug Issues* 35(2): 255–79 DOI: 10.1177/002204260503500203

Schulz, K.F. and D.A. Grimes (2002). Sample size slippages in randomised trials: exclusions and the lost and wayward. *Lancet* 359(9308): 781–85 DOI: 10.1016/S0140-6736(02)07882-0

Schwab, C. (1993). Cigarette advertising and quitting. New York: Philip Morris USA. https://www.industrydocuments.ucsf.edu/tobacco/docs/#id=ljgj0106

Scientific Committee on Health, Environmental and Emerging Risks (SCHEER) (2021). Final opinion on electronic cigarettes. Brussels: European Commission. https://ec.europa.eu/health/sites/default/files/scientific_committees/scheer/docs/scheer_o_017.pdf

Scollo, M. (2020). Chapter 13: Taxation. In Greenhalgh, E.M., M.M. Scollo and M.H. Winstanley (eds) *Tobacco in Australia: facts and issues*. Melbourne: Cancer Council Victoria. https://www.tobaccoinaustralia.org.au/chapter-13-taxation

Scollo, M., M. Bayly and M. Wakefield (2015). The advertised price of cigarette packs in retail outlets across Australia before and after the implementation of plain packaging: a repeated measures observational study. *Tob Control* 24(Suppl 2): ii82–ii89 DOI: 10.1136/tobaccocontrol-2014-051950

Segan, C.J., R. Borland and K.M. Greenwood (2002). Do transtheoretical model measures predict the transition from preparation to action in smoking cessation? *Psychol Health* 17: 417–35 DOI: 10.1080/0887044022000004911

Seidel, A.K., A. Pedersen, R. Hanewinkel and M. Morgenstern (2019). Cessation of cannabis use: a retrospective cohort study. *Psychiatry Res* 279: 40–46 DOI: 10.1016/j.psychres.2019.07.003

Self selection bias. (2020) *Wikipedia*. https://en.wikipedia.org/wiki/Self-selection_bias

Shaw, R.L., A. Booth and A.J. Sutton et al. (2004). Finding qualitative research: an evaluation of search strategies. *BMC Med Res Methodol* 4: 5 DOI: 10.1186/1471-2288-4-5

Shiffman, S. (2007). Nicotine replacement therapy for smoking cessation in the "real world". *Thorax* 62(11): 930–31 DOI: 10.1136/thx.2007.081919

Shiffman, S., S.E. Brockwell, J.L. Pillitteri and J.G. Gitchell (2008). Individual differences in adoption of treatment for smoking cessation: demographic and smoking history characteristics. *Drug Alcohol Depend* 93(1–2): 121–31 DOI: 10.1016/j.drugalcdep.2007.09.005

Shiffman, S., S.G. Ferguson, J. Rohay and J.G. Gitchell (2008). Perceived safety and efficacy of nicotine replacement therapies among US smokers and ex-smokers: relationship with use and compliance. *Addiction* 103(8): 1371–78 DOI: 10.1111/j.1360-0443.2008.02268.x

Shiffman, S., J.R. Hughes, J.L. Pillitteri and S.L. Burton (2003). Persistent use of nicotine replacement therapy: an analysis of actual purchase patterns in a population based sample. *Tob Control* 12(3): 310–16 DOI: 10.1136/tc.12.3.310

SHORE & Whariki Research Centre (2014). *Review of tobacco control services*. Auckland: College of Health, Massey University. https://www.health.govt.nz/system/files/documents/publications/review-of-tobacco-control-services-nov14.pdf

Shuttleworth, M. (2008). Scientific reductionism. *Explorable*. https://explorable.com/scientific-reductionism

Sjöström, H. and R. Nilsson (1972) *Thalidomide and the power of the drug companies*. London: Penguin.

Slutske, W.S. (2006). Natural recovery and treatment-seeking in pathological gambling: results of two US national surveys. *Am J Psychiatry* 163(2): 297–302 DOI: 10.1176/appi.ajp.163.2.297

Slutske, W.S. (2010). Why is natural recovery so common for addictive disorders? *Addiction* 105(9): 1520–21 DOI: 10.1111/j.1360-0443.2010.03035.x

Slutske, W.S., A. Blaszczynski and N.G. Martin (2009). Sex differences in the rates of recovery, treatment-seeking, and natural recovery in pathological gambling: results from an Australian community-based twin survey. *Twin Res Hum Genet* 12(5): 425–32 DOI: 10.1375/twin.12.5.425

References

Smedslund, G., K.J. Fisher, S.M. Boles and E. Lichtenstein (2004). The effectiveness of workplace smoking cessation programmes: a meta-analysis of recent studies. *Tob Control* 13(2): 197–204 DOI: 10.1136/tc.2002.002915

Smit, E.S., J.A. Fidler and R. West (2011). The role of desire, duty and intention in predicting attempts to quit smoking. *Addiction* 106(4): 844–51 DOI: 10.1111/j.1360-0443.2010.03317.x

Smith, A. and S. Chapman (2014). Quitting smoking unassisted: the 50-year research neglect of a major public health phenomenon. *JAMA* 311(2): 137–38 DOI: 10.1001/jama.2013.282618

Smith, A.L. (2020). Being serious about quitting: a qualitative analysis of Australian ex-smokers' explanations of their quitting success. *Int J Drug Policy* 86: 102942. DOI: 10.1016/j.drugpo.2020.102942

Smith, A.L., S.M. Carter, S. Chapman, S.M. Dunlop and B. Freeman (2015a). Why do smokers try to quit without medication or counselling? A qualitative study with ex-smokers. *BMJ Open* 5(4): e007301 DOI: 10.1136/bmjopen-2014-007301

Smith, A.L., S.M. Carter, S.M. Dunlop, B. Freeman and S. Chapman (2015b). The views and experiences of smokers who quit smoking unassisted: a systematic review of the qualitative evidence. *PLOS One* 10(5): e0127144 DOI: 10.1371/journal.pone.0127144

Smith, A.L., S.M. Carter, S.M. Dunlop, B. Freeman and S. Chapman (2017). Measured, opportunistic, unexpected and naive quitting: a qualitative grounded theory study of the process of quitting from the ex-smokers' perspective. *BMC Public Health* 17(1): 430 DOI: 10.1186/s12889-017-4326-4

Smith, A.L., S.M. Carter, S.M. Dunlop, B. Freeman and S. Chapman (2018). Revealing the complexity of quitting smoking: a qualitative grounded theory study of the natural history of quitting in Australian ex-smokers. *Tob Control* 27(5): 568–76 DOI: 10.1136/tobaccocontrol-2017-053919

Smith, A.L., S. Chapman and S.M. Dunlop (2015). What do we know about unassisted smoking cessation in Australia? A systematic review, 2005–2012. *Tob Control* 24: 18–27 DOI: 10.1136/tobaccocontrol-2013-051019

Smith, D.R., R.A. Imawana, M.N. Solim and M.L. Goodson (2021). Exposure–lag response of smoking prevalence on lung cancer incidence using a distributed lag non-linear model. *Nature Sci Rep* 11(14478) DOI: 10.1038/s41598-021-91644-y

Smith, E.A. and R.E. Malone (2020). An argument for phasing out sales of cigarettes. *Tob Control* 29(6): 703–08 DOI: 10.1136/tobaccocontrol-2019-055079

Smithers, R. (2016). Four in 10 retailers sell e-cigarettes and vaping liquids to under-18s. *Guardian*, 9 August. https://www.theguardian.com/society/2016/aug/09/four-in-10-retailers-sell-e-cigarettes-and-vaping-liquids-to-under-18s

Sobell, L.C. (2007). The phenomenon of self-change: overview and key issues. In Klingemann, H. and L.C. Sobell (eds) *Promoting self-change from addictive behaviors*. New York: Springer.

Sobell, L.C., J. Cunningham and M. Sobell (1996). Recovery from alcohol problems with and without treatment: prevalence in two population surveys. *Am J Public Health* 86(7): 966–72 DOI: 10.2105/ajph.86.7.966

Sollenberger R. and W. Bredderman (2022) Guess who's secretly backing this "anti-smoking" vape group. *The Daily Beast*, 11 January. https://tinyurl.com/yckukuj7

Solheim, K. (1989). The smoking cessation process. *J Holistic Nursing* 7(1): 26–33 DOI: 10.1177/089801018900700106

Song, Y., L. Zhao and K.M. Palipudi et al. (2016). Tracking MPOWER in 14 countries: results from the Global Adult Tobacco Survey, 2008–2010. *Glob Health Promot* 23(2 Suppl): 24–37 DOI: 10.1177/1757975913501911

Song, Y.M., J. Sung and H.J. Cho (2008). Reduction and cessation of cigarette smoking and risk of cancer: a cohort study of Korean men. *J Clin Oncol* 26(31): 5101–06 DOI: 10.1200/JCO.2008.17.0498

Springett, J., C. Owen and J. Callaghan (2007). The challenge of combining "lay" knowledge with "evidence-based" practice in health promotion: Fag Ends smoking cessation service. *Crit Public Health* 17(3): 243–56 DOI: 10.1080/09581590701225854

St Helen, G., K.C. Ross, D.A. Dempsey, C.M. Havel, P. Jacob and N. Benowitz (2016). Nicotine delivery and vaping behavior during ad libitum e-cigarette access. *Tob Regul Sci* 2(4): 363–76 DOI: 10.18001/TRS.2.4.8

Staff, J., B.C. Kelly, J.L. Maggs and M. Vuolo (2021). Adolescent electronic cigarette use and tobacco smoking in the Millennium Cohort Study. *Addiction* DOI: 10.1111/add.15645

Stafford, B. (2017). Case closed: study shows no lung damage from vaping. https://regulatorwatch.com/brent_stafford/case-closed-study-shows-no-lung-damage-vaping/

Stapleton, J.A. (2010). Commentary on Banham & Gilbody (2010): the scandal of smoking and mental illness. *Addiction* 105(7): 1190–91 DOI: 10.1111/j.1360-0443.2010.03025.x

Statista (2021a). Number of prescription items of bupropion (Zyban) to quit smoking in England from 2000 to 2020. https://www.statista.com/statistics/370277/prescription-of-bupropion-to-quit-smoking-in-england/

References

Statista (2021b). Number of prescription items of nicotine replacement therapies (NRT) to quit smoking in England from 2000/01 to 2019/20. https://www.statista.com/statistics/370253/nicotine-replacement-therapies-in-england-uk/

Statista (2021c). Number of prescription items of varenicline (Champix) to quit smoking in England from 2006/07 to 2019/20. https://www.statista.com/statistics/370285/prescription-items-of-varenicline-to-quit-smoking-in-england/

Statistics Canada (2021). Canadian Tobacco and Nicotine Survey: public use microdata file. https://www150.statcan.gc.ca/n1/pub/13-25-0001/132500012021001-eng.htm

Stead, L.F. et al (2012). Nicotine replacement therapy for smoking cessation. *Cochrane Database Syst Rev* Issue 11: Art. No.: CD000146 DOI: 10.1002/14651858.CD000146.pub4

Stead, L.F., R. Perera, C. Bullen, D. Mant and T. Lancaster (2013). Physician advice for smoking cessation. *Cochrane Database Syst Rev* (5): CD000165 DOI: 10.1002/14651858.CD000165.pub4

Stead, L.F., R. Perera and T. Lancaster (2007). A systematic review of interventions for smokers who contact quitlines. *Tob Control* 16 Suppl 1: i3–8 DOI: 10.1136/tc.2006.019737

Stewart, C. (1999). Investigation of cigarette smokers who quit without treatment. *J Drug Issues* 29: 167–85 DOI: 0.1177/002204269902900111

Stockwell, T. (2014). Minimum alcohol pricing: Canada's accidental public health strategy. *Conversation*, 4 August. https://theconversation.com/minimum-alcohol-pricing-canadas-accidental-public-health-strategy-25185

Streiner, D.L. (2002). The 2 "es" of research: efficacy and effectiveness trials. *Can J Psychiatry* 47(6): 552–56 DOI: 10.1177/070674370204700607

Sung, H., J. Ferley and R.L. Siegel et al. (2021). Global cancer statistics 2020: GLOBOCAN estimates of incidence and mortality worldwide for 36 cancers in 185 countries. *CA Cancer J Clin* 71(3): 209–49 DOI: 10.3322/caac.21660

Suzer-Gurtekin, Z.T., R. McBee, R. Curtin, J.M. Lepkowski, M. Liu and M. ElKasab (2016). Effect of a pre-paid incentive on response rates to an Address-Based Sampling (ABS) Web-Mail survey. *Survey Practice* 9(4): 1–8 DOI: 10.29115/SP-2016-0025

Syrjanen, K., K. Syrjänen and K. Eronen et al. (2017). Slow-release L-cysteine (Acetium®) lozenge is an effective new method in smoking cessation: a randomized, double-blind, placebo-controlled intervention. *Anticancer Res* 37(7): 3639–48 DOI: 10.21873/anticanres.11734

Tannenbaum, M.B., J. Hepler and R.S. Zimmerman et al. (2015). Appealing to fear: a meta-analysis of fear appeal effectiveness and theories. *Psychol Bull* 141(6): 1178–204 DOI: 10.1037/a0039729

Tanzania Invest (2018). Tanzania inaugurates USD 29 million cigarette factory. 19 March. https://www.tanzaniainvest.com/industry/new-philip-morris-cigarette-factory

Taylor, G.M.J., M.N. Dalili, M. Semwal, M. Civljak, A. Sheikh and J. Car (2017). Internet-based interventions for smoking cessation. *Cochrane Database Syst Rev* 9: CD007078 DOI: 10.1002/14651858.CD007078.pub5

Teague, S., G.J. Youssef, and J.A. Macdonald et al. (2018). Retention strategies in longitudinal cohort studies: a systematic review and meta-analysis. *BMC Med Res Methodol* 18(1): 151 DOI: 10.1186/s12874-018-0586-7

Tehrani, M.W., M.N. Newmeyer, A.M. Rule and C. Prasse (2021). Characterizing the chemical landscape in commercial e-cigarette liquids and aerosols by liquid chromatography-high-resolution mass spectrometry. *Chem Res Toxicol* DOI: 10.1021/acs.chemrestox.1c00253

Therapeutic Goods Administration. Accessing unapproved products. Canberra: TGA. https://www.tga.gov.au/accessing-unapproved-products

Therapeutic Goods Administration (2017). Scheduling delegate's interim decisions and invitation for further comment: ACCS/ACMS, November 2016. Canberra: TGA. https://www.tga.gov.au/book-page/21-nicotine

Therapeutic Goods Administration (2021a). Melbourne-based individual fined $7,992 for alleged unlawful importation of nicotine vaping products. https://tinyurl.com/93h3rsyr

Therapeutic Goods Administration (2021b). Nicotine vaping products: Information for prescribers. Canberra: TGA. https://www.tga.gov.au/nicotine-vaping-products-information-prescribers

Therapeutic Goods Administration (2021c). RV Global Ecommerce Pty Ltd fined $39,960 for alleged unlawful advertising of nicotine vaping products. https://tinyurl.com/mtjm76a9

Thomas, J. and A. Harden (2008). Methods for the thematic synthesis of qualitative research in systematic reviews. *BMC Med Res Methodol* 8: 45 DOI: 10.1186/1471-2288-8-45

Thompson, D.S. and T.R. Wilson (1966). Discontinuance of cigarette smoking: "natural" and with "therapy"—a ten-week and ten-month follow-up study of 298 adult participants in a five-day plan to stop smoking. *JAMA* 196(12): 1048–52 DOI: 10.1001/jama.196.12.1048

Thompson, E.M. (1995). A descriptive study of women who have successfully quit smoking. Georgia State University. PhD thesis.

References

Tierney, P.A., C.D. Karpinski, J.E. Brown, W. Luo and J.F. Pankow (2016). Flavour chemicals in electronic cigarette fluids. *Tob Control* 25(e1): e10–5 DOI: 10.1136/tobaccocontrol-2014-052175

TLB Productions (2007). Ghetto science: smoking. https://www.youtube.com/watch?v=IQ4n7g31RlE&t=5s

Tobacco Business (2021). Major flavored ends manufacturers receive FDA MDOs. https://tobaccobusiness.com/major-flavored-ends-manufacturers-receive-fda-mdos/

Tobacco Control Legal Consortium (2011). Cigarette minimum price laws. https://publichealthlawcenter.org/sites/default/files/resources/tclc-guide-cigminimumpricelaws-2011.pdf

Tobacco Tactics (2020a). E-cigarettes: Industry timeline. University of Bath. https://tobaccotactics.org/wiki/e-cigarettes-industry-timeline/

Tobacco Tactics (2020b). Tobacco smuggling. University of Bath. https://tobaccotactics.org/wiki/tobacco-smuggling/

Tobacco Tactics (2021). Next generation products: British American Tobacco. University of Bath. https://tobaccotactics.org/wiki/next-generation-products-british-american-tobacco/

Tocque, K., A. Barker and B. Fullard (2005). Are stop smoking services helping to reduce smoking prevalence? New analysis based on estimated number of smokers. *Tobacco Control Research Bulletin (Smoke Free Northwest, Department of Health, England)* (3): 1–13.

Tofler, A. and S. Chapman (2003). "Some convincing arguments to pass back to nervous customers": the role of the tobacco retailer in the Australian tobacco industry's smoker reassurance campaign 1950–1978. *Tob Control* 12 Suppl 3: iii7–12 DOI: 10.1136/tc.12.suppl_3.iii7

Tomioka, H., T. Wada, M. Yamazoe, Y. Yoshizumi, C. Nisho and G. Ishimoto (2019). Ten-year experience of smoking cessation in a single center in Japan. *Respir Investig* 57(4): 380–87 DOI: 10.1016/j.resinv.2019.01.007

Transparency International (2021). Corruption Perceptions Index 2020. https://www.transparency.org/en/cpi/2020/index/nzl

Triggle, N. (2013). NHS stop-smoking service "a success". *BBC News*, 21 August. http://www.bbc.co.uk/news/health-23766070

Truth Tobacco Industry Documents. https://www.industrydocuments.ucsf.edu/tobacco/

Tsai, M., M.K. Byun, J. Shin, and L.E. Crotty Alexander (2020). Effects of e-cigarettes and vaping devices on cardiac and pulmonary physiology. *J Physiol* 598(22): 5039–62 DOI: 10.1113/JP279754

Tuchfeld, B. (1981). Spontaneous remission in alcoholics: empirical observations and theoretical implications. *J Studies Alcohol* 626–41 DOI: 10.15288/jsa.1981.42.626

Tulloch, H.E., A.L. Pipe, C. Els, M.J. Clyde and R.D. Reid (2016). Flexible, dual-form nicotine replacement therapy or varenicline in comparison with nicotine patch for smoking cessation: a randomized controlled trial. *BMC Med* 14: 80 DOI: 10.1186/s12916-016-0626-2

Tverdal, A. and K. Bjartveit (2006). Health consequences of reduced daily cigarette consumption. *Tob Control* 15(6): 472–80 DOI: 10.1136/tc.2006.016246

Tyrrell, I. (1999). *Deadly enemies: tobacco and its opponents in Australia.* Sydney: UNSW Press.

United Nations Conference on Trade and Development (1985). United Nations guidelines on consumer protection. https://unctad.org/en/Pages/DITC/CompetitionLaw/UN-Guidelines-on-Consumer-Protection.aspx

United States Federal Trade Commission (2021). Cigarette report for 2020. https://ftc.gov/system/files/documents/reports/federal-trade-commission-cigarette-report-2020-smokeless-tobacco-report-2020/p114508fy20cigarettereport.pdf

United States Surgeon General (2020). *Smoking cessation: a report of the Surgeon General.* U.S. Department of Health and Human Services, Centers for Disease Control and Prevention, National Center for Chronic Disease Prevention and Health Promotion Office on Smoking and Health. https://www.hhs.gov/sites/default/files/2020-cessation-sgr-full-report.pdf

US Food and Drug Administration (2019). 2018 NYTS data: a startling rise in youth e-cigarette use. Washington DC: USFDA. https://bit.ly/3L15bL1

US Food and Drug Administration (2021a). FDA denies marketing applications for about 55,000 flavored e-cigarette products for failing to provide evidence they appropriately protect public health. Washington DC: USFDA. https://bit.ly/3CZrHRH

US Food and Drug Administration (2021b). FDA permits marketing of e-cigarette products marking first authorization of its kind by the agency. *Press Release.* Washington DC: USFDA. https://bit.ly/36w3dDr

Vaillant, G.E. (1995). *The natural history of alcoholism revisited.* Cambridge, MA: Harvard University Press.

Vangeli, E., J. Stapleton, E.S. Smit, R. Borland and R. West (2011). Predictors of attempts to stop smoking and their success in adult general population samples: a systematic review. *Addiction* 106(12): 2110–21 DOI: 10.1111/j.1360-0443.2011.03565.x

Vanyukov, M.M., R.E. Tarter and G.P. Kirillova et al. (2012). Common liability to addiction and "gateway hypothesis": theoretical, empirical and evolutionary

References

perspective. *Drug Alcohol Depend* 123 Suppl 1: S3–17 DOI: 10.1016/j.drugalcdep.2011.12.018

Various authors (2003). Insights from Australia's national tobacco campaign. *Tob Control* 12. https://tobaccocontrol.bmj.com/content/12/suppl_2

Vered, M.P., R. Kedem, D. Tzur, Y.H. Even and S. Chapman (2016). Self-reported difficulty of smoking cessation among ex-smokers in the Israel defense force career service personnel: observational study. University of Sydney e-Scholarship Respository. https://tinyurl.com/7e8fjkvw

Verrall, A. (2021). New Zealand voices shape vaping regulations. *Beehive*, 10 August. https://www.beehive.govt.nz/release/new-zealand-voices-shape-vaping-regulations

Viswam, D., S. Trotter, P.S. Burge and G.I. Walters (2018). Respiratory failure caused by lipoid pneumonia from vaping e-cigarettes. *BMJ Case Rep* 2018 DOI: 10.1136/bcr-2018-224350

Vogt, F., S. Hall and T.M. Marteau (2008). Understanding why smokers do not want to use nicotine dependence medications to stop smoking: qualitative and quantitative studies. *Nicotine Tob Res* 10(8): 1405–13 DOI: 10.1080/14622200802239280

Wakefield, M. and F. Chaloupka (1998). Improving the measurement and use of tobacco control "inputs". *Tob Control* 7(4): 333–35 DOI: 10.1136/tc.7.4.333

Wakefield, M., K. Coomber and S.J. Durkin et al. (2014). Time series analysis of the impact of tobacco control policies on smoking prevalence among Australian adults, 2001–2011. *Bull WHO* 92: 413–22 DOI: 10.2471/BLT.13.118448

Wakefield, M., D. Germain and L. Henriksen (2008). The effect of retail cigarette pack displays on impulse purchase. *Addiction* 103(2): 322–28 DOI: 10.1111/j.1360-0443.2007.02062.x

Wakefield, M., B. Loken and R.C. Hornik (2010). Use of mass media campaigns to change health behaviour. *Lancet* 376(9748): 1261–71 DOI: 10.1016/S0140-6736(10)60809-4

Wakefield, M., K.S. McLeod and K.C. Smith (2003). Individual versus corporate responsibility for smoking-related illness: Australian press coverage of the Rolah McCabe trial. *Health Promot Int* 18(4): 297–305 DOI: 10.1093/heapro/dag413

Wakefield, M., G. Szczypka and Y. Terry-McElrath et al. (2005). Mixed messages on tobacco: comparative exposure to public health, tobacco company- and pharmaceutical company-sponsored tobacco-related television campaigns in the United States, 1999–2003. *Addiction* 100(12): 1875–83 DOI: 10.1111/j.1360-0443.2005.01298.x

Wakefield, M.A., S. Durkin and M.J. Spittal et al. (2008). Impact of tobacco control policies and mass media campaigns on monthly adult smoking prevalence. *Am J Public Health* 98(8): 1443–50 DOI: 10.2105/AJPH.2007.128991

Wakefield, M.A., L. Hayes, S. Durkin and R. Borland (2013). Introduction effects of the Australian plain packaging policy on adult smokers: a cross-sectional study. *BMJ Open* 3(7) DOI: 10.1136/bmjopen-2013-003175

Walker, M.B. and M.G. Dickerson (1996). The prevalence of problem and pathological gambling: a critical analysis. *J Gambl Stud* 12(2): 233–49 DOI: 10.1007/BF01539176

Walker, R. (1984). *Under fire: a history of tobacco smoking in Australia*. Melbourne: Melbourne University Press.

Walsh, R.A. (2008). Over-the-counter nicotine replacement therapy: a methodological review of the evidence supporting its effectiveness. *Drug Alcohol Rev* 27(5): 529–47 DOI: 10.1080/09595230802245527

Walsh, R.A. (2011). Australia's experience with varenicline: usage, costs and adverse reactions. *Addiction* 106(2): 451–2 DOI: 10.1111/j.1360-0443.2010.03282.x

Walters, G.D. (2000). Spontaneous remission from alcohol, tobacco, and other drug abuse: seeking quantitative answers to qualitative questions. *Am J Drug Alcohol Abuse* 26(3): 443–60 DOI: 10.1081/ada-100100255

Wang, R.J., S. Bhadriraju and S.A. Glantz (2021). E-cigarette use and adult cigarette smoking cessation: a meta-analysis. *Am J Public Health* 111(2): 230–46 DOI: 10.2105/AJPH.2020.305999

Ward, J.E. and Sanson-Fisher, R. (1996). Accuracy of patient recall of opportunistic smoking cessation advice in general practice. *Tob Control* 5: 110–13 https://www.jstor.org/stable/20207168

Warner, K.E. (1977). The effects of the anti-smoking campaign on cigarette consumption. *Am J Public Health* 67(7): 645–50 DOI: 10.2105/ajph.67.7.645

Warner, K.E. and G.A. Fulton (1994). The economic implications of tobacco product sales in a nontobacco state. *JAMA* 271(10): 771–76 DOI: 10.1001/jama.1994.03510340061035

Warner, K.E. and J.L. Mackay (2008). Smoking cessation treatment in a public-health context. *Lancet* 371(9629): 1976–78 DOI: 10.1016/S0140-6736(08)60846-6

Weber, M.F., P.E.A. Sarich and P. Vaneckova et al. (2021). Cancer incidence and cancer death in relation to tobacco smoking in a population-based Australian cohort study. *Int J Cancer* DOI: 10.1002/ijc.33685

Ween, M.P., R. Hamon, M.G. Macowan, L. Thredgold, P.N. Reynolds and S. Hodge (2020). Effects of e-cigarette e-liquid components on bronchial epithelial cells: demonstration of dysfunctional efferocytosis. *Respirol* 25(6): 620–28 DOI: 10.1111/resp.13696

Wehrli, F.W., A. Caporale, M.C. Langham and S. Chatterjee (2020). New insights from MRI and cell biology into the acute vascular-metabolic implications of electronic cigarette vaping. *Front Physiol* 11: 492 DOI: 10.3389/fphys.2020.00492

Weiner, B. (1985). An attributional theory of achievement motivation and emotion. *Psychol Rev* 92(4): 548–73 https://psycnet.apa.org/buy/1986-14532-001

West, R. (2005). Time for a change: putting the transtheoretical (stages of change) model to rest. *Addiction* 100(8): 1036–39 DOI: 10.1111/j.1360-0443.2005.01139.x

West, R. and J. Brown (2012). Smoking and smoking cessation in England 2011. *Smoking in England*. https://tinyurl.com/2ccy3xeu

West, R., M.E. DiMarino, J. Gitchell and A. McNeill (2005). Impact of UK policy initiatives on use of medicines to aid smoking cessation. *Tob Control* 14(3): 166–71 DOI: 10.1136/tc.2004.008649

West, R., D. Kale, L. Kock and J. Brown (2021). Top-line findings on smoking in England from the Smoking Toolkit Study. *Smoking Toolkit Study*. https://smokinginengland.info/resources/latest-statistics

West, R., S. May, M. West, E. Croghan and A. McEwen (2013). Performance of English stop smoking services in first 10 years: analysis of service monitoring data. *BMJ* 347 DOI: 10.1136/bmj.f4921

West, R., A. McNeill and J. Britton et al. (2010). Should smokers be offered assistance with stopping? *Addiction* 105(11): 1867–69 DOI: 10.1111/j.1360-0443.2010.03111.x

West, R., L. Shahab and J. Brown (2016). Estimating the population impact of e-cigarettes on smoking cessation in England. *Addiction* 111(6): 1118–19 DOI: 10.1111/add.13343

West, R. and T. Sohal (2006). "Catastrophic" pathways to smoking cessation: findings from national survey. *BMJ* 332(7539): 458–60 DOI: 10.1136/bmj.38723.573866.AE

White, A.R., H. Rampes, J.P. Liu, L.F. Stead and J Campbell (2014). Acupuncture and related interventions for smoking cessation. *Cochrane Database Syst Rev*(1): CD000009 DOI: 10.1002/14651858.CD000009.pub4

White, V., N. Tan, M. Wakefield and D. Hill (2003). Do adult focused anti-smoking campaigns have an impact on adolescents? The case of the Australian National Tobacco Campaign. *Tob Control* 12 Suppl 2: ii23–9. http://www.ncbi.nlm.nih.gov/pubmed/12878770

WHO (2021). *WHO report on the global tobacco epidemic 2021: addressing new and emerging products*. Geneva: WHO.
https://www.who.int/publications/i/item/9789240032095
WHO Europe (2016). *Evidence brief: tobacco point-of-sale display bans*. Copenhagen: WHO. https://tinyurl.com/mv9tnxmk
WHO Study Group on Tobacco Product Regulation (2021). *Report on the scientific basis of tobacco product regulation: eighth report of a WHO study group*. Geneva: WHO. https://www.who.int/publications/i/item/9789240022720
Wickstrom, G. and T. Bendix (2000). The "Hawthorne effect": what did the original Hawthorne studies actually show? *Scand J Work Environ Health* 26(4): 363–67. http://www.ncbi.nlm.nih.gov/pubmed/10994804
Wilkinson, A.L., M.M. Scollo, M.A. Wakefield, M.J. Spittal, F.J. Chaloupka and S.J. Durkin (2019). Smoking prevalence following tobacco tax increases in Australia between 2001 and 2017: an interrupted time-series analysis. *Lancet Public Health* 4(12): e618-e27 DOI: 10.1016/S2468-2667(19)30203-8
Wills, T.A., R. Knight, J.D. Sargent, F.X. Gibbins, I. Pagano and R. Williams (2017). Longitudinal study of e-cigarette use and onset of cigarette smoking among high school students in Hawaii. *Tob Control* 26(1): 34–39 DOI: 10.1136/tobaccocontrol-2015-052705
Wilson, A., J. Hippisley-Cox, C. Coupland, T. Coleman, J. Britton and S. Barrett (2005). Smoking cessation treatment in primary care: prospective cohort study. *Tob Control* 14(4): 242–46 DOI: 10.1136/tc.2004.010090
Winick, C. (1962). Maturing out of narcotics addiction. *Bull Narcotics* 14: 1–7. https://www.unodc.org/unodc/en/data-and-analysis/bulletin/bulletin_1962-01-01_1_page002.html
Winnicka, L. and M.A. Shenoy (2020). EVALI and the pulmonary toxicity of electronic cigarettes: a review. *J Gen Intern Med* 35(7): 2130–35 DOI: 10.1007/s11606-020-05813-2
Wodak, A. (2020). Why Australia should make it as easy as possible for smokers to switch to vaping. *Sydney Morning Herald*, 26 June.
https://tinyurl.com/4nvmcdah
Woods, S.S. and A.E. Haskins (2007). Increasing reach of quitline services in a US state with comprehensive tobacco treatment. *Tob Control* 16 Suppl 1: i33–6 DOI: 10.1136/tc.2007.019935
World Bank (1999). *Curbing the epidemic: governments and the economics of tobacco control*. Washington DC: World Bank.
https://elibrary.worldbank.org/doi/pdf/10.1596/0-8213-4519-2
Wynder, E.L. and E.A. Graham (1950). Tobacco smoking as a possible etiologic factor in bronchiogenic carcinoma: a study of 684 proved cases. *J Am Med Assoc* 143(4): 329–36 DOI: 10.1001/jama.1950.02910390001001

References

Yach, D. (2019). Twitter. https://twitter.com/swimdaily/status/1098256065383358464

Yeomans, K., K.A. Payne and J.P. Marton et al. (2011). Smoking, smoking cessation and smoking relapse patterns: a web-based survey of current and former smokers in the US. *Int J Clin Pract* 65(10): 1043–54 DOI: 10.1111/j.1742-1241.2011.02758.x

Yingst, J., J. Foulds and S. Veldheer et al. (2020). Measurement of electronic cigarette frequency of use among smokers participating in a randomized controlled trial. *Nicotine Tob Res* 22(5): 699–704 DOI: 10.1093/ntr/nty233

Yoong, S.L., A. Hall and H. Turon et al. (2021). Association between electronic nicotine delivery systems and electronic non-nicotine delivery systems with initiation of tobacco use in individuals aged < 20 years: a systematic review and meta-analysis. *PLOS One* 16(9): e0256044 DOI: 10.1371/journal.pone.0256044

Young, J.M. and J.E. Ward (2001). Implementing guidelines for smoking cessation advice in Australian general practice: opinions, current practices, readiness to change and perceived barriers. *Family Practice* 18(1): 14–20 DOI: 10.1093/fampra/18.1.14

Zhang, Y.-Y., F.L. Bu and F. Dong et al. (2021). The effect of e-cigarettes on smoking cessation and cigarette smoking initiation: an evidence-based rapid review and meta-analysis. *Tob Induc Dis* 19: 04 DOI: 10.18332/tid/131624

Zhu, S.-H., M. Lee, Y.-L. Zhuang, A. Gamst and T. Wolfson (2012). Interventions to increase smoking cessation at the population level: how much progress has been made in the last two decades? *Tob Control* 21(2): 110–18 DOI: 10.1136/tobaccocontrol-2011-050371

Zhu, S.-H., B. Rosbrook, C. Anderson, E. Gilpin, G. and J.P. Pierce (1995). The demographics of help-seeking for smoking cessation in California and the role of the California smokers' helpline. *Tob Control* 4 S9–S15 https://tobaccocontrol.bmj.com/content/4/Suppl_1/S9

Zwar, N.A., A. Nasser, E.J. Comino and R.L. Richmond(2002). Short-term effectiveness of bupropion for assisting smoking cessation in general practice. *Med J Aust* 177(5): 277–78 DOI: 10.5694/j.1326-5377.2002.tb04772.x

Index

Action on Smoking and Health (ASH) England 89, 135
alcohol 2–5, 10, 21, 29, 114, 205, 272, 274, 276
American Cancer Society (ACS) 60, 83, 122
American Psychiatric Association 9, 77, 151
amphetamines 2, 57
anecdotes about quitting 13, 14–20
assisted quitting xxii–xxiv, 51–54, 72, 80, 125, 134
Australian Institute of Health and Welfare (AIHW) 2, 176, 233
AIHW National Drug Household Study 2019 8

Baden-Powell, Robert xix
Barthes, Roland xvi
Bates, Clive 152, 153, 173
Beaglehole, Robert 153
beliefs about quitting and personal responsibility 5, 216–217, 223
Benowitz, Neil 28, 122
Bevins, John xxi
Biernacki, Patrick 2, 5–7
Bittoun, Rene xxii–xxiv

blindness integrity in trials 19, 27–32
Borland, Ron 45, 48–50, 75, 117, 211–212
Brandt, Alan 58
Brereton, Laurie xxi
brief interventions 20, 52, 66, 93, 215
British American Tobacco (BAT) 147, 248, 290
British American Tobacco Australia (BATA) 260
British Household Panel Survey 46
Britton, John 123, 136, 153
bupropion xxxi, 19, 25, 31, 66–69, 71, 74, 77, 86, 87, 161, 195, 205, 215

Cambodia 76
Canada 3, 40, 45, 53, 82, 113, 115, 163, 273, 276, 279, 283
Cancer Council Victoria xx–xxi, 261–262
Cancer Institute NSW 75
cannabis 2, 8–9, 29
catastrophe theory 116
cessation *see* quit attempts
Champix *see* varenicline
China 76, 145
Choice magazine xx

354

Index

citation bias 37–38
Clarke, Chris xxii–xxiv
cocaine 2, 29, 114
Cochrane Collaboration 19, 32, 34, 66, 70, 92, 97, 98, 180, 193
cohort studies 4, 9, 26, 42–43, 59–60, 71, 81, 134, 150, 166–168, 178, 180, 184–189, 200, 201
commitment to quitting 71, 207, 209–210, 211–212
common liability theory 166–168
Commonwealth Scientific and Industrial Research Organisation (CSIRO) 180
competing interest bias 32–33, 34
concepts central to self-quitting 207–209, 211–213
consumer safety criteria and tobacco 292
contingency payments 97
cross-sectional surveys 39–42, 43, 46, 48, 81
cysteine 69

Daube, Mike 191
difficulty in quitting 28, 57, 118–122
Doll, Richard xix, 152
dominance of interventionism 125–127, 142, 230
"don't quit – switch" 111, 145, 235–236
Doron, Gideon 62
dual use (smoking and vaping) 148, 158–159, 174, 177, 184, 186, 187–189, 235
Durante, Nicandro 148, 291

e-cigarettes (ECs) *see* vaping
efficacy vs effectiveness 18, 123
electronic cigarettes (ECs) *see* vaping

endgame for combustible tobacco 285–289
English quit smoking services 86–91, 132, 135
ethics of scare messaging 252–257
ethics of tobacco control 141, 286
Europe, cessation in 42, 72
EVALI 154
evidence-based cessation xxxiii, 64, 70, 71, 123

Fagerström, Karl 111, 290
Fairness Doctrine USA 61–62
Fiore, Michael 63–64
Flavor and Extracts Manufacturing Association USA 170–171
flavours and vaping 164, 168–174, 284
folk remedies for quitting xviii, 57–58
Framework Convention on Tobacco Control (FCTC) 84, 143, 265, 271
Freeman, Becky 10, 242, 244, 250, 265, 289, 291

Gallup poll USA 71
gambling 9–10
gateway hypothesis 165–168
general practitioners and cessation 46, 92–96
GlaxoSmithKline Nicabate promotion 129–130
Goffman, Erving xvi, 255
Gray, Nigel xx, xxiv, 64

hardening hypothesis xxxii, 110–114, 139
Hart, Julian Tudor xxix
Hawthorne effects 23–24
health concerns and quitting, importance of 208, 251

health consequences of vaping
    150–156, 159, 161
heated tobacco products (HTP) 147,
    148, 178, 290; *see also* vaping
Heaviness of Smoking Index (HSI) 50,
    111
Henningfield, Jack 28
heroin 5–8, 29
Hill, David xxv, 64
Horn, Daniel 59
Hughes, Hollie 14, 16
Hughes, John 38, 43, 44, 47, 70, 112,
    246

Illich, Ivan xxv, 127
illicit tobacco trade (ITT) 261–262
impact of cessation medication a
    population level 68–69
indication bias 50–51, 63, 71, 134
Indonesia 142, 146–147
information campaigns xix, 135, 144,
    212, 234, 240, 252, 254, 257
inhalation frequency, smoking vs.
    vaping 153, 174–175
intention to treat analysis 36–37
Israel 120

Japan 85
Japan Tobacco International (JTI) 147

Klingemann, Harald 2, 132, 203

Larabie, Lynn 115
laser acupuncture 15, 16–18
lay knowledge about quitting 217, 224,
    225, 227
Le Houezac, Jacques 136
Lévi-Strauss, Claude xvi
Leymore, Varda Langholz xvi
licensing

limits on number of cigarettes sold
    277
loss of retail licence 279
    smokers 277–278
tobacco retailers 265–267, 271–273,
    278, 295
longitudinal cohort studies *see* cohort
    studies
loss to follow-up 4, 43
low income nations 76–77, 141–143,
    248
lung cancer 152, 201

Malone, Ruth 291
marijuana *see* cannabis
maturing out 8–9
Mayer, Henry xvi
McKay, Bernie xxi
McNeill, Ann 136, 191, 197
mechanisation of cigarette production
    56–57, 152, 270
medication in smoking cessation xxxiii,
    20, 25, 47, 65–74, 76–78, 117, 128,
    133, 135, 142, 237
mental health and smoking 23, 37
meta-analysis 41, 66, 69–71, 125, 166,
    226
Millennium Cohort Study UK 167
miracle smoking cures 16
motivation to quit 22, 41, 207–209,
    211–212, 236
Māori smoking cessation 84, 163

narcotics *see* opiates
National Academies of Science,
    Engineering and Medicine
    (NASEM) USA 161, 180
National Health and Medical Research
    Council (Australia) (NHMRC) xix,
    104

Index

National Institutes of Health, USA (NIH) 154
New Zealand 67, 84, 162, 198-199, 273
news coverage of tobacco control xix, xx-xxi, 59, 248-249
next generation products (NGP) 148
nicotine 27, 28, 58, 65, 164, 221, 225, 230, 280
nicotine addiction xxviii, 21, 27, 29, 65, 110, 150, 189, 230
nicotine replacement therapy (NRT) 27, 34, 47-48, 65-74, 76, 82, 126, 128, 142, 181-183, 214-216, 221, 225, 281
  NRT in Australia 74-75, 214
  promotions 128-130
nicotine vaping products (NVP) see vaping
North American Quitline Consortium 82
Nutt, David 149, 150

Ochsner, Alton 152
Office of Population Censuses and Surveys (UK) 118
online quit interventions 81, 96, 215
opiates 5-8

pack warnings xix, xxvii, 53, 55, 62, 69, 144, 240, 252, 256
Papua New Guinea (PNG) 247
PATH (US Population Assessment of Tobacco and Health) cohort study 72-74, 150, 157, 159, 184-189, 193, 200
Pavlov, Ivan xxiii
Peele, Stanton xxv, 2, 229-230
Peters, Matthew 153, 191, 197
Pharmaceutical Benefits Scheme (Australia) (PBS) 25, 66

pharmacists and smoking cessation 20, 87, 269
phasing out combustible tobacco sales 291-296
Philip Morris International (PMI) 56, 146, 162, 171, 238, 260, 262, 290
Pierce, John xxi
Pinney, John 83
plain tobacco packs xxvii, 45, 144, 238, 240-241, 249, 260
pleasure and smoking 28-30
population focus xxvii, 26, 49, 54-55, 68, 90, 95, 137, 139, 142, 232, 238
positive outcome bias 33-36
prescription access to NVPs 155, 160, 164, 269-270, 279-285
primary and secondary prevention of smoking 232-235
problem gambling see gambling
Prochaska, Judith 122
proximal and distal influences on quitting 63, 125, 238-241
public awareness see information campaigns
Public Health England (PHE) 90, 153, 170

qualitative research on smoking cessation xxxiv, 204-226
quality of evidence pyramid 14
quit and win lotteries 98-101
Quit. For Life campaign xxii, 90
quit attempts xxxiii, 13, 25, 43, 44-46, 49, 60, 64, 76, 112, 117, 138, 189, 192, 194, 236, 239, 277
  importance of 237
quit programs run by tobacco companies 143
quit smoking clinics xxii-xxiv, xxvi, xxviii, 17, 84, 85, 90

quit smoking services 52, 72, 80, 84, 86, 88-90, 132
quitlines 52, 72, 79-83, 239
quitting before advent of NRT xxxi, 59-63
QALY (Quality Adjusted Life Years) 87

randomised controlled trials (RCT) 18-24, 30-32, 36, 70, 125, 180-183
real world effectiveness 18, 25, 134
real world use 19, 25, 161, 181-183
recall bias 45, 48-50, 75, 134
reduced smoking frequency 62, 120, 199
regulation of NVPs, the case for 156, 160, 161, 175-177, 280-285, 296
regulation of other goods and services 169, 266, 267
regulation of pharmaceutical retailing 268, 271
relapse in cessation xxxii, 17, 44-48, 116, 186, 195, 196, 236
Roxon, Nicola 249
rule of rescue xxvi
Russell, Michael 92, 94, 280

salbutamol inhalers 169, 174
scare tactics 251-257
schizophrenia and smoking 37-38, 113
Scollo, Michelle 261
scream test 144
self-selecting motivated samples 40-42, 182
self-selection bias 15-18, 20
Senate Enquiry into Tobacco Harm Reduction 2019 13, 15, 191, 269
Seventh Day Adventist church 5-Day Plan xviii, 83
Shiffman, Saul 50, 81, 117
silver nitrate 58

SimSmoke simulation model 247
Smith, Andrea xxxiv, 51, 204
Smith, Elizabeth 291
smokers' agency xxv, xxxv, 108, 229
smokers licences *see* licensing
smoking cessation and vaping xxxiv, 149, 175-180, 183, 185, 187, 193, 199-202
smoking cessation services *see* quit smoking services
smoking frequency and reductions in lung cancer 201
smoking prevalence and social disadvantage 262
smuggling *see* illicit tobacco trade (ITT)
Sobell, Linda and Mark 2, 132, 203
social desirability effects 23, 177
Society for Research on Nicotine and Tobacco 153
sound bites 51
spontaneous unplanned quitting 60, 114-117
stages of change xxxii, 114-116
Stapleton, John 47, 70, 130
stigmatisation 11, 228, 255
success rates vs intervention and policy reach 54-55
systematic reviews 2, 64, 87, 97, 113, 115, 130, 166, 200, 204, 261, 272

Tanzania 146
tax rises as cover for extra retail prices rises 262
Thailand 76, 84, 85, 275
Therapeutic Goods Administration (Australia) (TGA) 66, 156, 160, 280, 284, 285
tobacco affordability 57, 152, 189, 191
tobacco control inputs 246

Index

Tobacco Control Scale 72, 247
tobacco industry investment in NVPs 146–148, 188, 234, 270, 289
tobacco retailing density, restricting 271–273
tobacco supply, controlling 276
Tobacco Tactics, University of Bath 261
tobacco tax 69, 144, 147, 194, 234, 240, 257, 259–262, 265, 287
toxicant exposure with vaping 157–161, 172, 235
trial exclusion criteria 21–23
trial participant retention strategies 24–27, 181

unassisted quitting xxix, xxx, xxxiii, xxxiv, 2, 52, 60, 64, 73, 74–75, 81, 117, 122–124, 125, 140, 203, 205, 206–210, 211, 215–221, 231, 236
and the 'right' choice 223
denigration of 130
United States Food and Drug Administration (USFDA) 160, 171
University of Newcastle, NSW 93
upscaled interventions 98, 101–106

Vaillant, George 2, 4, 7
value of NRT market 126

value of NVP market 145
vaping 149–156, 175–177
prescription access to 155
and smoking frequency 185–189, 194, 198, 199–202
varenicline xxxi, 19, 25, 66–69, 71, 74, 77, 161, 205, 215
victim blaming 254–256
Vietnam War 7

Walsh, Raoul 24
Warner, Ken 61–63, 141, 294
West, Robert 89, 114, 131, 138, 170, 201
WHO (World Health Organization) 84, 150, 247, 265
willpower and quitting 71, 90, 209, 212, 218
Wodak, Alex 162, 282
workplace smoking cessation 91
Wynder, Ernst xix, 59, 152

youth uptake of vaping 162–168, 171, 283

Zola, Irving xxv
Zyban *see* bupropion

Made in United States
Troutdale, OR
09/02/2025